AMBULATORY MONITORING

DEVELOPMENTS IN CARDIOVASCULAR MEDICINE

Lancée CT, ed: Echocardiology, 1979. ISBN 90-247-2209-8.

Baan J, Arntzenius AC, Yellin EL, eds: Cardiac dynamics. 1980. ISBN 90-247-2212-8.

Thalen HJT, Meere CC, eds: Fundamentals of cardiac pacing. 1970. ISBN 90-247-2245-4.

Kulbertus HE, Wellens HJJ, eds: Sudden death. 1980. ISBN 90-247-2290-X.

Dreifus LS, Brest AN, eds: Clinical applications of cardiovascular drugs. 1980. ISBN 90-247-2295-0.

Spencer MP, Reid JM, eds: Cerebrovascular evaluation with Doppler ultrasound. 1981. ISBN 90-247-2348-1.

Zipes DP, Bailey JC, Elharrar V, eds: The slow inward current and cardiac arrhythmias. 1980. ISBN 90-247-2380-9.

Kesteloot H, Joossens JV, eds: Epidemiology of arterial blood pressure. 1980. ISBN 90-247-2386-8.

Wackers FJT, ed: Thallium-201 and technetium-99m-pyrophosphate myocardial imaging in the coronary care unit. 1980. ISBN 90-247-2396-5.

Maseri A, Marchesi C, Chierchia S, Trivella MG, eds: Coronary care units. 1981. ISBN 90-247-2456-2.

Morganroth J, Moore EN, Dreifus LS, Michelson EL, eds: The evaluation of new antiarrhythmic drugs. 1981. ISBN 90-247-2474-0.

Alboni P: Intraventricular conduction disturbances. 1981. ISBN 90-247-2484-X.

Rijsterborgh H, ed: Echocardiology. 1981. ISBN 90-247-2491-0.

Wagner GS, ed: Myocardial infarction: Measurement and intervention. 1982. ISBN 90-247-2513-5.

Meltzer RS, Roelandt J, eds: Contrast echocardiography. 1982. ISBN 90-247-2531-3.

Amery A, Fagard R, Lijnen R, Staessen J, eds: Hypertensive cardiovascular disease; pathophysiology and treatment. 1982. ISBN 90-247-2534-8.

Bouman LN, Jongsma HJ, eds: Cardiac rate and rhythm. 1982. ISBN 90-247-2626-3.

Morganroth J, Moore EN, eds: The evaluation of beta blocker and calcium antagonist drugs. 1982. ISBN 90-247-2642-5.

Rosenbaum MB, ed: Frontiers of cardiac electrophysiology. 1982. ISBN 90-247-2663-8.

Roelandt J, Hugenholtz PG, eds: Long-term ambulatory electrocardiography. 1982. ISBN 90-247-2664-8.

Adgey AAJ, ed: Acute phase of ischemic heart disease and myocardial infarction. 1982. ISBN 90-247-2675-1.

Hanrath P, Bleifeld W, Souquet, J. eds: Cardiovascular diagnosis by ultrasound. Transesophageal, computerized, contrast, Doppler echocardiography. 1982. ISBN 90-247-2692-1.

Roelandt J, ed: The practice of M-mode and two-dimensional echocardiography. 1983. ISBN 90-247-2745-6.

Meyer J, Schweizer P, Erbel R, eds: Advances in noninvasive cardiology. 1983. ISBN 0-89838-576-8.

Morganroth J, Moore EN, eds: Sudden cardiac death and congestive heart failure: Diagnosis and treatment. 1983. ISBN 0-89838-580-6.

Perry HM, ed: Lifelong management of hypertension. 1983. ISBN 0-89838-582-2.

Jaffe EA, ed: Biology of endothelial cells. 1984. ISBN 0-89838-587-3.

Surawicz B, Reddy CP, Prystowsky EN, eds: Tachycardias. ISBN 0-89838-588-1.

Spencer MP, ed: Cardiac Doppler diagnosis. 1983. ISBN 0-89838-591-1.

Villarreal H, Sambhi MP, eds: Topics in pathophysiology of hypertension. 1984. ISBN 0-89838-595-4.

Messerli FH, ed: Cardiovascular disease in the elderly. 1984. ISBN 0-89838-596-2.

Simoons ML, Reiber JHC, eds: Nuclear imaging in clinical cardiology. 1984. ISBN 0-89838-599-7.

Ter Keurs HEDJ, Schipperheyn JJ, eds: Cardiac left ventricular hypertrophy. 1983. ISBN 0-89838-612-8.

Sperelakis N, ed: Physiology and pathophysiology of the heart. ISBN 0-89838-612-2.

Messerli FH, ed: Kidney in essential hypertension. ISBN 0-89838-616-0.

Sambhi MP, ed: Fundamental fault in hypertension. ISBN 0-89838-638-1.

Marchesi C, ed: Ambulatory monitoring: Cardiovascular system and allied applications. ISBN 0-89838-642-X.

Kupper W, MacAlpin RN, Bleifeld W, eds: Coronary tone in ischemic heart disease. ISBN 0-89838-646-2.

Sperelakis N, Caulfield JB, eds: Calcium antagonists: Mechanisms of action on cardiac muscle and vascular smooth muscle. ISBN 0-89838-655-1.

Godfraind T, Herman AS, Wellens D, eds: Calcium entry blockers in cardiovascular and cerebral dysfunctions. ISBN 0-89838-658-1.

Morganroth J, Moore EN, eds: Interventions in the acute phase of myocardial infarction. ISBN 0-89838-659-4.

AMBULATORY MONITORING

Cardiovascular system and allied applications

Proceedings of a workshop held in Pisa, April 11–12, 1983.
Sponsored by the Commission of the European Communities, as advised by
the Committee on Medical and Public Health Research.

edited by

CARLO MARCHESI

CNR Institute of Clinical Physiology
Pisa, Italy

1984 **MARTINUS NIJHOFF PUBLISHERS**
a member of the KLUWER ACADEMIC PUBLISHERS GROUP
BOSTON / THE HAGUE / DORDRECHT / LANCASTER
for the Commission of the European Communities

Distributors

for the United States and Canada: Kluwer Boston, Inc., 190 Old Derby Street, Hingham, MA 02043, USA
for all other countries: Kluwer Academic Publishers Group, Distribution Center, P.O.Box 322, 3300 AH Dordrecht, The Netherlands

Library of Congress Cataloging in Publication Data

Main entry under title:

Ambulatory monitoring.

    (Developments in cardiovascular medicine)
    1. Electrocardiography, Ambulatory--Congresses.
2. Cardiovascular system--Diseases--Diagnosis--Congresses.
3. Patient monitoring--Congresses. 4. Ambulatory medical
care--Congresses. I. Marchesi, Carlo. II. Commission
of the European Communities. Committee on Medical and
Public Health Research. III. Series. [DNLM: 1. Cardiovascular diseases--Congresses. 2. Monitoring, Physiologic
--Congresses. 3. Ambulatory care--Congresses.
W1 DE997VME / WG 140 A4985 1983]
RC683.5.A45A43 1984   616.1'207547   84-4011

ISBN-13: 978-94-009-6014-5   e-ISBN-13: 978-94-009-6012-1
DOI: 10.1007/978-94-009-6012-1

Book information

Publication arranged by: Commission of the European Communities, Directorate-General Information Market and Innovation, Luxembourg

Copyright/legal notice

FOREWORD

Ambulatory monitoring of signals, related to cardiovascular system performances, is one of the biomedical technologies of wider interest.

This interest is well documented by the literature, by the number of instruments available on the market and by the increasing diffusion of this technique at routine clinical level. The wide distribution of ambulatory monitoring is however not yet well supported by commonly accepted criteria of clinical interpretation, by an assessment of the minimal requirements for instrumentation performances, or by indications of cost/benefit figures in relation to different situations.

Several European centres have a recognized expertise and are well suited to the examination of the problem of defining common guidelines and of making recommendations so as to stimulate an improvement of the clinical usage and of the performance of the instrumentation.

The Biomedical Engineering Standing Group of the Committee for Medical and Public Health Research approved the organization of this workshop which had as its aims the assessment of the state-of-the-art of different aspects of ambulatory monitoring and the discussion within a group of experts of the feasibility and interest in promoting the coordination in Europe of these activities in the framework of a "concerted action".

The workshop was held in Pisa over two full days (April 11-12, 1983). The participants were physicians and engineers, experts in their fields.

The sessions were organized around four main topics : 34 papers were presented and discussed and 30 of them are published in this book. A final session was devoted to discussion of the proposal for a concerted action.

The opinion of the participants was that coordinated efforts could be extremely useful in investigating the problems of the effective role of ambulatory monitoring and of common criteria for minimal requirements for clinical applications of the instrumentation. My hope is that this book will be an appropriate reference for future cooperation.

Pisa, November 12, 1983   Carlo Marchesi

CONTENTS

X

ACKNOWLEDGEMENTS

The Workshop and the publication of this book have been possible by the support of the Commission of the European Communities. The members of the Bio-medical Engineering standing group gave their approval and contributed to the general planning of the Workshop.

Dr. K. Gerbaulet, Mr. G. Evrard and Dr. W. Skupinsky gave their effective support to solve the organizational and financial problems.

The organization of the Workshop in Pisa has been cared by the CNR Institute of Clinical Physiology, with the skillful personal help of Mr. G. Magni of the "tre emme" agency.

A particular gratitude has to be rendered to Miss Graziella Distante for her continuous, proficient help throughout all the steps of the Workshop organization.

CONTRIBUTORS

P.Attuel, Department of Cardiology, Lariboisier Hospital, Paris Cedex, France.

V.Bala Subramanian, Brunel University, Uxbridge, Middx, England.

R.Balzarotti, Centro di Teoria dei Sistemi, Department of Electronics, Politecnico di Milano, Milano, Italy.

M.Baratto, Clinical Physiology Institute, National Research Council of Italy, and Department of Medicine, University of Pisa, Pisa, Italy.

F.Bartoli, Centro di Teoria dei Sistemi, Department of Electronics, Politecnico di Milano, Milano, Italy.

G.Baselli, Centro di Teoria dei Sistemi, Department of Electronics, Politecnico di Milano, Milano, Italy.

J.H.Van Bemmel, Department of Medical Informatics, Vrije Universiteit, Amsterdam, The Netherlands.

G.Bertinieri, Istituto di Clinica Medica IV, University of Milano and Center of Clinical Physiology and Hypertension, Ospedale Maggiore, Milano, Italy.

A.Biagini, Clinical Physiology Institute, National Research Council of Italy, and Department of Medicine, University of Pisa, Pisa, Italy.

P.Bjerregaard, University Department of Cardiology, Aarhus Kommunehospital, Aarhus C, Denmark.

M.Bobelyn, Department of Cardiology, University Hospital, Gent, Belgium.

M.G.Bongiorni, Clinical Physiology Institute, National Research Council of Italy, and Department of Medicine, University of Pisa, Pisa, Italy.

C.Carpeggiani, Clinical Physiology Institute, National Research Council of Italy, and Department of Medicine, University of Pisa, Pisa, Italy.

P.M.M.Cashman, Clinical Research Centre, Harrow, England.

S.Cerutti, Centro di Teoria dei Sistemi, Department of Electronics, Politecnico di Milano, Milano, Italy.

L.R.Cicchiello, Istituto di Fisica, Facolta' di Ingegneria, Universita', Napoli, Italy.

D.L.Clement, Department of Cardiology, University Hospital, Gent, Belgium.

C.Contini, Clinical Physiology Institute, National Research Council of Italy, and Department of Medicine, University of Pisa, Pisa, Italy.

P.Coumel, Department of Cardiology, Lariboisiere Hospital, Paris Cedex, France.

J.Damgaard Andersen, Medical Department B, Rigshospitalet, Copenhagen, Denmark.

M.Di Rienzo, Centro di Bioingegneria, Politecnico e Fondazione Don Gnocchi, Milano, Italy.

A.Ferrari, Istituto di Clinica Medica IV, University of Milano and Center of Clinical Physiology and Hypertension, Ospedale Maggiore, Milano Italy.

G.Grassi, Istituto di Clinica Medica IV, University of Milano and Center of Clinical Physiology and Hypertension, Ospedale Maggiore, Milano, Italy.

E.Gymoese, Medical Department B, Rigshospitalet, Copenhagen, Denmark.

G.Kraft, Clinical Physiology Institute, National Research Council of Italy, and Department of Medicine, University of Pisa, Pisa, Italy.

A.L'Abbate, Clinical Phsyiology Institute, National Research Council of Italy, and Department of Medicine, University of Pisa, Pisa, Italy.

L.Landucci, Clinical Physiology Institute, National Research Council of Italy, and Department of Medicine, University of Pisa, Pisa, Italy.

J.F.Leclercq, Department of Cardiology, Lariboisiere Hospital, Paris Cedex, France.

D.Levorato, Clinical Physiology Institute, National Research Council of Italy, and Department of Medicine, University of Pisa, Pisa, Italy.

D.Liberati, Centro di Teoria dei Sistemi, Department of Electronics, Politecnico di Milano, Milano, Italy.

A.Macerata, Clinical Physiology Institute, National Research Council of Italy, and Department of Medicine, University of Pisa, Pisa, Italy.

G.Mancia, Istituto di Clinica Medica IV, University of Milano and Center of Clinical Physiology and Hypertension, Ospedale Maggiore, Milano, Italy.

C.Marchesi, Clinical Physiology Institute, National Research Council of Italy, Pisa, Italy.

R.G.Mark, Biomedical Engineering Center for Clinical Instrumentation, Harward-MIT Division of Health Sciences and Technology, Massachusetts Institute of Technology, Cambridge Massachusetts, USA.

M.G.Mazzei, Clinical Physiology Institute, National Research Council of Italy, and Department of Medicine, University of Pisa, Pisa, Italy.

G.F.Mazzocca, Clinical Physiology Institute, National Research Council of Italy, and Department of Medicine, University of Pisa, Pisa, Italy.

G.B.Moody, Biomedical Engineering Center for Clinical Instrumentation,

Harward–MIT Division of Health Sciences and Technology, Massachusetts Institute of Technology, Cambridge Massachusetts, USA.

S.Moulopoulos, Medical Department Clinical Therapeutics, Athens University, Alexandra Hospital, Athens, Greece.

A.Murray, Regional Medical Physics Department, Freeman Hospital, Newcastle upon Tyne, England.

L.Packet, Department of Cardiology, University Hospital, Gent, Belgium.

O.Pahlm, Department of Clinical Physiology, University Hospital, Lund, Sweden.

C.Palombo, Clinical Physiology Institute, National Research Council of Italy, and Department of Medicine, University of Pisa, Pisa, Italy.

G.Parati, Istituto di Clinica Medica IV, University of Milano and Center of Clinical Physiology and Hypertension, Ospedale Maggiore, Milano, Italy.

M.Pauletti, Clinical Physiology Institute, National Research Council of Italy, and Department of Medicine, University of Pisa, Pisa, Italy.

P.Petrou, Medical Department Clinical Therapeutics, Athens University, Alexandra Hospital, Athens, Greece.

G.Pomidossi, Istituto di Clinica Medica IV, University of Milano and Center of Clinical Physiology and Hypertension, Ospedale Maggiore, Milano, Italy.

K.L.Ripley, Thoraxcentrum, Erasmus University, Rotterdam, The Netherlands.

A.Rosenfalck, Institute of Electronic Systems, Aalborg University Centre, Aalborg, Denmark.

E.Sandoe, Medical Department B, Rigshospitalet, Copenhagen, Denmark.

W.Sansen, Katholieke Universiteit Leuven, Elektrotechniek, Leuven Heverlee, Belgium.

B.McA Sayers, Imperial College, London, England.

L.Sornmo, Department of Telecommunication Theory, University of Lund, Lund, Sweden.

S.Stamatelopoulos, Medical Department Clinical Therapeutics, Athens University, Alexandra Hospital, Athens, Greece.

F.D.Stott, Clinical Research Center, Harrow, Middlesex, England.

A.Taddei, Clinical Physiology Institute, National Research Council of Italy, Pisa, Italy.

J.L.Talmon, Department of Medical Informatics, Vrije Universiteit, Amsterdam, The Netherlands.

R.Testa, Clinical Physiology Institute, National Research Council of Italy, and Department of Medicine, University of Pisa, Pisa, Italy.

G.O.Van Maele, Department of Cardiology, University Hospital, Gent, Belgium.

M.Varanini, Clinical Physiology Institute, National Research Council of Italy, Pisa, Italy.

N.Yannopoulos, Medical Department Clincal Therapeutics, Athens University, Alexandra Hospital, Athens, Greece.

C.Zeelenberg, Thoraxcentre Erasmus University, Rotterdam, The Netherlands.

C.Zyweitz, Arbeitsbereich Biosignalverarbeitung im Zentrum Biometrie, Medizinische Hochschule Hannover, Bundesrepublik, Duetschland.

CHAPTER 1

TRANSDUCERS AND ANALYSIS SYSTEMS FOR AMBULATORY MONITORING

TOPIC 1.1

Sensors for Electrophysiological signals monitoring

SILICON SENSORS FOR ELECTROPHYSIOLOGICAL
SIGNALS MONITORING

W. Sansen

Katholieke Universiteit Leuven, Elektrotechniek
94 K. Mercierlaan, B-3030 Leuven-Heverlee, Belgium

ABSTRACT

Silicon technology has emerged as a new technology for the fabrication of sensors with low cost and high quality. Silicon sensors are therefore essential for the development of multi-sensor ambulatory monitoring systems which include data reduction and storage.

The state of the art is given of sensors which are all compatible with silicon technology. They are pressure sensors, accelerometers, chemical sensors, flow sensors and biopotential measurement electrodes.

INTRODUCTION

Monitoring physiological parameters requires data acquisition systems in which sensors are of primary importance. Even for the measurement of biopotentials such as ECG, EMG, EEG etc. the sensing electrodes play a vital role in the quality of the signal obtained.

Sensors have traditionally been realized in many different materials such as platinum, silver, gold etc. Also they are a result of piece-by piece fabrication where they are costly.

On the other hand silicon has emerged as a material which can be used for the realization of sensors. The main advantage of silicon however, is that silicon is the material in which most of the micro electronics chips are realized. By means of advanced photolithographic techniques, complex functions can be integrated in silicon chips. Moreover the integration is carried out by planar processing ie on the surface of the silicon wafers, which allows mass production at a low cost.

This text illustrates how the silicon technology has invaded the world of sensors. As a result silicon sensors have emerged which combine high quality and low cost [2].

Moreover the addition of sensor compatible circuitry on the same chip allows the enhance the quality of the sensor ie its selectivity and its level of intelligence.

Ambulatory monitoring has mainly been limited to ECG and heart pressure recording. As soon as other sensors can be integrated with circuits, they will be included in ambulatory monitoring. Full systems can easily

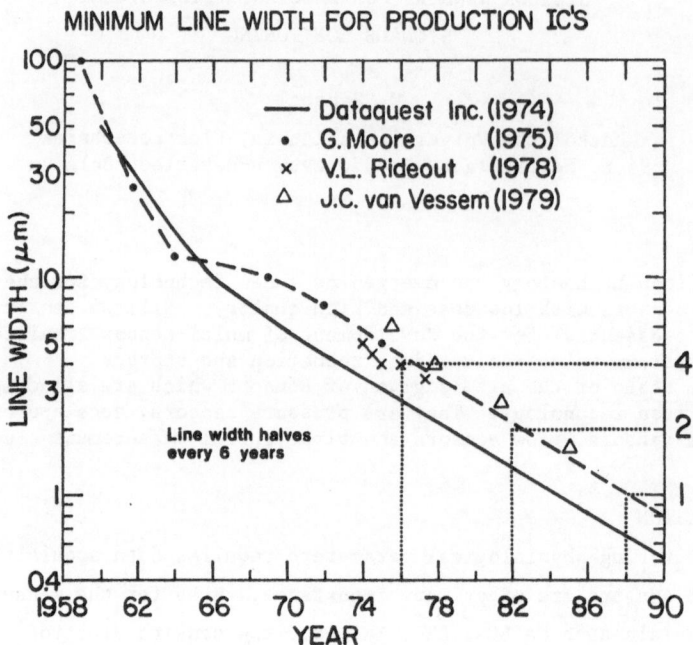

Fig.1 : The evolution of the minimum linewidth which is inversely proportional to complexity on one chip [1].

be devised where a large number of sensor signals and biopotentials are
multiplexed on one line linked to a microcomputer for real time processing.

   This text pays attention to a number of sensor principles which can
all be realized in silicon technology and which may play a rule in future
ambulatory monitoring systems. They are pressure sensors, accelerometers,
chemical sensors, flow sensors and biopotential measurement electrodes.

PRESSURE SENIORS

a. Piezo resistive

   Silicon has been used for the fabrication of pressure sensors since
1973 [3,4]. A silicon wafer is etched out to about 10 μm (see fig.1).
Four resistances on the edges of the so formed membrane are in desequili-
brium as soon as a pressure difference is applied across the membrane.
This is the piezoresistive effect, which actually occurs in any solid
material with a crystal structure. The resistances can easily be diffused

or ionimplanted, which is a standard processing step.

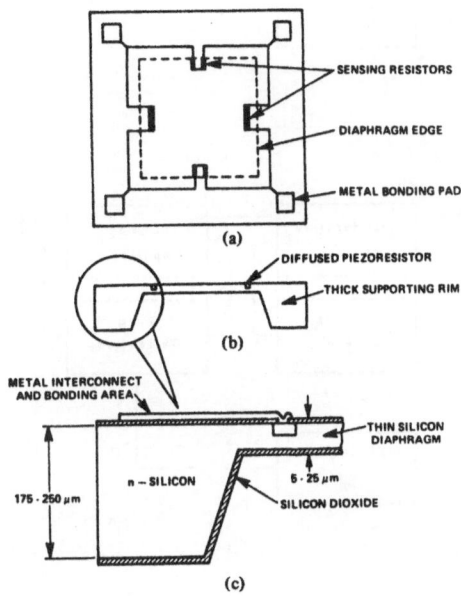

Fig.2 : Piezo resistive pressure sensor [4].

The most difficult step is the etch of membrane. The sensitivity is
inversely proportional to its thickness squared. Reproducibility is therefore difficult to achieve.

The sensitivity of this sensor is quite low. Typically the differential voltage generated is 10 μV/V/mm Hg. The efficiency is of the order
of 10^{-5}. As a result many other effects are as important. Temperature is
one of them and the influence of the packaging is another. Compensation
is provided by adding additional circuitry to the output amplifier (fig.3)
which is easy to implement on the same chip.

The influence of packaging is not so easy to remedy. The package
applies a pressure on the membrane by itself. This offset voltage drifts
in time. As a result the long term drift of the pressure sensor is one
of the most critical parameters to specify. It is a result of highly proprietary fabrication techniques, which considerably increase the cost of
the device.

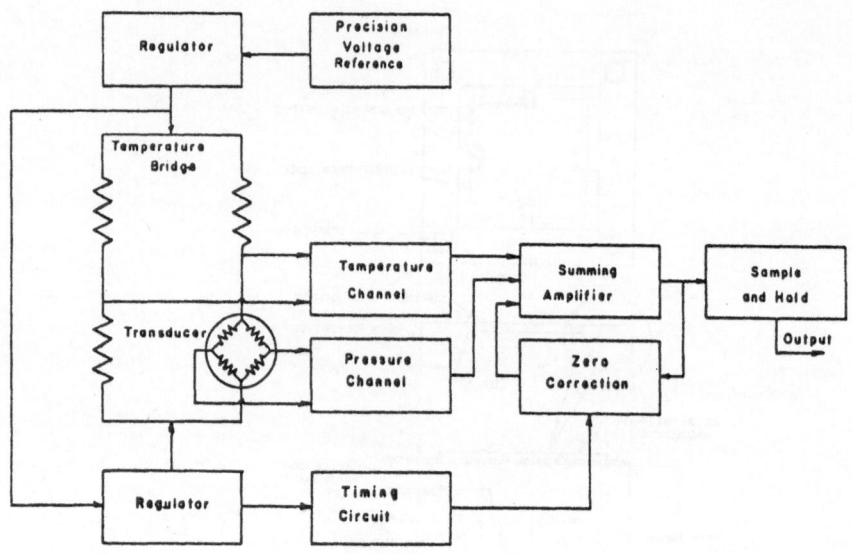

Fig.3 : Block diagram of interface circuit for pressure transducers[5].

b. Capacitive

More recently capacitive pressure sensors have been introduced [6]. They require the same membrane as for piezoresistive pressure sensors. The deflection of the membrane causes the distance between the plates of a capacitance to change. This results in a change in capacitance which is a measure of the pressure applied.

The capacitance has air as a dielectricum (fig.4), the silicon membrane as one plate and a metal layer on the glass cover as the other. The capacitance is nonlinear and needs a lot of circuitry to provide a linear output voltage. Therefore integration on one chip is mandatory again.

The capacitive pressure sensor is expected to have a lower drift component than the piezoresistive one.

c. Other

A very simple pressure sensor is realized by application of pressure on the emitter of a bipolar transistor (fig.5). The change of the saturation current of the transistor is a measure for the applied pressure [7].

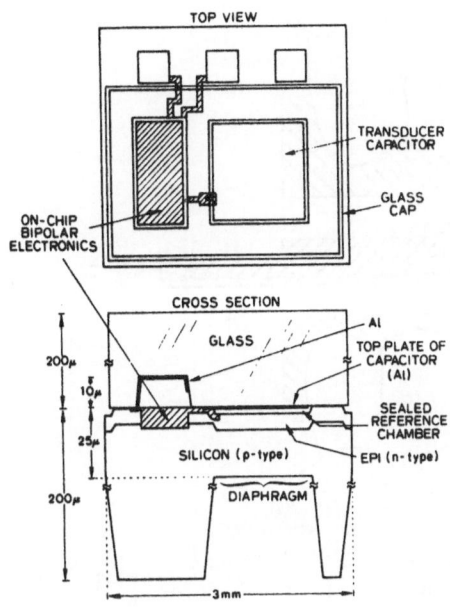

Fig.4 : Capacitive pressure transducer [6].

A recent realization is shown in figure 6 and was used to measure differential force between teeth. The device has a low sensitivity. Moreover
the need for a mechanical contact makes this device extremely difficult to
package.

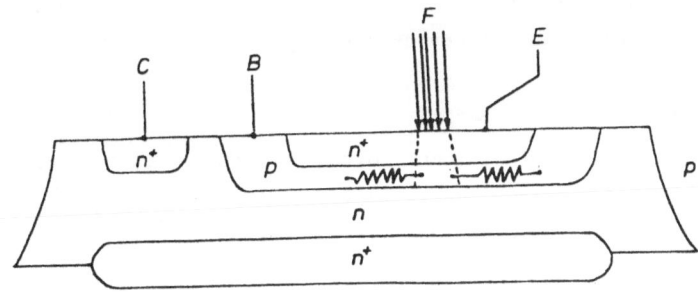

Fig.5 : Piezo effect of bipolar transistor [7].

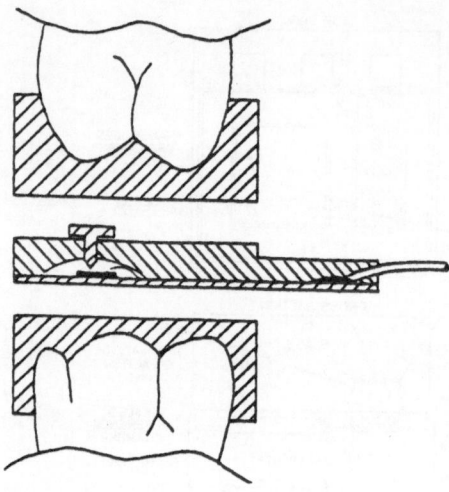

Fig.6 : Measurement of teeth force [7].

ACCELEROMETERS

Accelerometers are usually bulky devices. A recent development has made it possible to integrate such a device in silicon [8]. The resultant area is a mere 2 x 2 mm (fig.7). It consists of a mass of silicon which is suspended at a thin bridge of silicon. Vertical acceleration deflects the bridge which causes an assymmetry in the resistances diffused in the bridge. Since it involves the same principle as in the piezoresistive pressure sensor, it only provides low sensitivity. Also it is by no means a trivial task to etch out the silicon mass despite the availability of this etch procedure in silicon processing.

CHEMICAL SENSORS

The measurement of hydrogen, oxygen and CO_2 concentration is of crucial importance in an ambulatory monitoring system. In general a selective sensor is required for each chemical product of importance. Some of them have been studied quite extensively for at least 10 years. Yet very few seem to be commercialized. Packaging is certainly one of the main obstacles. But stability and selectivity are also very much absent. It will now be examined how the implementation in silicon can improve the performance of this kind of device.

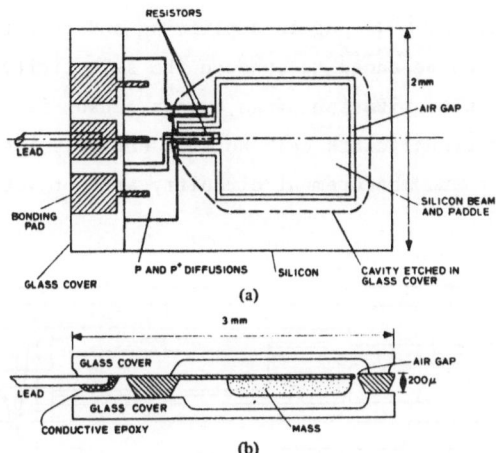

Fig.7 : Top and cross-section view of the
accelerometer [8].

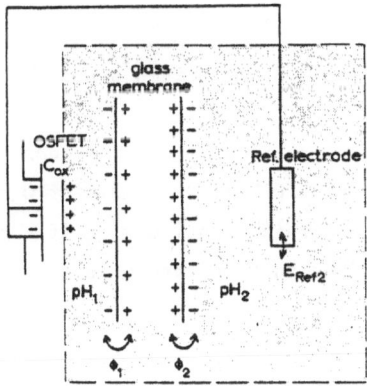

Fig.8 : Glass membrane with one reference electrode
and an ISFET [9].

The best known chemical sensor is doubtless an ISFET (Ion Sensitive FET). The coating on top of the gate of this FET absorps ions out of the solution (see fig.8), which changes the induced charge and hence the current through the transistor [9]. Again amplifying and temperature compensating circuitry is to be added to enhance the selectivity.

A good example of planarization of an oxygen sensor is given in fig. 9 [10]. It is a conventional clark cell but has entirely been integrated. The polarographic drive and measurement circuitry are not yet on chip.

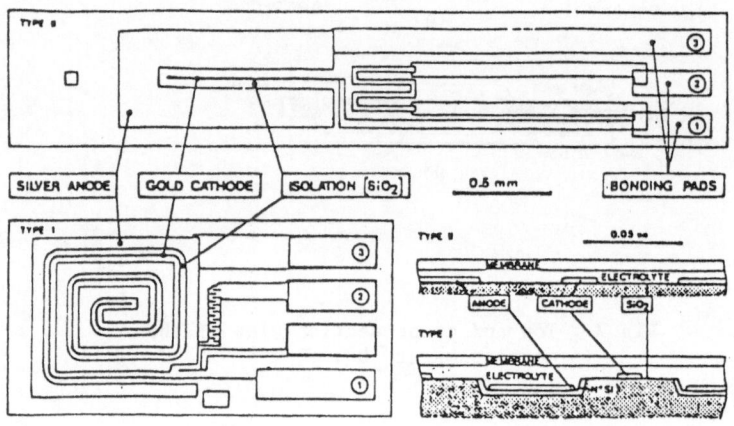

Fig.9 : Solid State oxygen sensor [10].

FLOW SENSORS

In order to detect a gas flow along a silicon chip, the differential stage can be used of figure 10 [11]. Transistor Q_3 is heated and will warm up transistor Q_2 more than transistor Q_1 if a gas flow is present as indicated. This difference in temperature is converted into a difference in input voltage (2mV/°C), which is easily measured. Again this sensor is to be combined with a conventional integrated circuit, which again illustrates the powerful potential of the combination of sensor principles with IC processing.

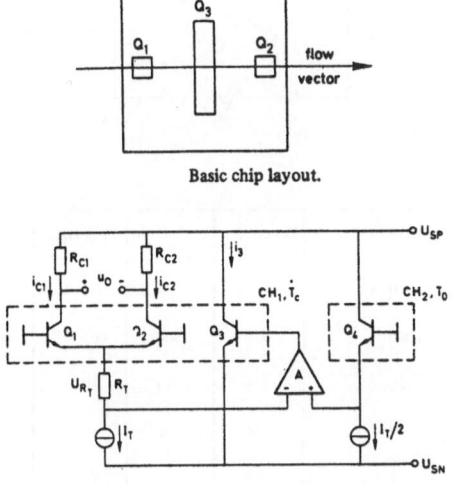

Basic chip layout.

Fig.10 : Direction sensitive flow sensor [11].

BIOPOTENTIALS

In order to measure ECG, EMG, EEG etc. conventional electrodes in platinum, stainless steel etc. are used. However in order to avoid the effect of the transition impedances between the electrode material and tissue, four-point measurements have to be carried out [12]. In figure 11 a model is given for this transition impedance including the values for some conventional electrode materials. As a result additional circuitry is required to realize this measurement procedure. Silicon technology allows to integrate and miniaturize the circuits such that they can be positioned very closely to the top of the electrode.

CONCLUSION

This text has illustrated that the application of silicon technology may start a renewed developement of sensors with more sensitivity and selectivity and lower price. Pressure sensors, accelerometer, chemical sensors, flow sensors and biopotential electrode have been described in detail.

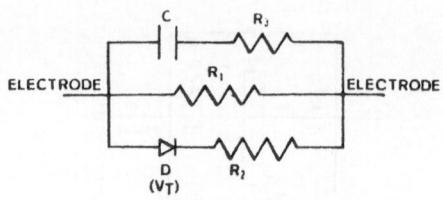

		Stainless Steel	Tantalum	Tivanium	Platinum	Skin, St St
V_T	V	0.9	9	4	1.7	0.5
R_1	kΩ	·1000	500	3500	165	650
R_2	kΩ	20	9	73	10	25
R_3	kΩ	20	30	30	10	30
C	μF	20	25	26	10	25

Fig.11 : Model of transition impedance electrode-
          tissue.

REFERENCES

1 Painke, H. 1981. Digital Technology Status and Trends, Oldenbourg,
   p. 14.
2 Solid-State Tranducers Conference, June 1983, Delft.
3 Gieles, A., Somers G. 1973. Miniature pressure tranducers with a
   silicon diaphragm, Philips Techn. Review, 33, N°1.
4 Wolber, W., Wise, K. December 1979. Sensor development in the microcomputer age, IEEE Trans. Electron Devices, ED-26, p. 1864-1874.
5 Ko, W., Hynecek, J.,Boettcher,S.December 1979, Development of a miniature pressure transducer for biomedical applications, IEEE Trans.
   Electron Devices, ED-26, p. 1896-1905.
6 Sander, C., Knutti, J., Meindl, J. May 1980. A monolithic capacitive
   pressure sensor with pulse-period output, IEEE Trans. Electron Devices
   ED-27, p. 927-930.
7 Sansen, W., Vandeloo, P. Puers, R. 1983. A force transducer based on
   stress effects in bipolar transistors, Sensors and Actuators, Vol. 3,
   N°4, p. 343-354.
8 Roylance, L., Angell, J. December 1979. A batch-fabricated silicon
   accelerometer, IEEE Trans. Electron Devices, ED-26, p. 1911-1917.
9 Bergveld, P., de Rooij, N. 1979. From conventional membrane electrodes
   to ionsensitive field-effect transistors, Med. & Biol. Eng. & Comput. 17, p. 647-654.
10 Engels J. et al. A disposable oxygen sensor for biomedical applications, Honeywell & Philips Medical Electronics, Best, Netherlands.
11 Huijsing, J., Schuddemat, J., Verhoef, W. January 1982. Monolithic

Integrated Direction-sensitive flow sensor, IEEE Trans. Electron
Devices, ED-29, p. 133-136.

12 Sansen, W., De Dijcker, F. 1976. The four-point probetechnique to
    measure bio-impedance, Electromyography clin. Neurophys., p. 509-510.

DISCUSSION

Chairman: C. Zeelenberg

1.1 - Sensors for Electrophysiological signals monitoring.

WOLFF: You have misled us to some extent. That is almost every transducer you have mentioned can in fact be made better, not in the way in which you have suggested. You can make better pH electrodes, you can make silicon integrated transducers which are very much more sensitive. Separate transducers, are more sensitive than normal strain gauge transducers because the pH resistive effect in silicon is greater than in metals. I think the only merit of using the technology which you've described is if one expects to want large quantities of some particular transducer electronic combination, as one might indeed do in the motor-car industry. I think the case is not proven in the relatively speaking hard-fulls of transducers which one might require for the purpose of medical research, and I am not convinced about the disadvantages of making a transducer on the same chip, having to take into account things like lack of sensitivity, and lack of selectivity, because your gas tranducers, for example, are very unselective; it may 100 to 1 between methane and air, but it's too sensitive if you're only trying to detect 1% in air, you aren't going to do so well. What you say is interesting, but I'm not sure it is as interesting for its relatively small quantity-high quality market which we're looking at as you pretend.

SANSEN: There are two points I'd like to make on that. First of all, my experience is that when you make a device or sensor in the laboratory, you face the problem of continuity, that is you make one device, and two devices; as soon as somebody has five of those device you have a problem. I mean it's nice to know that a company or another group is interested in those, and they will do it if there is a mass-production possibility. I won't say that there is mass production, but there is a possibility of mass production, that means that a larger quantity of devices are only possible if the device is standardized and if it's used as standard technology. That is why I do believe in the use of silicon for sensors. I have no belief in sensors of which there are only a few made in a laboratory. And the second point is that whatever device you make, the addition of some electronics will always, in some sense, add to the selectivity or add the sensitivity or maybe add to the stability of it. That means that if you prefer a technology in which electronics can be added I think you will always be better. But of course this could be a point of discussion.

ZYWIETZ: I was missing some information about electrical sensors, that means electrodes. Can you give some idea of what happens in that area at this time?

SANSEN: If you ar more specific, then I can be more specific. But, just quoting in general, electrodes is not a problem to be discussed at this first discussion. If you take the right material, like for example, platinum or iridium and you add the right electronics most of the problems are solved. But I will say more about that tomorrow.

TOPIC: 1.2

Transducers for long term hemodynamic signals monitoring.

SOURCES OF ERROR IN DIRECT AND INDIRECT
BLOOD PRESSURE MEASUREMENTS

F.D. Stott
Watford Road, Harrow, Middlesex, UK.

ABSTRACT

Factors governing the accuracy of direct blood pressure measurement
are considered, and the order of magnitude of the errors to be expected is
estimated. Errors in indirect measurements as compared with simultaneous
direct measurements are examined and an attempt is made to understand the
sources of these errors; finally a possible approach the improving the
accuracy of indirect measurement of Blood Pressure is suggested.

INTRODUCTION

Both direct and indirect methods of measuring Blood Pressure are
subject to errors, both random and systematic. To use the results of these
measurements with confidence, it is necessary to know the probable magnitude
of these errors; an over-optimistic assessment of the accuracy of the
measurement could lead to incorrect and unjustified conclusions.

DIRECT SYSTEMS

All methods of direct measurement of BP use some form of transducer
connected to a hydraulic system terminating in a cannula in the artery.
The sources of error can be divided into those governing static accuracy
(steady pressures), which are dependent only on the transducer, and those
governing dynamic accuracy, which depend on the combination of transducer
and the hydraulic system.

STATIC ACCURACY

Errors due to lack of stability (drift) can be largely eliminated if
the system is calibrated often enough. Errors due to hysteresis are
difficult to compensate, but are negligible with nearly all modern transducers.

DYNAMIC ACCURACY

The accuracy measurement of rapidly changing pressures is determined
by the frequency response of the measuring system as a whole, which in turn
is determined by the compliance of the transducer and the length and
diameter of the cannula and connecting tubing. For any given compliance,
there is an optimum diameter of connecting tubing which will give a
critically damped system; if the tubing is too large in diameter the system
will resonate; if too small, the maximum usable frequency will be reduced.
The system must therefore be designed as a whole to give the best perform-

ance, but in general the lower the compliance of the transducer the less critical is the design and the easier it becomes to achieve satisfactory frequency response.

It has been shown (Wood 1950a) that in the absence of resonance systolic and diastolic pressure will be correctly recorded if the response is uniform to about the 5th harmonic of the pulse frequency; and the waveform will be reproduced with no measurable error if the response extends to about the 10th - 15th harmonic. Any high-Q resonance even at much higher frequencies will however introduce large errors. It is therefore always safer to err on the side of overdamping rather than underdamping. These experimental results are confirmed by the analysis of peripheral artery waveforms carried out by Womersley and McDonald, (McDonald 1974) which show negligible energy present in harmonics above the 10th.

It is imperative that if the potential performance of a system is to be be realised in practise, that it should be completely fluid-filled; the presence of even a very small bubble raises the compliance of the system to such an extent that low-frequency resonance may occur, with gross distortion of waveforms. Some systems used in invasive cardiology are very difficult to fill properly, because the method of interconnection of the various parts has not been properly thought out. A system which is transparent throughout, as is that used for ambulatory monitoring, is much easier to fill properly, and this system has been found on repeated tests to perform very consistently.

As in indication of the magnitude of possible errors, a good properly filled system under laboratory conditions should be accurate to about 1% of full scale; under ambulatory conditions with less frequent calibration, errors should still not exceed 2%. Some additional error is introduced by the tape record/replay system noise and drift, and individual readings may be subject to errors of the order of 3% of full scale, though averages over a number of cycles, say 1-minute averages, should be better.

If one works on the basis that any individual reading may be in error by 5mm either way, then one is unlikely to be misled.

INDIRECT SYSTEMS

Before discussing errors in indirect BP measurements, it is necessary to decide on the standard of comparison.

There is no laboratory method available to us whereby we can make an absolute determination of the characteristic of an indirect system, because the artery and the limb form essential parts of the measuring system. The direct system on the other hand can be tested in the laboratory to ensure accurate measurements. We can therefore only determine the accuracy of the indirect system by comparing the results it gives with simultaneous direct measurements. The measurements must be simultaneous, as the pressure varies from beat to beat; ideally they should be made in the same artery but this is not possible in practice. The presence of the cannula in the artery must modify the properties of the artery and the blood flow in it, to an unknown and unpredictable extent. If we apply the cuff to the brachial artery and cannulate the radial artery on the same side, then the direct pressure recording is obliterated or greatly modified during inflation and deflation of the cuff, which is just the time when we need it. It is perfectly possible to cannulate the brachial artery and apply the cuff to the radial artery, but this is not the standard technique which we wish to test.

The best option is to apply the cuff to one brachial artery and cannulate the other, provided we can be sure that the pressure in the two brachial arteries is the same. This has been studied very carefully by Harrison (1960), and he concluded that the differences are small (ca± 5mm) for systole and zero within the limits of experimental error for diastole, except in a small proportion of people who have vascular disease, when the differences are large. If there are no clinical signs of vascular disease, the armcuff measurements are similar (say ± 10mm) on the two arms, it is safe to use readings in the two brachial arteries to compare two different methods of measurement.

A number of such studies have been carried out comparing the arm-cuff method, using the Korotkoff sounds as end points, with direct measurements, but not all these studies are sufficiently fully reported for us to be sure that the direct measurements were acceptably accurate. Three studies which meet all the criteria for reliability are those of Van Bergen (1954), Raftery & Ward (1968), and Bruner (1981). The results are very similar in respect of the scatter of the paired measurements, but there are differences in the mean errors found, both Raftery & Ward and Bruner

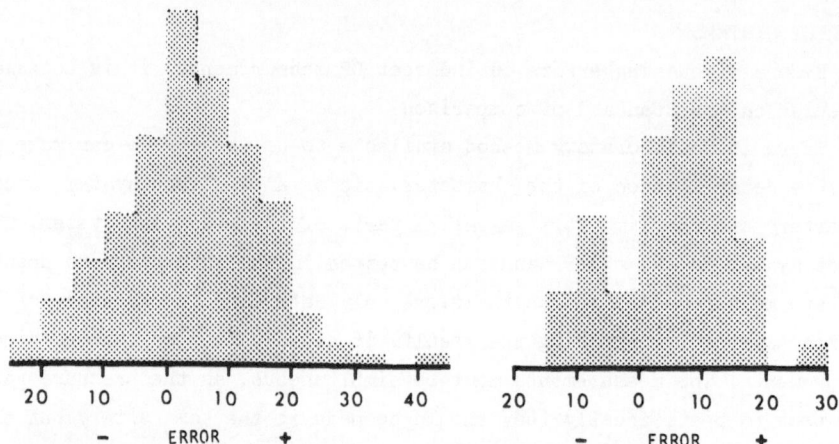

Fig. 1   Diastolic pressure error histograms, left Bruner et al,
right Raftery & Ward.

finding that the indirect method over-reads diastolic pressure while Van
Bergen found it to under-read. More recently, comparisons have been made
by several authors between the standard Oxford ambulatory direct system and
both manual and automatic indirect methods. These studies too show
comparable scatter, and all lead to the conclusion that although the mean
difference between paired points is probably less than 5mm Hg, the standard
deviation is of the order of 10-12 mm Hg, with a significant number of
errors exceeding 20 mm Hg in either direction.

What are the causes of these errors; are they due to imperfect equipment, the way the equipment is used, or unavoidable anatomical or physiological factors? It has been suggested that indirect BP is a different
physiological measurement from direct BP, but equally valid. I do not
believe this; the distribution of errors is too close to that to be expected
when comparing an accurate instrument with one subject to random errors,
but both measuring the same parameter, to allow me to believe they are
actually measuring correctly two different but related parameters.

The use of Korotkoff sounds to determine the systolic and diastolic end
points in conjunction with an arm cuff vests on the following assumptions:
1. The hydrostatic pressure in the volume of tissue contained by the cuff
   is equal to the air pressure in the cuff.
2. The artery closes (is collapsed) when the external pressure exceeds

(however slightly) the internal pressure, and opens when the internal pressure exceeds (however slightly the external pressure.

3. The opening of the artery at systole as the cuff is gradually deflated can be detected by listening for, or feeling the pulse at a point downstream from the cuff.

4. There is an identifiable change in the sound or feel of the pulse at the downstream point when the artery no longer closes at any point in the cycle; and this corresponds to diastole.

(1) can be accepted as valid, to the accuracy required, provided the cuff is long enough to wrap fully around the arm, and wide enough to ensure that edge effects are not significant, so that at least some part of the artery is in a region of zero pressure gradient.

(2) Is demonstrably not true in general. A healthy artery is a highly compliant, but fairly thick walled tube, and the external pressure must appreciably exceed the internal pressure fully to collapse it. A hardened artery (arteriosclerosis) is less compliant, and less easy to collapse fully. Arbitrarily, it might make better sense to take the external pressure needed to reduce the cross-sectional area by say 50% as equal to the internal pressure.

(3) If the above qualification to (2) is accepted, the first appearance of sound or pulse, which is easily and unambiguously determined, is not in fact the required point.

(4) A change certainly does occur, but exactly how the sounds are produced and why they change is not understood, and the relationship to diastolic pressure is empirical only.

That errors of considerable magnitude are caused by using the wrong size of cuff has long been known (Pickering (1968), Karvonen (1964)). A recent study by Maxwell (1982) based on over 80,000 readings, has qualified this; Fig 2 is plotted from his data, and shows the magnitude of the corrections to diastolic pressure readings which are required. It is worth noting that the least variation in error with arm size is obtained with the largest cuff, which is what would be expected on physical grounds.

Raftery & Ward (loc cit) showed that the first Korotkoff sound heard is not consistently related to the first appearance of the distal pulse, as sensed by direct pressure measurement distal to the cuff. This may well be a source of random error in systolic measurements, and it is probable that

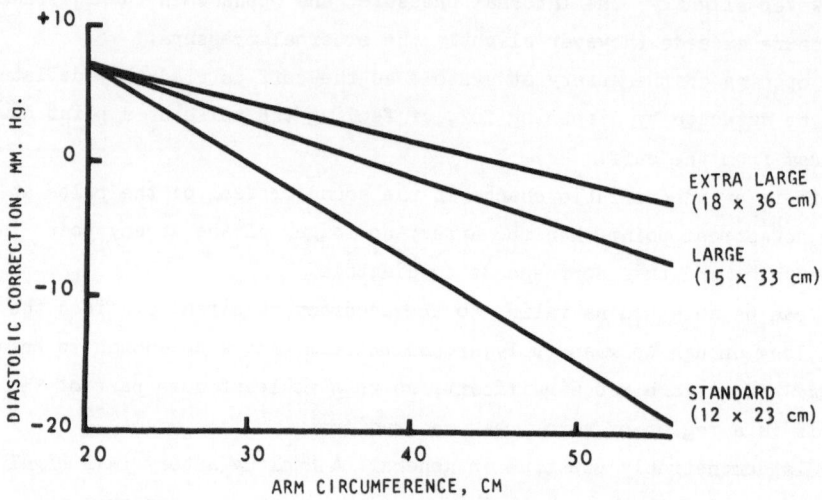

Fig. 2   Diastolic pressure correction required in relation to arm
circumference, for 3 different cuff sizes. Plotted from data by
Maxwell et al (Loc cit.)

the same lack of consistency may exist between the Korotkoff diastolic end
points and the physical events in the artery.

Is any alternative approach possible which will reduce the errors? is
it possible to obtain accurate blood pressure measurements indirectly? I
believe it can be done, though the evidence is as yet far from conclusive,
and the techniques not fully developed. Aaslid & Brubakk (1981) have used a
vascular unloading technique (first suggested I believe by Shirter (1962))
on the brachial artery, and on a small group of subjects obtains results
agreeing with direct measurements within about 2 mm. A similar method
applied to the digital artery (proposed by Penaz (1973)) has been developed
by Yamakoshi (1980) and again the results are good; SD about 5 mm, but a
non-normal distribution of errors, in that there are no gross errors, all
readings are within about 10 mm of direct measurements. Some of the scatter
here must be due to genuine differences between the direct and indirect
measurement sites. These vascular unloading methods are complex and not very
easy to use and are very unlikely ever to be practicable as the basis for
an ambulatory measuring system.

At the Clinical Research Centre, we have followed up earlier work by
Earl Wood (1950b) at the Mayo Clinic who showed that it was possible to
measure BP on the dilated vessels of the ear, using a modified ear oximeter

to apply pressure by an inflatable capsule, and follow changes of blood
volume in the vessels by photoelectric densitometry. This is essentially
the same as the photoelectric plethysmographic technique which is the basis
of the vascular unloading methods of Penaz and Yamakoshi referred to above.

We were able to verify Woods results, but also concluded from studies
on a number of subjects that the systolic readings are unreliable by this
method, and that it is unworkable on a significant proportion of subjects.
Maintaining the blood vessels sufficiently dilated for long periods also
presents problems.

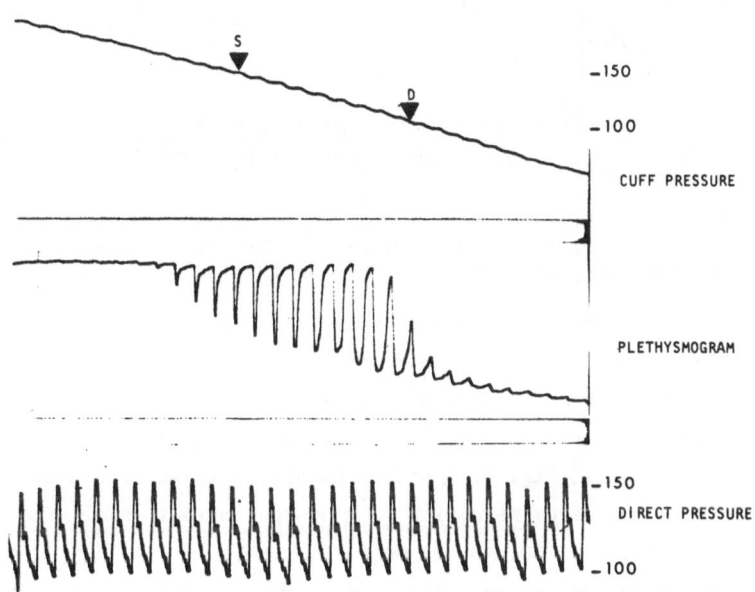

Fig. 3   Simultaneous recording of Brachial Artery Pressure (lower
tracing), Radial artery volume (centre), and Cuff Pressure (upper).
Note that in R.A. volume tracing bloodless level is at the top.

We therefore decided to carry out a series of measurements by the same
method on the radial artery, with the light source (an infra-red LED) and
photocell placed on opposite sides of the line of the artery about 1 to 2 cm
apart, in the centre of the area to which the cuff was applied.

The resultant tracings of the cuff pressure, plethysmogram and Brachial
artery pressure are shown in Fig. 3. This tracing was used to determine the

correct systolic and diastolic end points for this subject; cuff pressure
and direct pressure were found to be the same when the blood volume shown

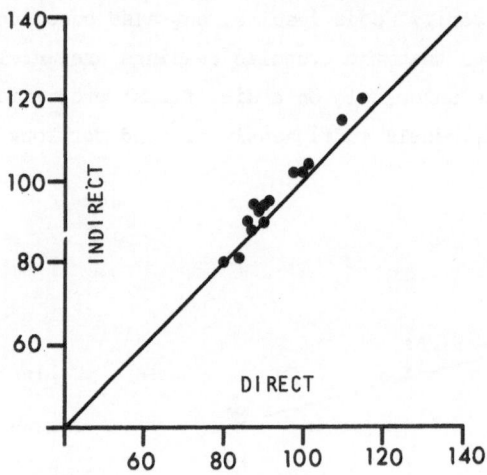

Fig. 4   Diastolic pressure, Direct and Indirect Methods, using the
photo-electric plethysmogram method on the Radial Artery.

by the plethysmograph departed from the bloodless level by half the maximum
amplitude of pulsation. (The points marked S and D in the figure).

The same criteria for determining systolic and diastolic pressures were
then applied to the tracings from the rest of the subjects. The results for
diastole are shown in Fig. 4. Systole was not quite so accurately recorded;
9 out of the 13 readings were with 7 mm of the correct value, the remaining
4 were in error by 10, 10, 13, 14 mm respectively.

These may however represent real differences; the advantage of concent-
rating on diastolic reading is that the diastolic pressure is much the same
in all arteries, whereas systolic pressures differ widely at different
sites.

This small study, like those of Aarslid and Brubakke and Yamakoshi,
are, even taken together, not conclusive proof that accurate pressure
measurements can be made by indirect methods, but they are enough to
suggest that further development is justified, when we compare the results
with the proven inaccuracy of the traditional method.

REFERENCES

Aaslid, R. and Brubakk, A.O. 1981. Circulation 64, 4, 753
Bruner, J. et al, 1981. Medical Instrumentation 14, 3, 182; 15, 1, 11;
    15, 2, 97.
Harrison, E.G. et al, 1960. Circulation 22, 419.
Karvonen, M.J. et al, 1964. Medicor, 4, 27-35.
McDonald, D.A. 1974, Blood Flow in Arteries, 2nd Ed. Arnold, London.
Maxwell, Morton, H. et al, 1982. Lancet, July 3, 33.
Penaz, J. 1973. Dig. 10th Int. Conf. Med. Biol. Eng. Dresden, Germany, 104.
Pickering, G. 1968. High Blood Pressure, 10.12, Churchill, London.
Raftery, E.B. and Ward, A.P. 1968. Cardiovasc. Res. 2, 210-218.
Shirer, H.W. 1962. IRE TRans. Biomed. Electron. BME 9, 116-125.
Van Bergen, F.H. et al, 1954. Circulation, 10, 4, 481.
Wood, E.H. 1950. Am. J. Physiol. 163, 762.
Wood, E.H. 1950. Staff Meetings of Mayo Clinic, July 5, 398.
Yamakoshi, et al. 1980. IEEE Trans. Biomed. Eng. BME 27, 3, 150.

AIR-CHAMBER SENSING FOR BLOOD PRESSURE MONITORING

P. Petrou, N. Yannopoulos, S. Stamatelopoulos, S. Moulopoulos

Medical Department Clinical Therapeutics,
Athens University , Alexandra Hospital,
V. Sofias - K. Lourou street,
Athens - Greece

ABSTRACT

A non-invasive method for blood pressure (BP) monitoring, by using a continuously inflated air-chamber, positioned against the area of either brachial or radial artery pulsation is tested. Tracings obtained via conventional pressure trans-ducers or a catheter-tip-manometer through 5 types of air-cham-bers are compared to simultaneously obtained tracings, via an intraarterial catheter. The pulse tracings obtained via an air-chamber of 2.0x2.5x4.0 cm, positioned into the empty case of a wrist watch and placed against the area of the radial artery pulsations showed a highly significant correlation (p varying from p<0.01 to p<0.001, in 20 patients, 10 hyperten-sives and 10 normotensives) to the simultaneously recorded intraarterial BP tracings for a time period of 2 hours.

INTRODUCTION

Effective reduction of increased BP lessens the risk of premature death even in mild hypertension (Hypertension Detec-tion and Follow up Program Cooperative Group, 1979). However, the BP level at which treatment should be initiated remains still (Alderman and Madhavan, 1981; Caplan, 1981; Freis, 1981) uncertain. It seems highly improbable to establish a critical pressure level for the initiation of treatment based only on casual BP readings by the sphygmomanometer, since a wide ran-ge of often unpredicted BP variations (Clement, 1979) exists during the day. Recent evidence (Millar-Craig et al., 1981 and 1982; Takeda et al., 1981; Tochikubo et al., 1981; Petrou et al., 1982) indicates the possibility of using data from 24 hr BP monitoring for the assessment of the need and/or the effectiveness of antihypertensive treatment. Under their pre-sent form, the methods of continuous BP recording are not ve-ry suitable for everyday clinical application. An attempt to use air-chamber sensing for blood pressure monitoring, from either the brachial or the radial artery is presented.

METHODS AND PATIENTS

Five types of non-invasive, air-chamber arterial sensing devices (A to E, Fig. 1) were tested for 2 hours in 10 hypertensive and 10 normotensive subjects during intraarterial BP recording. The same devices were further tested in 10 hypertensive and 10 normotensive subjects while BP reading were obtained by the sphygmomanometer at every 2 min for 1 hour.

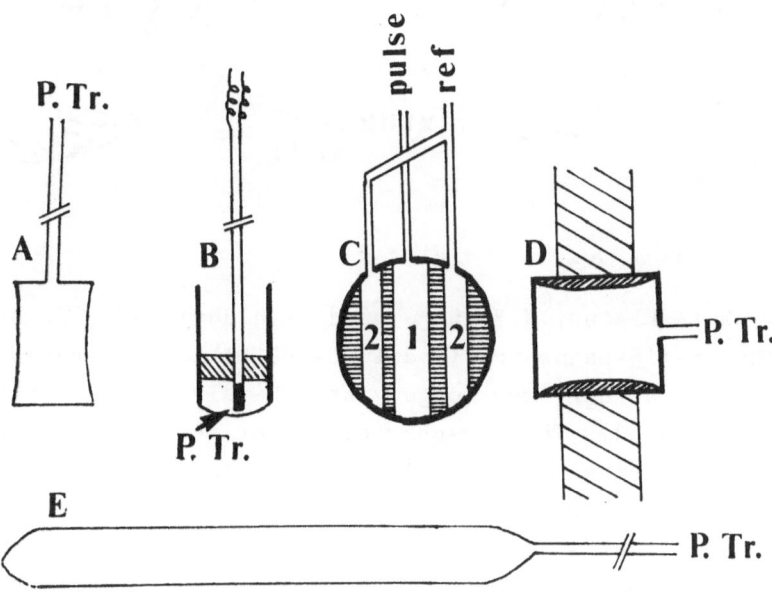

Fig. 1

The devices A to D were applied against the area of radial artery pulsation, as shown in fig. 2. The device E was applied against the area of brachial artery pulsation with its long axis being parallel to the artery. Recordings were made at bed rest and in sitting position, as well as during isometric exercise and movements of the arm on which the device was positioned. The wrist was immobilized by a sling when the devices A to D were tested.

All air-chambers were made from polyurethane in tetrahydrofuranium and connected to polyethylene tubes (fig. 1). Statham, inductance type transducers (Electronics for Medicine

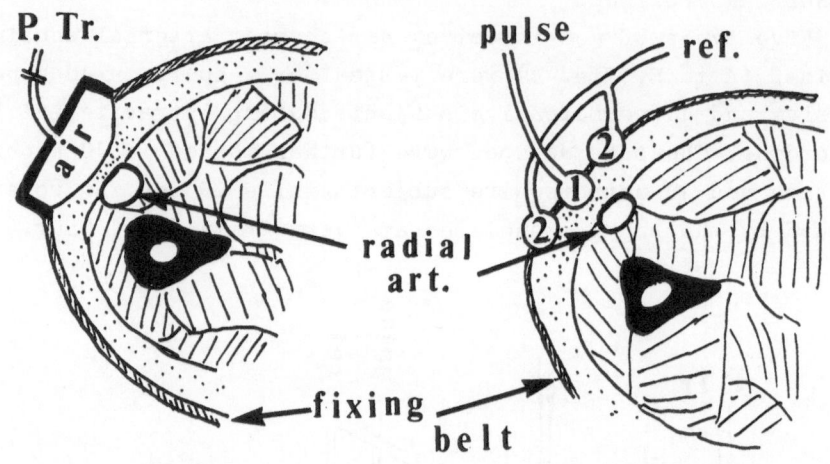

Fig. 2

Inc., White Plains, N.Y) were used with devices A, C, D and E.
A catheter-tip-manometer (Model PC-460 Millar Instruments,
Houston, Texas USA) was lodged into the air-chamber of the device B (Fig. 1). The air-chamber "1" of the device C (Figs.
1 and 2) was sensing the radial artery pulse ("pulse",Figs.1,2).
while the air-chambers "2", connected to a second pressure
transducer ("ref", Figs. 1, 2) were used for the recordings
of probable baseline fluctuations during monitoring. The air-
chambers (2.0x2.5x0.4 cm) of the device D was positioned into
the emptly case of a wrist-watch (Figs. 1 and 2).

The inflation of the air-chambers was initiated, via a
stopcock, as soon as the devices were positioned against the
arterial pulsation. The inflation continued until the arterial
pulse waveform obtained was matched, as close as possible,with
the simultaneously recorded intraarterial one from the opposite side. The pressure applied to that effect did never exceed
a limit causing discomfort to the subject. All subjects
were selected to have the same BP in both arms. Informed con-
cent was obtained from the subjects submitted to simultaneous
intraarterial BP recording.

The frequency response was tested with each one of the
devices connected to the recording apparatus. It was found

satisfactory following the applications of intermittent positive pressure to the air-chamber at a rate up to 50 Hz.

RESULTS

The stablest non-invasive pulse recordings, showing a
highly significant (r varying from 0.96 to 0.99 and p from $<$
0.05 to $<$ 0.001 in the 10 hypertensives and r from 0.89 to
0.99 and p from $<$0.01 to $<$ 0.001 in the 10 normotensives) correlation with the intraarterial ones were obtained by using
device D against the area of the radial pulsation. Valsava ma-
neuver caused (Fig. 3) identical changes in both the non-invasive and the intraarterial pulse tracings. No baseline correct-

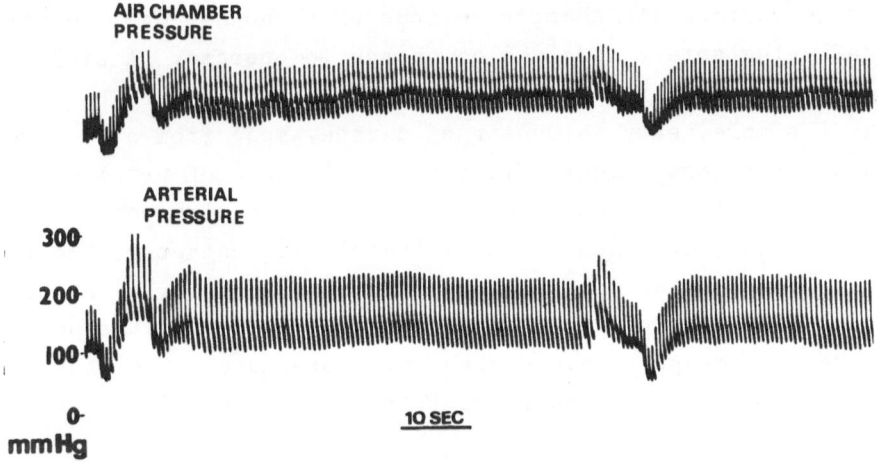

Fig. 3

ions were needed during the two-hour period of observation,
though transient distortions were noted on the non-invasive
recordings during movements of the forearm.

The baseline monitoring via the lateral ("reference") air-
chambers of the device D,did not provide more accurate tracings: In several instances baseline fluctuations were recorded
without any appreciable changes on the pattern of non-invasive
pulse tracing.

The sensors can be used in connection to a transducer-
amplifier-tape recorder portable system.

COMMENT

The non-invasive methods in use for BP monitoring are safer but less accurate (Clement, 1979) compared to the invasive ones, which are associated with the potential risks of a prolonged arterial catheterization. Furthermore, the apparatuses for non-invasive BP monitoring are often (Horan et al., 1981) complex or their operation involves frequent periodical arterial obstructions, which might affect the BP level obtained since they can cause discomfort to the subject examined. Still, some of these apparatuses remain quite expensive. It has to be stressed that what really differs between the invasive and the various non-invasive methods is the sensor device. This work deals with the idea of obtaining arterial pulse recordings through various air-chamber devices which do not occlude periodically the artery and need no energy to operate. A simple calibration to mercury manometer readings would suffice.

A simple, easy to construct device, made from a polyurethane air-chamber located into the empty case of wrist watch provided pressure recordings, which showed a high correlation with the ones obtained via an intraarterial catheter. The frequency response of the system was satisfactory for a rate up to 50 Hz and the correlation between intraarterial and non-invasive recordings remained high for a pressure range from 60 to 260 mmHg. A sling can prevent from recording distortions during the usual movements of the arm.

The sensor device described here has to be considered as an attempt to offer a simple and accurate, as possible, approach to solve the problems of sensing during non-invasive BP recording. It can operate in connection to any of the existing portable transducer-amplifier-recording systems.

REFERENCES

Alderman, M.H., Madhavan, S. 1981. Management of the hypertensive patient: A continuing dilemma. Hypertension, 3, 192.
Clement, D.L. 1979. Blood Pressure Variability. MTP Press Limited, Lancaster, England.
Freis, E.D. 1981. Treatment of hypertension in 1981. Hypertension (Suppl. II), 11-230.
Horan, M.J., Padgett, N.E., Kennedy, H.L. 1981. Ambulatory blood pressure monitoring: Recent advances and clinical

applications. Am. Heart J., <u>101</u>, 843-848.

Hypertension Detection and Follow-up Program Cooperative Group 1979. Five year findings of the Hypertension Detection and Follow-up Program. I. Reduction in mortality of persons with high blood pressure, including mild hypertension. J.A.M.A., <u>242,</u> 2562.

Kaplan, N.M. 1981. Whom to treat. The dilemma of mild hypertension. Am. Heart J., <u>101</u>, 867-870.

Millar-Craig, M.W., Manus, S., Balasubramanian, V., Cashman, P., Raftery, E.B. 1981. Effects of chronic beta blockade on intra-arterial blood pressure during motor car driving. Brit. Heart J., <u>45</u>, 645-648.

Petrou, L.P., Georgilis, A.C., Contoyannis, A.D., Yannopoulos, N.M., Elias, C.J., Maintas, G.P., Antonatos, P.S., Stamatelopoulos, F.S., Moulopoulos, D.S. 1982. Continuous blood pressure recording for the diagnosis of borderline hypertension. Hellenic Cardiol. Review (In Press).

Takeda, T., Nishiyama, K., Hirata, Y. 1981. Blood pressure variations to be considered in the treatment of hypertension. JPN Circ. J., <u>45</u>(7), 800.

Tochikubo, O., Umermura, S., Noda, K., Kaneko, Y. 1981. Variability of arterial blood pressure and classification of essential hypertension by multivariate statistical analysis. JPN Circ. J., <u>45</u>(7), 781.

TOPIC: 1.3

Review of existing systems for ECG ambulatory monitoring.

REVIEW OF COMMERCIALLY AVAILABLE SYSTEMS
FOR AMBULATORY MONITORING *

C.Marchesi, A.Taddei, M.Varanini, A.Macerata

CNR Institute of Clinical Physiology, Pisa

ABSTRACT

Instrumentation for ambulatory monitoring is presently available on the market in more than 20 different models.

This wide choice can make it difficult to adopt a particular solution. In order to investigate the existence of common criteria used in the design of the different systems, an inquiry has been made among most of the manufacturers of Ambulatory Monitoring systems. By the analysis of the questionnaires it is possible to conclude that very few components of the systems are carried out following the same approach, and that the problem of the evaluation of the performances is not approached in a uniform way. Thus the user has no objective elements suited to operate rational choices.

INTRODUCTION

This review has been based on a questionnaire forwarder to all the available addresses of manufacturers of ambulatory monitoring systems. The questionnaire, which is a modified version of one already published (Ripley, 1980), includes more than 100 questions grouped in several topics: recording unit, hardware structure, general characteristics, algorithms, performance evaluation.

Seventeen manufacturers have limited their answers, to 22 models. A number of questionnaires was not filled out completely; when possible the answers have been derived from appropriate data sheets.

All the material is presented in the format of tables, allowing a comparison between the different types of systems.

In view of the relevant differences between the real time portable analyzers and the more traditional playback scanners, they have been considered separately.

* Partly supported by CNR special project on Biomedical and Clinical Engineering.

1. PLAY-BACK SCANNERS

Figure 1 shows the general scheme of an analyzer for the play-back analysis. Obviously the recording process is separate from the analysis, which is accomplished in accelerated time.

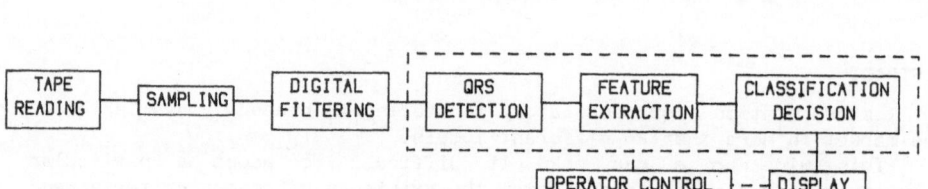

Fig.1

TABLE I.1

AMERICAN EDWARDS	(USA)	ELIMINATOR	A
CLINICAL DATA	(USA)	THE REPORTER	B
DEL MAR AVIONICS	(USA)	HEART SCREEN	C
		TREND SETTER	D
ELA MEDICAL	(F)	ANATEC S	E
HELLIGE	(D)	MEMOPORT C	F
ICR	(USA)	EVENT MASTER IV	G
		6201-G3	H
MARQUETTE	(USA)	8000	I
OXFORD	(GB)	MEDILOG MA14	J
		MEDILOG MA20	K
		MEDILOG PMD12	L
		MEDILOG 9000	M
REMCO ITALIA	(I)	ETALONG	N
REYNOLDS	(GB)	PATHFINDER	O
SIEMENS	(D)	SIRETAPE 824	P

Table I.1 reports the list of the systems which have been considered.

The letters in the column on the right will be used to identify the different systems throughout the text.

1.1 Recorders

Table I.2 shows that some features of the recorders have to be considered as a standard: the number of leads (2), the medium (cassette), the duration of the recording (24 hours).

TABLE I.2

SIGNALS:	2 ECG LEADS	12	ABCDEFGJKNOP
	2 ECG LEADS + 1 (AV.)	1	I
	PACEMAKER ANALYSIS	3	DFO
	CUFF PRESSURE	2	BD
	RESPIRATORY SIGNALS	2	BO
	8 EEG LEADS	1	M
	4 EEG LEADS	1	L
MEDIUM:	CASSETTE	13	BDEFGIJKLMNOP
	REEL (+ CASSETTE)	2	AC
METHOD:	DIRECT	6	FGJLMO
	FM	6	BEIKNP
	PCM	2	CD
	PWM	1	A
DURATION:	24 HOURS	10	ABEFJKLMNP
	26 "	2	CD
	48 "	2	GI
	32.5 "	1	O
BANDWIDTH:	0.05–100 Hz	8	ACDEGIKO
	0.05–40	1	B
	0.05–60	1	P
	0.05–70	1	N
	0.08–70	1	J

The method of recording is not always the frequency modulation; probably this choice, while preferable as far as signal to noise ratio and low frequency responce are concerced has some limitations because it requires a more sophisticated tape speed control. The data about the bandwidth should be considered carefully. In fact the standard recommended by the American Heart Association (0.05–100Hz) is often satisfied only by the electronics; the true bandwidth, available at the reproducing head, could be far lower (Bragg Remschel et al. 1982, Boter and Van Keulen 1981)

1.2 Acquisition

TABLE I.3

SAMPLING RATE: 100 SPS		3	BNO
(REAL TIME) 256		2	CD
240		1	I
200		1	G
PRECISION: 8 BITS		5	BCDHN
10 BITS		2	IO
7 BITS		1	E

1.3 Scanners

Most of the systems are carried out with a multi–micro processors structure, in order to achieve the necessary processing speed. In fact the mean interbeat interval is only 5 msec. (for a heart rate of 100 beats per minute at 120 times the real time speed).

The scanners can be grouped in 3 categories (Table I.4).

TABLE I.4

VISUAL ANALYSIS	4	ABCN
INTERACTIVE ANALYSIS	9	DEFGHJKOP
AUTOMATIC ANALYSIS	1	I

Table I.5 shows the different playback speeds. In most of the systems the analysis is performed during the acquisition, thus the speed factor is not greater than 120.

Factors greater than 120 also imply very simple operations or only acquisition on mass storage (like system I), for subsequent analysis.

TABLE I.5

PLAYBACK SPEED: X 60–120	4	HJKO
240	2	CG
60	2	F
240–480	1	A
60–120–240	1	D
120	1	B
1–30–60	1	P
32–64	1	N
100	1	E
500	1	I
20–60	1	L
20–40–60	1	M

Table I.6 reports the number of leads analyzed and the processing time required. Practically all the systems analyze only one channel.

TABLE I.6

ECG LEADS ANALYZED: 1		13	ABCDEFGHJKNOP
2		1	I
TIME REQUIRED	6 min.	1	G
FOR ANALYSIS	12	1	H
OF 24 HOUR TAPE	15 (+10 OP.EDIT.)	1	I
	20	3	ACD
	24 (2 hours in man.)	1	F
	24	1	P
	30	2	BN
	40	1	O

The problem of the time required for the analysis is quite controversial. Manufacturers usually refer to automatic (unsupervised) analysis, which is usually of poor quality. Probably a typical figure for operator assisted analysis is about 1 hour.

1.3.1. QRS detection

We can distinguish analog and digital detectors (Table I.7): digital ones are software or hardware implemented. The trend is toward the software implementation because of the large diffusion of more powerful and low cost microprocessors. The software implementation allows a more complex structure, great flexibility and controlled accuracy.

TABLE I.7

IMPLEMENTATION:	SOFTWARE	4	ADEI
	SOFTWARE +DIG. HARD.	2	GH
	DIGITAL HARDWARE	1	C
	ANALOG	4	BNOP
AUTOADAPTABILITY:		10	ACDEFGHIOP
CIRTERION BASED ON:	AMPLITUDE	4	ACDP
	FIRST DIFFERENCE	4	BGHN
	SECOND DIFF.	2	AO
	WAVE SHAPE	4	EIOP
	DURATION	1	P
FIDUCIAL POINT			
	R WAVE PEAK	3	AEF
	CENTER OF GRAVITY	2	GH
	FOURIER ANALYSIS	1	I
	SLOPE CHANGE	2	CD
	DEFLECTION AN.	1	O

However, the limiting factor is represented by the algorithm execution time, to be kept low particularly in accelerated time analysis. Sometimes hardware is associated to software for saving computer time. Auto adaptability is an important feature for the detectors used to scan the long term ECG tracings, because the signal is affected by a large variability in the amplitude, rhythm and morphology.

The detection algorithm is generally based on the analysis of some parameters derived from the ECG signal, such as a time derivative or some particular transformation which enhances the QRS features in the context of the other ECG cycle events.

Sometimes a combination of more parameters is used in the detection process as the amplitude combined with the second derivative (A) or with a shape parameter (P).

An accurate identification of a fiducial point within the QRS complex is important for the further operation of beat classification.

Therefore, after the QRS complex detection, a search is started for a reference point which has to be stable even in presence of noise and signal variations.

1.3.2 Classification

All systems perform the analysis of RR intervals, which often consists only in the comparison between two consecutive RR intervals. A more sophisticated analysis based on the morphology is accomplished with a variety of methods (Table I.8).

An approach is based on the extraction of features from the signal (such as: duration, offset, areas, etc) and on their comparison with reference values.

TABLE I.8

CLASSIFICATION:

RR ANALYSIS	13	ACDEFGHIJKNOP
SHAPE ANALYSIS		
FEATURE EXTR.	5	FGJKP
TEMPLATE ANALYSIS		
SINGLE TEMPL.	1	O
MULTIPLE TEMPL.	4	CDFI
CORRELATION	3	CDF
DIFFERENCE AREA	1	O

ST ANALYSIS: 7   DEHIJKO

A second approach consists in the definition of one or more templates as references for the comparison, which is usually performed through the correlation coefficients and sometimes with other criteria such as some kind of distance measure.

When the processing speed is crucial, only two classes are defined (normal-abnormal). Of course only the systems using a multiple templates approach are able to classify the events in several classes.

Most of the systems are interactive (Table I.4) and the definition of the typical templates is done by the operator.

Recently ST-T analysis has been added to the system functions. This is simply performed by measuring the ST changes in some predetermined time instants.

1.3.3 Data Presentation.

Since the systems usually require an interaction with the operator, the presentation of the results is an important function to be considered (Table I.9). There is usually a combination of techniques both on hard copy and on visual display units used by all the systems. We can observe that the so called full disclosure technique has been adopted by 6 manufactures and the dynamic contourography by one. This last method seems particularly suited to the morphological changes detection.

TABLE I.9

```
HARD COPY: FULL DISCLOSURE            6     ACDGHO
           TREND PLOTS
           STRIPS                          in combination
           NUMERICAL PRINTOUT


LABILE DISPLAY: SUPERIMPOSED (SINGLE, MULTIPLE)
                JOG
                SLIDE SERIAL            in combination
                PAGE
                DYNAMIC CONTOUROGRAPHY 1    N
```

---

2. REAL TIME SYSTEMS

Table II.1 reports the list of the real time systems which have been considered in this review.

TABLE II.1

CIRCADIAN	(USA)	CIRCAMED	A
COM	(ISR.)	CARDICOM	B
CUSTOMED	(D)	CUSTOPORT	C
DATAMEDIX	(USA)	PECGASYS	D
IMC	(USA)	HOLTER II	E
MEDICAL CONCEPTS	(USA)	AEGIS	F

Figure 2 shows the typical structure of a real* time portable analyzer.

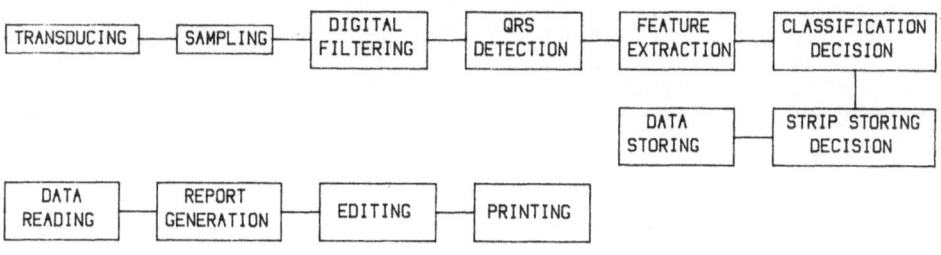

Fig.2

2.1 Recording

A group of real time systems still make use of cassette recording to allow the storage of a large number of ECG strips. Others use only a solid state memory thereby allowing a reduced space for ECG records (Table II.2).

TABLE II.2

NUMBER OF LEADS: 2	5	ACDEF
3	1	B
PACEMAKER CONTROL:	2	CDBE
MASS STORAGE: ON CASSETTE	3	CF
SOLID STATE	2	CD
BOTH	1	AB
REC. METHOD: FM	2	AE
DIGITAL	2	BF
ECG STORAGE: 120 SEC	1	C
256 SEC	1	D
2880 SEC	1	F
14400 SEC	1	E
21600 SEC	1	B
SINGLE STRIP DURATION: 10 SEC	2	AE
6-10 SEC	1	F
8-10 SEC	1	B
8 SEC	1	D
8-2 SEC	1	C

2.2 Analysis

As a general comment we can state that the design of the real time systems is based on a compromise among various factors, such as: cost, power consumption, weight, physical dimensions and reliability of the analysis. Of course the last is the most important feature, since the system allows only a partial verification of the analysis, based on the abnormal events recorded. In principle the real time systems should offer a more sophisticated analysis than playback scanners, because their computing power is distributed over 24 hours. From this point of view they take advantage of the decreasing cost and dimensions of LSI technology. In fact we can see from Table II.3 that sampling rate is usually larger than in playback scanners, two leads are analyzed and the detection and analysis algorithms are software implemented. Manufacturers did not give satisfactory information about the algorithms used for signal processing.

TABLE II.3

SAMPLING RATE:	400 SPS	1	A
	256	1	E
	250	1	D
	125	1	F

CONTINUOUS ANALYSIS:	24 HOURS	4	BCDF
	48	1	A
	VARIABLE TO 72	1	E

NUMBER OF LEADS ANALYZED:	1	3	DEF
	2	2	AC
	3	1	B

QRS DETECTION:

SOFTWARE IMPL.	3	ADE
AUTOADAPTABILITY	2	AE
CRITERION BASED:		
ON AMPLITUDE	2	AE
FIRST DIFFERENCE	1	E
WAVESHAPE	2	AE

FIDUCIAL POINT:

| GEOMETRIC ANALYSIS | 1 | A |
| MAX NEG SLOPE | 1 | E |

CLASSIFICATION:

RR ANALYSIS	6	ABCDEF
SHAPE ANALYSIS		
FEATURE EXTRACTION	1	A
SINGLE TEMPLATE	1	E
MULTIPLE TEMPLATE	1	D

| ST LEVEL: | 4 | BCDE |

As far as the display of the data is concerned, we can observe that different solutions have been realized. In particular some systems allow both a graphical and numerical presentation of the results on the visual screen. Thus an editing is possible and the copy of only interesting data is obtained on a hard copy device. A useful solution consists in printers with graphic and alphanumeric capabilities, allowing a compact and uniform reporting.

TABLE II.4

DATA PRESENTATION:	ON A SINGLE PRINTER PLOTTER	2	CD
	PRINTER + STRIPS	4	ABEF
	ECG DISPLAY	4	BCDE

As a concluding remark we can say that the operator time required to obtain the final report is not much reduced in real time systems in comparison with playback scanners. In fact additional time consuming operations, such as initialization procedures and editing, or "post-processing", should be taken into account.

3. EVALUATION

The performance evaluation of the instrumentation should be made according to the definition of standard criteria about reference data, events of clinical importance and statistical indicators to be used to assess or compare the results of the evaluation. Unfortunately such a complete golden standard does not exist. Therefore MIT and AHA have made available reference data useful to test the algorithms at least as regards most of the important rhythm abnormalities. Table III shows the list of all the systems which have been submitted to some form of performance evaluation. Some manufacturers did not communicate how the evaluation was performed and/or the results of the evaluation. Many others used their own data base and communicated only partial results of the evaluation. Thus data available at the time of the inquiry (April 1983) does not allow a choice based on the performances of the systems, neither in absolute nor in relative terms.

TABLE III

MANUFACTURER	HOW	RESULTS	
AVIONICS	?	?	
HELLIGE	?	?	
ICR	ICR DATA BASE	?	
MARQUETTE	MIT/BIH DATA BASE (48 HOURS)	QRS SENS.	99%
	AHA (PLANNED)	PVC SENS.	99%
		PVC PRED.	92-95%
ELAMEDICAL	UNSPECIFIED DATA BASE	?	
REMCO ITALIA	QUALITATIVE COMPARISON	HIGH MORPH. SENS	
REYNOLDS	MANY COMPARISONS BY INDEPEN-	PVC CORR.	0.89
	DENT INSTITUTIONS	COUPL.	0.95
		TACH.	0.98
CIRCADIAN	UNIV. OF MINNESOTA DATA BASE	?	
COM	AHA DATA BASE (PLANNED)	?	
DATAMEDIX	MIT + UNIV. OF ALABAMA		
	42 PATIENTS X 1 HOUR	QSR SENS	99%
		TYP. BEAT	99%
		ATYP. BEAT	96-98%
IMC	10 TAPES X 2 HOURS	PVC SENS	94%
		(72%-100%)	
		COUPL.	100%
		RUNS	100%
		PAUSES	96%
AEGIS	154 CONSECUTIVE PATIENTS	SENS	SPEC
	(799 HOURS)	PVC 92%	92%
		TACH 81%	92%
		SVP 81%	82%
		SVT 76%	85%

REFERENCES

Boter, J. and Van Keulen, G.J. 1981. In "Ambulatory Electrocardiographic Recording" (Ed. N.K. Wenger, M.B. Mock and R. Ringqvist) (Year Book Medical Publishers). pp. 23-32.

Bragg-Remschel, D.A. et al. 1981. New Methods to evaluate the frequency response and ST segment reproducibility of ambulatory ECG systems. Computers in Cardiology, IEEE Computers Society, pp. 91-96, Long Beach.

Ripley, K.L. and Murray A. 1980. Introduction to automated arrhythmia detection, IEEE Computer Society, Long Beach.

APPENDIX: Addresses of manufacturers

PLAYBACK SYSTEMS

MANUFACTURER	SYSTEM DESIGNATION
AMERICAN EDWARDS LABORATORIES DIVIS. OF AMER. HOSP. SUPPLY CORP. 17221 RED HILL AVENUE (IRVINE) P.O. BOX 11150, SANTA ANA CA 92711, USA	ELIMINATOR
CLINICAL DATA, INC. 1371 BEACON STREET BROOKLINE, MASS. 02146 U.S.A.	THE REPORTER
DEL MAR AVIONICS 1601 ALTON AVENUE IRVINE, CA. 92714 U.S.A.	HEART SCREEN TREND SETTER
ELA MEDICAL – MICROMED 98–100 RUE MAURICE ARNOUX 92541 MONTROUGE CEDEX FRANCE	ANATEC 'S'
HELLIGE GMBH HEINRICH VON STEPHAN STRASSE 4 D–7800 FREIBURG IM BREISGAU WEST GERMANY	MEMOPORT C
INSTRUMENTS FOR CARDIAC RESEARCH, INC. 6057 CORPORATE DRIVE EAST SYRACUSE, NEW YORK 13057 U.S.A.	EVENT MASTER IV 6201–G3
MARQUETTE ELECTRONICS, INC. P.O. BOX 23181 8200 W. TOWER AVE. MILWAUKEE, WIS. 53223 U.S.A.	8000
OXFORD ELECTRONIC INSTRUMENTS LTD. MEDICAL SYSTEMS DIVISION NUFFIELD WAY ABINGDON, OXON OX14 1 BZ ENGLAND	MEDILOG MA14 '' MA20 '' PMD12 '' 9000

REMCO ITALIA S.p.A.   ETALONG
STRADA RIVOLTANA NUOVA
20060 S. PEDRINO DI VIGNATE
MILANO
ITALY

REYNOLDS MEDICAL LIMITED   PATHFINDER
CAWTHORNE HOUSE
51 ST. ANDREW STREET
HERTFORD SG14 1HZ
ENGLAND

SIEMENS AG   SIRETAPE 824
HENKESTRASSE 127
8520 ERLANGEN
WEST GERMANY

REAL TIME SYSTEMS

CIRCADIAN INC.   CIRCAMED
777 PALOMAR AVENUE
SUNNYVALE, CALIFORNIA 94086
U.S.A.

C.O.M. MEDICAL SYSTEMS LTD   CARDICOM
P.O. BOX 9292, HAIFA 31 092
ISRAEL

CUSTOMED   CUSTOPORT
CLEMEN STRASSE 17
8000 MUNCHEN 40
WEST GERMANY

DATA MEDIX, INC.   PECGASYS
ARVIDA PARK OF COMMERCE
1001 NW 58 STREET
BOCA RATON, FLORIDA 33431
U.S.A.

INTERNATIONAL MEDICAL CORPORATION   HOLTER II
64 INVERNESS DRIVE EAST
ENGLEWOOD, COLORADO 80112
U.S.A.

MEDICAL CONCEPTS, INC.   AEGIS
137 GAITHER DRIVE
MT. LAUREL, NEW YERSEY 08054
U.S.A.

REVIEW OF AMBULATORY MONITORING SYSTEMS
DEVELOPED AT RESEARCH INSTITUTES

C. Zeelenberg

Thoraxcentre
Erasmus University
Rotterdam, The Netherlands

ABSTRACT

Over the past decade a number of research institutions have developed computer based systems for the analysis of Longterm Ambulatory Continuous Electrocardiographic Recordings (LACER). Some of these systems derive from earlier coronary care monitoring systems and share basic detection and classification algorithms. While differing widely in detail, the broad outlines of these systems show many common features. The paper describes these common aspects and then compares the main features of several such systems. It remains hard to compare system performance and although recent development of standard databases and evaluation techniques show promise they are not yet widely used. New developments in real-time monitors and further clinical research using the LACER analysis systems themselves seem likely to change this field radically over the next decade.

INTRODUCTION

The electrocardiogram (ECG) was one of the first biological signals to be analysed using a digital computer. The early work was directed towards diagnostic interpretation of very short segments of either orthogonal lead or twelve-lead ECGs. The characteristics of this type of analysis are that the input signal is relatively clean, the processing time is, even today, usually long in comparison to acquisition time and the algorithms delineate and measure ECG features in a detail analogous to that of a human observer. Additionally, since the diagnostic ECG is essentially a snapshot process, the emphasis lies on the morphological features of the P-QRS-T complex rather than on the rhythm. Recently, considerable research effort has been devoted to serial ECGs taken in the same subject over long periods. The emergence of the Coronary Care Unit (CCU) in the early sixties (Lown et al., 1967) with the requirements for determining the ventricular arrhythmias coincided with the appearance of the first 'cheap' minicomputers. Although all early CCUs employed analog ECG monitors which provided little more than (often inaccurate) rate alarms, there were soon a number of institutions working on sophisticated monitoring systems using hybrid or digital processors. The characteristics of this type of system are the use of a single lead, the ability to handle noise contaminated input, processing time which is always less than the acquisition time (much less in the case of parallel processing of multiple beds) and algorithms which are normally confined to recognition only of the QRS and which make little attempt to delineate all features in detail. The analysis is directed towards recognition of rhythm disturbances and for the latter part of the seventies at least has been almost exclusively directed towards the recognition and counting of ventricular extrasystoles.

Presentation of the data brought with it the problem of summarising the situation over relatively long periods (upto 24 hrs or more), trend determiniation and techniques for ensuring that rare events are not lost in the large quantities of data available.

Concurrent with the development of the CCU, Holter (1961), introduced the concept of long-term ambulatory recording of one or two ECG leads using magnetic tape as medium. The resultant tapes were analysed manually using analog systems which presented the ECG to the operator either 60 or 120 times real-time. It soon became clear to researchers that the analysis of these tapes presents many of the same problems, and was susceptible to many of the same solutions, as the CCU ECG-monitoring. The data (one or two, often very 'noisy' leads), the information required (primarily incidence of ventricular arrhythmias) and many of the presentation aspects (summarising long periods containing a large number of events) are all similar. Work started at various institutions on applying the algorithms developed for monitoring to the analysis of ambulatory tapes. The interest in this work increased considerably as the emphasis moved during the early and mid seventies from treatment to prevention of cardiac arrhythmias, requiring more research into the efficacy of anti-arrhythmic drugs, and as more research was done into the significance as a precursor of sudden death of ventricular arrhythmias in post myocardial infarction outpatients. Existing (analog) scanning techniques were not accurate enough for such research applications (Stein et al., 1980). At the same time, the number of tapes to be processed increased. There was thus a great inducement to introduce accurate, automated systems for tape analysis and many of the institutions previously active in the area of CCU monitoring shifted much of their development effort to ambulatory monitoring.

Despite many different approaches chosen by different institutions, they exhibit many common aspects and use similar methods to overcome technical constraints. Since data acquisition (and processing in one-pass systems) must be many times the recording speed if satisfactory frequency

characteristics are to be obtained and since processing in multipass systems must clearly be nearly as fast if analysis time is not to be much
greater than that of a manual system, there are considerable constraints on
the hardware design.

A further point in this area is the high sampling rate, and hence data
transfer rate, needed. A sampling rate of 4-30 kHz per channel is needed to
obtain an effective sampling frequency of 60-250 Hz at playback speeds of
60-120 times the recording speed. In any multipass system, this also implies the existence of sufficient mass storage to buffer the data during
further processing. For a system where the raw data will later be needed
for strip-charts or other purposes, this means a considerable on line data
storage requirement. Various solutions have been tried such as special-
purpose data compression and tape storage while many systems use analog
preprocessors. Some systems use only the R-R intervals derived from such
preprocessors. The wider availability and lower price of both powerful
microprocessors and bulk mass storage (such as very large Winchester-
technology disks) is gradually changing this aspect of many analysis systems.

Most investigators considered fully automated systems not reliable
enough. This led to the introduction of multipass algorithms where the
decision as to the morphological classification of a given beat could be
deferred until more beats of a similar morphology were found and also to
the idea of 'editing' whereby a further pass could for instance be used to
amalgamate closely-related clusters. This latter was also combined with a
degree of operator interaction, enabling clusters of mislabelled beats to
be correctly reclassified once the operator had indentified one member. In
order to make multipass processing faster while still retaining enough data
to present the ECG to the operator for final decision, present-day systems
mostly retain the original (compressed) digitised data on a buffer storage
while working with beat descriptions containing an index to the raw data.

Data acquisition is almost entirely automatic in the majority of systems. It may be followed by, parallel to or include the data reduction
phase, whose output is the beat description, and which in its turn may precede or include a beat classification step. Systems using analog preprocessors (such as QRS detectors) combine acquisition and description and, sometimes classification as well.

Exceptions to almost all the above points are formed by the more recently developed, truly automated, real-time ambulatory monitors which use

powerful microprocessors. These are covered fully elsewhere in this volume and will therefore be omitted from the remainder of this review.

In some systems the beat descriptions and classifications can then be edited with more or less operator intervention. The final result in all systems is a stream of classifications which describes the recording. This is then used as the raw material for a summarised report which in most cases contains a tally of PVCs, and often other rhythm patterns as well, together with time-trend graphics of heart rate and PVC occurrence.

One very important aspect of LACER analysis systems which is common only insofar as it is a problem in all systems is the question of artifact rejection. This plays a role at all points in the process, starting from electrode placement through filtering (digital or analog) and QRS detection to beat classification and the final report, in which many systems give an indication of the degree of artifact encountered. Although most authors agree that this is a question best tackled at the front end of the system (careful skin-cleaning, good electrodes, proper placement, suitable recorder characteristics), it is accepted that many tapes will be inadequate in quality. Feedback from the analysis system to the originating physician is sometimes used to improve consistently poor quality recordings. However, artifact recognition is still a very important part of any system, fully automated or interactive. Although beat description and classification algorithms have been considered in detail elsewhere in this volume, a short overview may be useful when contrasting analysis systems.

The majority of systems use either a correlation technique or feature extraction for beat description and classification. The former method is a single stage process, the latter may use two steps. Correlation, whereby the complete signal is compared with one or more templates (which may or may not be produced as the average of all previously classified beats in a given family) is computationally expensive. New hardware developments may, however, make this the technique of choice. Feature extraction, on the other hand, reduces a beat to a set of measurements (typically some or all of QRS height, QRS offset, QRS duration, QRS area, together with timing information). A variant of this method represents a QRS as a set of orthonormal polynominals. The feature space then consists of the set of weight factors associated with the representation. Clusters are then formed in this feature space of similar beats using a distance measure. Many different combinations are possible and can be combined with a variety of clustering techniques. With either correlation or feature extraction, certain basic criteria are then used to classify the underlying rhythm and the various clusters into normal, doubtful or PVC. Some systems provide a more detailed classification of non-PVCs (supra ventricular, fusion etc). Other techniques which have been applied are syntactic analysis and Markov chain methods. These are, however, confined to experimental or special-purpose systems as yet.

PERFORMANCE EVALUATION

Formal evaluation of the performance of an analysis system is far from simple and interpretation of the results can be extremely difficult, particularly for systems with a high degree of operator interaction. Even in the case of fully automated systems it is rarely possible to compare results directly as until recently there was no standardised database to use as a yardstick and there is still little agreement as to the best methods of presenting the results although several approaches have been proposed (Hermes and Cox, 1980). In addition, most systems can be 'tuned' to fit certain requirements (e.g. screening systems which require a very low false negative rate but will accept a high rate of false positives) and centers seldom specify identical system characteristics. The increasing use of Receiver Operator Characteristics (ROC curves) is helping to clarify this and the existence of two standard (and reasonably compatible) arrhythmia databases should make it easier to compare results in future (Ripley and Oliver, 1977; Schluter et al., 1980). In the case of interactive systems (and the majority of non-commercial analysis systems are to a greater or lesser degree interactive) the evaluation becomes one of comparing system/operator combinations. There are as yet no satisfactory techniques for extracting the operator component of the total systems performance.

Another aspect which is important but is certainly not present in many systems is that of quality control. This is implemented in different ways depending on the degree of operator interaction. In a fully interactive system, for example, this might take the form of either a randomly selected block or one selected according to a suitable strategy (e.g. the block containing the most non-PVC premature beats) which is presented to the operator for beat by beat examination (Zeelenberg et al., 1982). The results of such quality control would then be stored for later analysis.

SYSTEMS

There are approximately 20-30 LACER analysis systems which have been developed within research institutions. A few of these are no longer operational. Few of the systems can be considered portable and most require special-purpose hardware. Very few of the systems are operational outside the originating institution. Most systems have a large research component and reporting is often tailored to the requirements of the researchers. The following section reviews a few of the representative systems and their history and describes the highlights of a number of other systems. The list is certainly not exhaustive. More detailed reviews of some of these systems have been published earlier (Ripley and Murray, 1980; Oliver et al., 1977; Thomas et al., 1979).

ARGUS was originally developed as a computer system for CCU monitoring at Washington University, St. Louis. In 1973 a modified version termed ARGUS/H (highspeed) was introduced to analyse LACER tapes (Nolle at al., 1974; Oliver at al., 1974). Three steps are involved in processing a recording: data acquisition, automatic scanning and manual editing. Data acquisition was done using special purpose hardware, whereby a single channel ECG is digitized 60 times real-time at 250 Hz effective sampling frequency. The second difference of this signal was compressed and written out onto digital magnetic tape. In the second pass, this tape was scanned at highspeed by the ARGUS rhythm algorithms, implemented on an IBM System/7. These algorithms are the well known Aztec, Primitive and Cycle processors (Cox et al., 1968; Nolle and Clark, 1971). Aztec transforms the original ECG samples into a series of line segments. This yields a considerable compression and also provides the input for the next processing step, Primitive, which performs QRS detection and feature extraction. After determining begin and end of a QRS complex, four features are extracted to characterize the complex: duration, height, offset and absolute area. Together with timing information these features are passed to the Cycle processor which maintains clusters ("families") of QRS complexes with similar features. New beats are either entered into an existing family or a new family is started if no good match can be found. Beats are classified into normal, borderline, abnormal and PVC depending on prematurity, width and family morphology. The datastream produced by the Cycle processor is saved for operator review. During this editing phase, the operator is shown each detected PVC within its context and can thus eliminate all false positive PVCs. Finally, the system produces summary plots of heartrate and PVC rate and a numerical summary of various measures and rates. In 1975 the system was modified to increase the use of waveform context information and machine learning through editor interaction. This led to reduced human editing times of at least a factor four, and corrected most false positive PVCs due to misclassified T-waves (Mead at al., 1975). In 1977 the IBM system was replaced with a dual processor PDP-11 system with sufficient on-line storage to keep 24 hours of 2 channel ECG data on-line. This also eliminated the expensive special purpose digitizing and compression hardware (Clark et al., 1977). Since that time many improvements and extensions of the system have been published such as the detection of ST-changes (Clark et al., 1980), the approach to supraventricular arrhythmias (Clark et al., 1981) and the use of a frequency domain based algorithm for processing difficult waveforms (Mead at al., 1981). Also a multi-user version of the system was introduced at another institution (Ripley et al., 1980). The performance of ARGUS has been evaluated at various stages of its live, the most recent one (Mead at al., 1982) reported a better than 99% PVC sensitivity and only one false positive PVC on 15 half-hour sections of the AHA database. This evaluation was done prior to human editing, and thus represents the performance of an entirely automated ARGUS system.

In 1973 Stanford developed a system based on a PDP-12 minicomputer and a special-purpose analog preprocessor (Fitzgerald et al., 1974; 1975). During the first pass of a two pass process, the analog tape is read at 60 times real-time and 3 features are collected and stored for each QRS complex: R-R interval, QRS duration and the area under the first major deflection of the QRS. At the end of this pass, time plots of these parameters are made on an electrostatic plotter. Arrhythmias are identified by the operator by variations from the normal sinus rhythm in these plots. In the second pass printouts of areas of abnormality are made. PVCs may be defined in terms of upper and lower limits on each of the three features. In 1976 a successor to this system was introduced, based on a HP2112 computer and a hardware QRS-detector (Spitz et al., 1977). During the first processing step, a single channel ECG is digitized at 60 times real-time with an effective sampling frequency of 100 Hz and stored on a digital magnetic tape. In the second step, correlation relationships are used to classify QRS complexes into dynamically created families, whereby each complex is classified into one of three groups: the operator selects it as a template for a new family, it is classified as a member of the family with which it has the highest correlation or the beat is rejected as noise and not analysed. In 1980 several modifications were made to both hardware and software of the system to move from single channel to two channel processing (Anderson et al., 1980; Bragg-Remschel and Harrison, 1980). A special two channel ECG preprocessor was constructed to provide two channel filtering, sampling and QRS detection. The operator may decide to digitize either channel or both and perform QRS detection on either channel or a summed channel. Also for classification the operator may choose to classify either channel or both. The algorithm for beat classification is a cross-correlation technique using the Fourier transform of a difference function. The program requires no further operator interaction other than setting up a correlation treshold level. After that data are automatically separated into different families. When two-channel analysis is selected, a primary ("best quality") channel is appointed and classification in families is done using an OR condition of the individual channels and templates with priority for the primary channel.

In 1973 the Rigshospitalet in Copenhagen introduced a system whereby ECG tracings are presented on a screen to the editor as a sequence of computer generated static pictures (Gymoese at al., 1975). Each page holds about 20 seconds of ECG and is shown about one second. They can be frozen for further investigation or copied to a plotter or a stripchart recorder. In 1977 a new system (RAMSES) was developed which includes automatic analysis and operator editing facilities (Gymoese at al., 1978). The beat classification algorithm uses a correlation technique based on 8 points before and 9 after a fiducial point to compare each beat with a maximum of 200 stored templates. A new template is created if correlation with all existing templates does not exceed a preset limit. Once templates are created, they are fixed, and not updated during the analysis. Merging of templates is done under operator supervision at the end of the analysis. At this point each template is also given a descriptive label, which is then used in the final documentation.

Columbia University, New York, in 1975 described a LACER analysis system which, like the ARGUS system, is based on a number of cascaded program modules (Florenz et al., 1975). Some of these modules are implemented as finite state machines, which are table driven algorithms, that allow complex analysis at very high processing speeds. This system had an average sensitivity of 97% and an average specificity of 99,9%. In 1978 a new system was reported that used a new QRS shape classification algorithm, whereby each complex is seen as a point in a multi-dimensional shape space

(Birman et al., 1978). This shape information is used for PVC identification, to define a notion of typical QRS complex, and as the basis of the interactive editing system.

In 1976 the Krannert Institute of Cardiology, Indianapolis, introduced a fully automated analysis system on a Honeywell 716 computer (Lovelace at al., 1976). It uses a single channel ECG, which is sampled at an effective sampling rate of 60 Hz. A maximum negative slope technique is used for QRS detection. Beat classification is based on R-R interval, QRS amplitude and a parameter representing T-wave morphology. Normal limits for these parameters are learned from the beginning of the recording and automatically redefined at least every 200 R-R intervals.

North Charles hospital, Baltimore, based a system on an Interdata 7/16 minicomputer (Bradley and Tabatznik, 1977). In a first pass, the data is read back at 120 times real-time, sampled at 225 Hz effective sampling rate and written to digital tape. The second pass attempts to classify QRS complexes in one of nine fimilies, depending on its morphology. A QRS complex is characterized by four features: sum of the first derivative, sum of the absolute derivative and maximum and minimum deflections. Upon detection of a QRS complex, the computer presents a rhythm strip to the system operator who must determine into which family the complex best fits. The action redefines the parameter units for that family and progressively reduces operator interactions.

The ATREC system from the hopital Lariboisiere, Paris, is based on a MITRA 15/35 minicomputer, and uses a hardware pre-processing unit to acquire the R-R-interval, QRS-duration and QRS-polarity (Coumel et al., 1977). The tape is played back at 60 times real-time, and the data is analysed in terms of rhythm disturbances, premature beats and heartrate trends. The system has extensive numerical and graphical reporting facilities.

In 1978 Yale university introduced a LACER analysis system based on a time shared dual processor PDP11/45-05 configuration (Gradman and Lewis, 1978). The YALECG system uses a statistical comparison technique based on a width-sensitive peak detector for QRS location and a dual width correlation factor algorithm for waveform comparison. Incoming beats are matched with up to 20 templates from a shape library. Three criteria are used to compare waveforms: the sign of peak polarity, which must match the area, which must be within 80% and a correlation factor, which must exceed a fixed threshold. The correlation factor is taken as the smallest of the correlation coefficients calculated over the QRS interval and the wider PT interval. A high performance graphics system is used for operator intervention and editing. The system was validated on 20 different one-hour segments yielding a PVC sensitivity of 99.2% and a specificity of 99.9%. In 1980 modifications to the algorithm provided a more accurate R-R interval estimation for studying PVC coupling intervals (Gradman et al., 1980).

The system developed at Lund University uses predictive coding to obtain a 2:1 compression ratio for storing the digitized ECG (Pahlm et al., 1978; 1980). On an inkt-jet recorder a report is generated containing graph of heartrate and the R-R interval distribution with event markers for tachycardia, prolonged intervals, premature beats, bigeminy and noise. This report is used to examine selected sections of the ECG on a screen, or make annotated recordings on the inkt-jet recorder.

The TELAVIV system provides fully automated analysis of three channel ECG records (Rosenberg et al., 1979; 1981; Tartakovsky et al., 1980). For each of the three channels templates of normal QRS-complexes are kept. After an initial learning phase, a beat is termed 'dominant' in shape if at least two channels show a high correlation with their normal templates. If a beat has a dominant shape, it is coded PAC, normal or dropped depending on its R-R timing. If the shape is non-dominant, the equivalent codings are PVC, fusion or escape beat. An evaluation performed on 45 patients ($\pm$ 40000 beats) showed above 98% specificity and above 95% sensitivity in separately identifying the different beat classifications, automatically rejecting 5% of signals for poor quality.

The system developed at the University of Iowa, processes two channels of ECG information, a conventional surface lead and an esophageal lead (Collins et al., 1979). A special esophageal electrode was developed which is enclosed in an ordinary pharmaceutical capsule and can be easily swallowed (Arzbaecher, 1978). The electrode is positioned in the esophagus by the two thin flexible wires it is attached to. On this channel, the atrial complex is typically 3-4 times as large as the ventricular complex. In conjunction with the surface lead it is therefore extremely usefull to classify both ventricular and supraventricular arrhythmias. The system uses a PDP11/45 minicomputer with hardware triggers for A-waves and QRS-complexes.

The ASTRI system was developed at the clinical physiology laboratory in Pisa for fast automatic rhythm analysis and the analysis of the ST-T interval (Biella et al., 1979). In a first pass the ECG is sampled and recorded on magnetic tape at 60 times real-time. At the start of the second pass, the operator adjusts a number of tresholds for the particular ECG. The system then proceeds to perform QRS detection, feature extraction, ST analysis, QRS classification and report printing in a fully automatic way. A better than 95% sensitivity and 99% specificity is reported for both PAC and PVC classification.

The Linkoping system performs a preliminary arrhythmia analysis of the entire recording without manual interventions (Nygards et al., 1979). Each QRS complex is approximated whith a weighted sum of four orthonormal functions. The parameters of this representation together with the preceding R-R interval form the basis for QRS classification. Waveforms of similar shape are grouped into families. Based on this grouping, beats are classified as normal, premature supraventricular, aberrant non-ventricular, or ventricular. When the automatic analysis is ready results are examined and edited from a graphic terminal.

GRETA, from the Clinical Research Centre in Harrow, is based on a small minicomputer and uses no mass storage (Cashman and Stott, 1979). A single lead ECG is replayed at 25 times real-time and is fed parallel into a hardware QRS-detector and through 5 kHz AD-conversion into a 10 second shift register. Detected beats are compared with four templates. If an insufficient match is found, it is stored as a fifth template, otherwise the best matching template is updated by partially averaging in the new complex. All five templates are continuously displayed to the operator. The system uses a fast best fit algorithm based on integer arithmetic (Cashman, 1978).

CONCLUSIONS

A large number of research institutions have contributed to the development of analysis systems. Despite the difficulty of comparing performance figures, most research systems appear to have ventricular arrhythmia detection rates of the order of 95% or better. This is very much better than a human scanner operator. This type of system is obviously essential to any institution wishing to perform drugstudies or other research requiring tallies of ventricular events from long-term electrocardiographic recordings. The lack of portability of most research systems may be compensated by the availability of extremely sophisticated commercial systems whose results are similar or better than of the research systems. In terms of ordinary clinical routine, however, the situation is far from clear. It seems likely that real-time portable monitors are in some ways both simple and more cost-effective than the big central systems. Summaries are still available for the patient dossier and for research. Future developments in this area are likely to make the systems still more attractive financially and as to performance.

One area which has not received quite as much attention as the performance criteria of these systems is their clinical relevance outside the area of research. It is infact necessary to have a system in order to investigate the problem at all and that may be a reason why there are today occasional question marks being placed against the analysis systems almost exclusive attention to ventricular events. Some research systems do provide more sophisticated arrhythmia analysis by using more or specialised ECG leads and it is possible that further work in this area will provide the questions leading to the next generation of computer-aided electrocardiographic analysis.

REFERENCES

Anderson, C.M., Sanders, W.J. and Harrison, D.C. 1980. Comparing the morphologies of ECG waveforms in frequency space. Proc. Computers in Cardiology, IEEE Computer Society, Long Beach, Calif., pp. 15-19.

Arzbaecher, R. 1978. A pill electrode for the study of cardiac arrhythmia. Medical Instrumentation, 12, 277-281.

Biella, M., Contini, C., Kraft, G., Marchesi, C., Mazzocca, G.F. and Taddei, A. 1979. A minicomputer based system for automatic analysis of 24 hour ECG and its evaluation. Proc. Computers in Cardiology, IEEE Computer Society, Long Beach, Calif., pp. 201-204.

Birman, K.P., Rolnitzky, L.M. and Bigger, J.T. 1978. A shape oriented system for automated Holter ECG analysis. Proc. Computers in Cardiology, IEEE Computer Society, Long Beach, Calif., pp. 217-220.

Bradley, J.B. and Tabatznik, B. 1977. A new computer system for processing of Holter recordings. Proc. Computers in Cardiology, IEEE Computer Society, Long Beach, Calif., pp. 187-189.

Bragg-Remschel, D. and Harrison, D.C. 1980. A computerized two channel ambulatory arrhythmia analysis system. Proc. Computers in Cardiology, IEEE Computer Society, Long Beach, Calif., pp. 197-356.

Cashman, P.M.M. and Stott, F.D. 1979. GRETA - A low cost arrhythmia analyser for Holter ECG recordings. Proc. Computers in Cardiology, IEEE Computer Society, Long Beach, Calif., pp. 457-460.

Cashman, P.M.M. 1978. A pattern-recognition program for continuous ECG processing in accelerated time. Computers and Biomedical Research, 11, 311-323.

Clark, K.W., Hitchens, R.E., Ritter, J.A., Rankin, S.L., Oliver, G.C. and Thomas, L.J. 1977. Argus/2H: A dual-channel Holter-tape analysis system. Proc. Computers in Cardiology, IEEE Computer Society, Long Beach, Calif., pp. 191-198.

Clark, K.W., McLear, P.W., Kortas, R.G., Mead, C.N. and Thomas, L.J. 1980. Argus/2H detection of ST-segment changes in ambulatory ECG recordings. Proc. Computers in Cardiology, IEEE Computer Society, Long Beach,

Calif., pp. 27-31.

Clark, K.W., Hermes, R.E., McLear, P.W., Mead, C.N. and Thomas, L.J. 1981. The Argus/2H approach to supraventricular arrhythmia analysis. Proc. Computers in Cardiology, IEEE Computer Society, Long Beach, Calif., pp. 165-168.

Collins, S., Jenkins, J., Brown, D, Dean, R. and Arzbaecher, R. 1979. Rapid analysis of supraventricular arrhythmia from long-term esophageal recordings. Proc. Computers in Cardiology, IEEE Computer Society, Long Beach, Calif., pp. 189-192.

Coumel, Ph., Attuel, P., Leclercq, J.F. and Flammang, D. 1977. Computerized quantitative evaluation of cardiac arrhythmias. Proc. Computers in Cardiology, IEEE Computer Society, Long Beach, Calif., pp. 571-577.

Cox, J.R., Nolle, F.M., Fozzard, H.A., et al. 1968. AZTEC, a preprocessing program for real-time ECG rhythm analysis. IEEE Trans. Biomed. Eng., 15, 128-129.

Fitzgerald, J.W., Clappier, R.R. and Harrison, D.C. 1974. Small computer processing of ambulatory electrocardiograms. Proc. Computers in Cardiology, IEEE Computer Society, Long Beach, Calif., pp. 31-36.

Fitzgerald, J.W., Winkle, R.A., Alderman, E.L. and Harrison, D.C. 1975. Computer analyzed ambulatory electrocardiograms for predicting and evaluation responses to antiarrhythmic agents. Proc. Computers in Cardiology, IEEE Computer Society, Long Beach, Calif., pp. 151-154.

Florenz, M.K., Rolnitzky, L.M. and Bigger, J.T. 1975. A rapid ECG processing computer program using the finite state machine approach. Proc. Computers in Cardiology, IEEE Computer Society, Long Beach, Calif., pp. 145-150.

Gradman, A.H. and Lewis, J.W. 1978. YALECG: A new system for computer analysis of ambulatory electrocardiograms. Proc. Computers in Cardiology, IEEE Computer Society, Long Beach, Calif., pp. 211-214.

Gradman, A.H., Lewis, J.W. and Mayer, J.L. 1980. An improved method for computer measurement of the R-R interval on the ambulatory electrocardiogram. Proc. Computers in Cardiology, IEEE Computer Society, Long beach Calif., pp. 213-216.

Gymoese, E., Larsen, I.A., Damgaard Andersen, J. and Sandoe, E. 1975. A system for high speed scanning of electrocardiographic tapes based on sequence of computer generated sratic TV pictures. Proc. Computers in Cardiology, IEEE Computer Society, Long Beach, Calif., pp. 3-6.

Gymoese, E., Damgaard Andersen, J. and Sandoe, E. 1978. Random access mass storage ECG-analysis system (RAMSES): A new system for quantitative analysis of long-term ECG's. 1978. Proc. Computers in Cardiology, IEEE Computer Society, Long Beach, Calif., pp. 221-224.

Holter, N.J. 1961. New method for heart studies. Science, 134, 1214-1120.

Lown, B., Fakhro, A.M., Hood, W.B. et al. 1967. The coronary care unit. New perspectives and directions. J. Amer. Med. Assoc., 199, 188-198.

Lovelace, D.E., Knoebel, S.B. and Zipes, D.P. 1976. Recognition of ventricular extrasystoles in sedentary versus ambulatory populations. Proc. Computers in Cardiology, IEEE Computer Society, Long Beach, Calif., pp. 9-11.

Mead, C.N., Ferriero, T., Clark, K.W., Thomas, L.J., Cox, J.R. and Oliver, G.C. 1975. An improved Argus/H system for high-speed ECG analysis. Proc. Proc. Computers in Cardiology, IEEE Computer Society, Long Beach, Calif., pp. 7-13.

Mead, C.N., Pull, H.R., Cheng, J-S, Clark, K.W. and Thomas, L.J. 1981. A frequency-domain-based QRS classification algorithm. Proc. Computers in Cardiology, IEEE Computer Society, Long Beach, Calif., pp. 351-354.

Mead, C.N., Pull, H.R., Clark, K.W. and Thomas, L.J. 1982. Expanded frequency-domain ECG waveform processing: integration into a new version of Argus/2H. Proc. Computers in Cardiology, IEEE Computer Society, Long Beach, Calif., pp. 205-208.

Nolle, F.M., Oliver, G.C., Kleiger, R.E., Cox, J.R., Clark, K.W. and Ambos, H.D.. 1974. The Argus/H system for rapid analysis of ventricular arrhythmias. Proc. Computers in Cardiology, IEEE Computer Society, Long Beach, Calif., pp. 37-42.

Nolle, F.M. and Clark, K.W. 1971. Detection of premature ventricular contractions using an algorithm for cataloging QRS complexes. San Diego Biomed. Symposium, 10, 85-97.

Nygards, M.E., Ahren, T., Tranesjo, J. and Wigertz, O. 1979. A computer program for analysis of long-term ECG recordings. Proc. Computers in Cardiology, IEEE Computer Society, Long Beach, Calif., pp. 429-432.

Oliver, G.C., Kleiger, R.E., Krone, R.J., Martin, T.F., Miller, J.P., Nolle, F.M. and Cox, J.R. 1974. Application of high speed analysis of ambulatory electrocardiography. Proc. Computers in Cardiology, IEEE Computer Society, Long Beach, Calif., pp. 43-46.

Oliver, G.C., Ripley, K.L., Miller, J.P. and Martin, T.F. 1977. A critical review of computer arrhythmia detection. Computer Electrocardiography: Current Status and Criteria. (Futura). pp. 267-308.

Pahlm, O., Borjesson, P.E., Johansson, K., Jonson, B., Petersson, K, Sornmo, L and Werner, O. 1978. Efficient data compression and arrhythmia detection for long term ECGs. Proc. Computers in Cardiology, IEEE Computer Society, Long Beach, Calif., pp. 395-396.

Pahlm, O., Jonson, B., Petersson, K and Eriksson, L. 1980. Computer-aided visual of long-term ECG recording. Proc. Computers in Cardiology, IEEE Computer Society, Long Beach, Calif., pp. 123-125.

Ripley, K.L. and Oliver, C.G. 1977. Development of an ECG database for arrhythmia detector evaluation. Proc. Computers in Cardiology, IEEE Computer Society, Long Beach, Calif., pp. 203-209.

Ripley, K.L., Okkerse, R.J., Engelse, W.A.H., Vinke, R.V.H. and Zeelenberg C. 1980. Implementation of Argus/2H at the Thoraxcentre. Proc. Computers in Cardiology, IEEE Computer Society, Long Beach, Calif., pp. 135-138.

Ripley, K.L. and Murray, A. 1980. Introduction to arrhythmia detection. (IEEE Computer Society, Long Beach, Calif.)

Rosenberg, N.W. and Tartakovsky, M.B. 1979. The TELAVIV system - Three-channel Evaluation of Long-term ECG Records for Atrial and Ventricular Identification and Verification of Arrhythmia. 1979. Proc. Computers in Cardiology, IEEE Computer Society, Long Beach, Calif., pp. 29-32.

Rosenberg, N., Tartakovsky, M., Elkin, S., Shabtai, I. and Ron, S. 1981. Automated analysis of three-channel Holter records taken in a factory environment. Proc. Computers in Cardiology, IEEE Computer Society, Long Beach, Calif., pp. 177-180.

Schluter, P., Mark, R., Moody, G., Olson, W. and Peterson, S. 1980. Performance measures for arrhythmia detectors. Proc. Computers in Cardiology, IEEE Computer Society, Long Beach, Calif., pp. 267-270.

Spitz, A.L., Fitzgerald, J.W. and Harrison, D.C.. 1977. Ambulatory arrhythmia quantification by a correlation technique. Proc. Computers in Cardiology, IEEE Computer Society, Long Beach, Calif., pp. 225-231.

Stein, I.M., Plunkett, J. and Troy, M. 1980. Comparison of techniques for examining long-term ECG recordings. Medical Instrumentation, 14, 69-72.

Tartakovsky, M.B., Rosenberg, N., Ron, S., Shabtai, I., Elkin, S. and Cocos, M. 1980. Unsupervised template construction for QRS classification in Holter tape analysis. Proc. Computers in Cardiology, IEEE Computer Society, Long beach, Calif., pp. 9-14.

Thomas, L.J., Clark, K.W., Mead, C.N., Ripley, K.L., Spenner, B.F. and Oliver, G.C. 1979. Proc. of the IEEE, 67, 1322-1337.

Zeelenberg, C., Ripley, K.L. and Okkerse, R. 1982. Equipment specifications and performance criteria: clinical evaluation. In "Long Term Ambulatory Electro-cardiography" (Ed. J. Roelandt and P.G. Hugenholtz). (Martinus Nijhoff, The Hague). pp.6-15.

DISCUSSION

Chairman: C. Zeelenberg

1.3 - Review of existing systems for ECG ambulatory monitoring.

CASHMAN: Could you be more specific about the mechanical signals which you advocate for improving the specificity of the ambulatory ECG?

MARCHESI: What I mean is the combination of contractility information and the behaviour of the electrical field on the surface. It seems that from our experience in the Coronary Care Unit that it's possible to solve, at least in part, the problems of obtaining more specificity for the diagnosis of ischemia based on ECG, when indicators of LV function performance are available. Hopefully these results obtained with direct methods in CCU will be achievable also in ambulant patients as soon as practical indirect methods to monitor LV function will be available.

BALASUBRAMANIAN: Taking the last point of mechanical signals, we have just analyzed blood pressure and ECG on the same tape, and we were rather disappointed to find that blood pressure does not add any significant information to ECG in ischemic patients.

MARCHESI: It would be interesting to go in details into this problem. Perhaps the discussion is open, I suppose.

ZEELENBERG: Do some of the manufacturers use the MIT data base to calculate QRS specificity and sensitivity rather than only test PVC?

MARCHESI: Only one uses the MIT database, both for QRS detection performances and for PVC.

CHAPTER 2

CLINICAL APPLICATIONS

TOPIC: 2.1

Ambulatory monitoring of arrhythmias

THE CLINICAL USE OF AMBULATORY MONITORING IN ARRHYTHMIA
EVALUATION

Erik Sandøe, J.D. Andersen and E. Gymoese
Medical Department B, Rigshospitalet Copenhagen, Denmark

ABSTRACT

A review of current clinical use of ambulatory monitoring
in arrhythmia evaluation is presented. Ambulatory monitoring
is particularly useful for evaluating the role played by
known or syspected cardiac arrhythmias in patient symptomatology. Ambulatory monitoring can be useful in the evaluation of the clinical significance of conduction defects or
complex ventricular arrhythmias observed in the ECG-recording
of the asymptomatic patient. Its role in the evaluation of
risk of sudden death in the asymptomatic patient is doubtful
at present. Other parameters such as ventricular failure and
exercise ECG seem more useful. Improved technology can remove
most present drawbacks and increase utility of the technique.

INTRODUCTION

Ambulatory ECG monitoring, originally performed by one
lead reel tape recorders which were heavy and uncomfortable
to the patient, has undergone considerable technical improvement since the introduction of the technique. Present systems
use a small, lightweight 2 channel recorder which records 24
hours of ECG on a standard Compact casette. After recording,
the ECG is played back into a dedicated analysis system,
frequently a minicomputer, and analyzed off-line. The patient
notes any incidents or symptoms in a diary with the time of
occurrence, so that symptoms may be correlated with the
findings of the analysis. Much improvement can be achieved in
ambulatory recordings technology because of the current
evolution in electronics towards higher density electronic

circuits. It is important that this improvement should be exploited for better arrhythmia diagnosis and research.

CLINICAL USE OF AMBULATORY MONITORING IN ARRHYTHMIAS

Ambulatory ECG monitoring is used clinically for establishing the diagnosis in the symptomatic patient suffering from syncope, palpitations or other symptoms which may be of cardiac origin. It is also used for evaluation of the clinical significance of conduction defects or ventricular ectopy, and to assess the risk of sudden death in the asymptomatic patient with coronary artery disease. Furthermore, it has a role in the selection and control of an antiarrhythmic drug regime, and finally to control pacemaker patients.

1. Diagnostically in the symptomatic patient

In the symptomatic patient ambulatory ECG is used to confirm or exclude possible arrhythmogenic origin of symptoms such as presyncope (near fainting) or syncope, palpitations or a feeling of racing or pounding heart action (Johansson, 1982; Antman et al., 1982; Josephson, 1981).

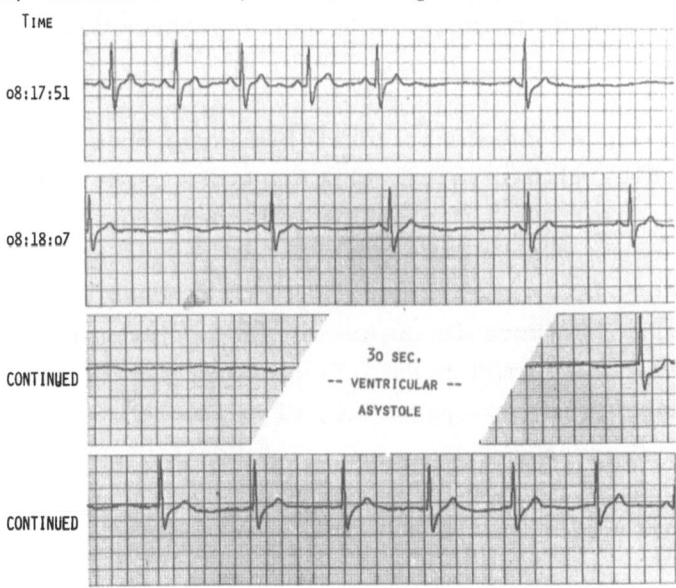

FIGURE 1. Ambulatory ECG monitoring in presyncope/syncope. Fainting due to SA block and ventricular asystole.

Thus, if the ECG tracing shows sino-atrial block with ventricular asystole of longer duration during a fainting attack, the attack may be due to the prolonged period of ventricular standstill (Fig. 1).

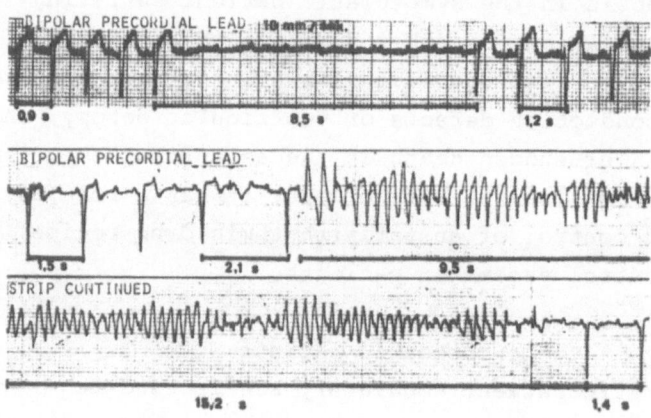

FIGURE 2. Ambulatory ECG monitoring in presyncope/syncope. Fainting due to AV-block and ventricular asystole (upper tracing), or torsades de pointes ventricular tachycardia (lower tracing).

Fainting may also be due to attacks of third degree AV block complicated by either ventricular asystole or by torsade de pointes ventricular tachycardia (Fig. 2). Besides such confirmative evidence of arrhythmic origin of presyncope/ syncope, ambulatory ECG monitoring can in other cases give evidence against arrhythmogenic origin of the symptoms by the recording of unchanged normal heart rhythm during an attack of fainting or near fainting. Recording of episodes of third degree AV-block, of advanced AV-block or of Mobitz type 2 block will be accepted by most clinicians as convincing evidence of arrhythmogenic origin of a patient's fainting attack, calling for a pacemaker implantation. But detection of first degree AV-block, of bundle branch block, AV-junc- tional escape rhythm, sinus bradycardia, or attacks of supra-

ventricular tachycardia and complex ventricular arrhythmias
are usually considered to serve more as circumstantial
evidence for an arrhythmogenic background to syncope or near
syncope than as the substantiated cause.

Case history

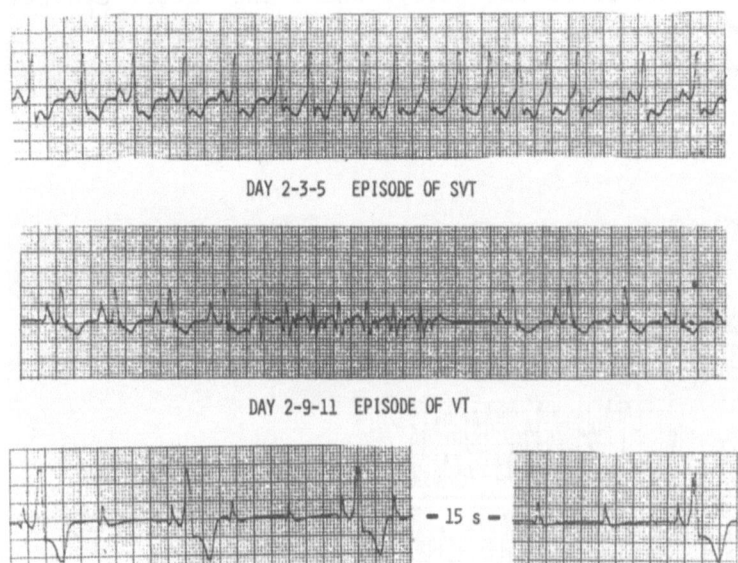

DAY 2-3-5   EPISODE OF SVT

DAY 2-9-11 EPISODE OF VT

DAY 11   AV BLOCK/FAINTING

FIGURE 3. Outcome of 11 days of continuous ECG monitoring in
an 16-year-old male with hypertrophic cardiomyopathy and
fainting.

A 16-year-old male was monitored continuously during 11
days (Fig. 3). The patient had hypertrophic cardiomyopathy
and was investigated due to repeated attacks of syncope
occurring at intervals of weeks to months. During the first
10-11 days the patient had no fainting attacks but several
symptomless episodes of supraventricular and ventricular
tachycardia which might confer the impression of a tachy-
arrhythmia. However, by the end of the 11th day the patient
suddenly fainted, and it appeared that the fainting was due

to an episode of AV-block complicated by ventricular asystole. A pacemaker was implanted and there have been no new fainting attacks.

The arrhythmias causing fainting may be evaluated either by ambulatory monitoring in the out-hospital patient or when the patient is admitted to a Coronary Care Unit and monitored, for example by wireless telemetry. While the latter evaluation method makes it possible to intervene with resuscitation if required, attacks of malignant arrhythmia occurring during ambulatory ECG monitoring are liable to result in sudden death.

Case history

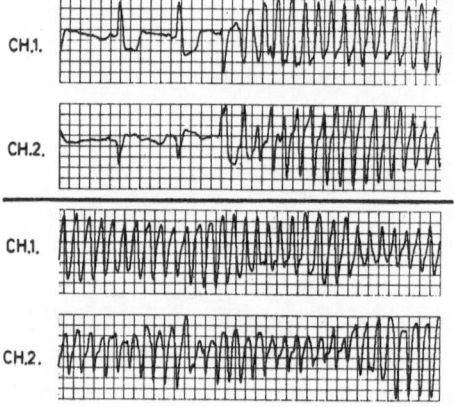

FIGURE 4. Ambulatory monitoring of death in an 80-year-old male suffering from fainting attacks.

The patient, an 80-year-old man had suffered from fainting attacks during a 3-month period. He was not interested in being admitted to hospital, and was therefore investigated by ambulatory ECG-monitoring. The ECG initially showed sinus rhythm, but later during his sleep the patient developed ventricular flutter and slept on into his death.

Eight patients suffering cardiac death during ambulatory recording have been described in the literature (Winkle,

1980). Six of them had ventricular fibrillation initiated in all cases by what appeared to be R-on-T ventricular complexes.

In general, ambulatory ECG-monitoring should be continued until the patient has had one of his typical episodes of symptoms. Because there can be long time intervals between attacks, ambulatory ECG monitoring can be an extremely time consuming task. For this reason, the patient should always be questioned about provocative factors and symptoms. Thus if he should faint in connection with exercise, then he or she should always first be challenged by heavy exercise on a bicycle ergometer.

Case history

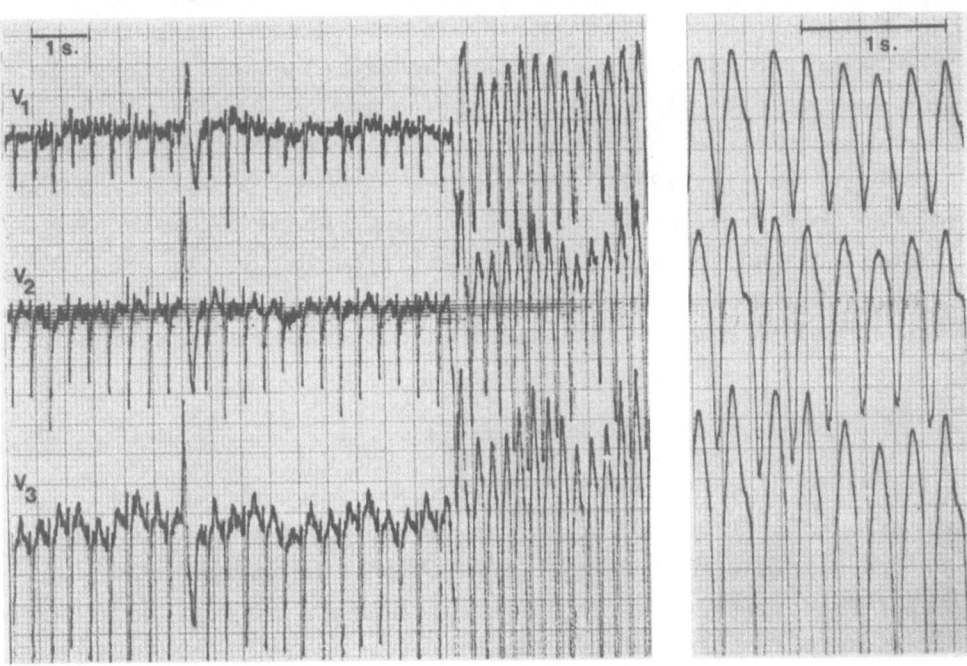

Rate: 180/min   240/min   240/min

FIGURE 5. Ergometer test in 19-year-old male with fainting in relation to effort. The reading shows onset of ventricular tachycardia at an workload of 230 Watts.

The ECG-recordings (Fig. 5) are from an 19-year-old youth who was a very able football player, but who during the previous year had been withdrawn from the offensive position to that of a defensive back because he always fainted when he had to run with the ball. With a smaller load on the bicycle ergometer only a few ventricular ectopics were recorded, but with increasing exercise load to 230 Watts he suddenly developed ventricular flutter and fainted.

Thus in patients with fainting or near-fainting episodes, ambulatory ECG-monitoring is contraindicated if there is any reason to believe that the fainting attacks have caused life threathening arrhythmias such as ventricular fibrillation or bifascicular or trifascicular AV-block. In such cases, the patient should be hospitalized and monitored by cable or telemetry in the Coronary Care Unit. Furthermore, the first choice of ECG recording should be an exercise-ECG. A possible but serious pitfall in the diagnositc use of ambulatory monitoring is that of the recording of artefact arrhythmias (Andersen et al., 1977). The problem has been somewhat reduced by the introduction of two-channel tape recorders which have also increased the accuracy of identification of the site of origin of ectopic complexes, and decreased the chance of technical failure of the recording and subsequent data loss due to electrode malfunctioning.

2. Evaluation of the clinical significance of conduction
   defects or ventricular arrhythmias

Ambulatory ECG monitoring may be useful in the evaluation of the clinical significance of a conduction defect or of complex ventricular arrhythmias recorded in the routine ECG of an asymptomatic patient (Jensen et al., 1972; Jensen et al., 1973; Sandøe et al., 1973).

Case history

The upper part of figure 6 shows a routine ECG recording from a 29-year-old man admitted to the hospital because of a leg fracture. The ECG shows as the only abnormal finding a PR

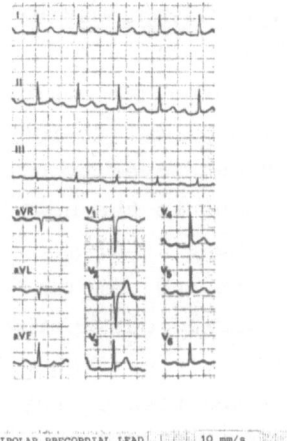

BIPOLAR PRECORDIAL LEAD   10 mm/s

FIGURE 6. 29-year-old male with leg fracture and no cardiac
symptoms. For explanation see text.

interval of about 0.03 s. The simultaneous finding of a
normal width QRS complex favored a diagnosis of monofascicular
atrial ventricular block. The patient presented no additional
signs of cardiac disease. The lower part of the figure shows
a strip from a continuous ECG monitoring performed during
early morning just before the patient woke up. There is a
period of 10 s with third degree AV-block and ventricular
asystole. When queried the patient denied ever having fainted,
but he had for years suffered from nightmares in the early
morning just before he woke up. Similar episodes of third
degree atrial ventricular block and ventricular standstill
lasting from 6 to 14 s were recorded on several occasions in
the early morning. They were always associated with bad
dreams. It was finally decided to implant a pacemaker in the
patient. After implantation the nightmares stopped. The
implantation may have saved the patient from sudden death at
an early age, but this cannot of course be proved.

3. Evaluation of the risk of sudden death in asymptomatic coronary artery disease patients

Large scale investigations have been performed to evaluate the risk of sudden death in the post-myocardial infarction patient by using as criteria the frequency and severity of ventricular ectopic beats classified according to the Lown scale (Lown, 1980; Rubermann et al., 1977; Moss et al., 1979). These studies have shown that frequent and complex ectopic activity in ambulatory recording carried out approximately 3 to 4 weeks after an acute myocardial infarction will identify a group of patients with an increased risk of subsequent sudden death (Møller, 1981; Rhenquist, 1978). The risk of death may be two to four times higher than in a similar patient population without these arrhythmias. However, additional and more easily handled predictors of sudden death are left ventricular function and ST-depression exercise ECG (Møller, 1981; Schulte et al., 1977).

4. Antiarrhythmic drug therapy

The clinician's choice of possible therapeutic interventions in patients with cardiac arrhythmias has widened rapidly during the past three decades. New possibilities include pacemaker treatment (Wiener, 1980), surgery (Waldo et al., 1981) and a much expanded armory of antiarrhythmic drugs (Sandøe et al., 1983). Access to a larger number and more efficacious treatments has imposed a greater demand on selecting the patients who may benefit from the treatment.

Ambulatory monitoring has been used to select an antiarrhythmic drug for use in a given patient or to control the treatment once it is established (Winkle, 1980). It has been widely assumed that the suppressive effect of antiarrhythmic drug therapy on attacks of ventricular fibrillation and tachycardia would be reflected by the suppressive effect of the drug on the frequency and complexity of ventricular extrasystoles. Since a serious life threatening attack of ventricular tachycardia and fibrillation can occur at wide time intervals, while the occurrence of ventricular extrasystoles is more or less a constant phenomenon, it should be possible to assess the efficacy of a drug treatment by finding the frequency of extrasystoles via ambulatory monitoring. Unfortunately, there is a considerable spontaneous variability in the number of ventricular extrasystoles over time (Fig. 7).

We performed repeated 24-hour Holter monitoring in a series of 28 clinically stable patients (Fig. 7). The selection criterion was an average ventricular ectopic count of 200 per hour or more at a previous 24-hour Holter monitoring. The spontaneous variation from the first to the second investigation is shown in the figure (Fig. 7). It was found by means of regression analysis that a reduction of at least 80 per cent in the average number of ectopics per hour was required to confirm drug efficacy. Figures between 65 to 83 per cent have been reported by previous investigators. Last but not least there is a great problem of whether there really is any relationship between the suppressive effect of a drug on ventricular extrasystoles and that of efficacy of

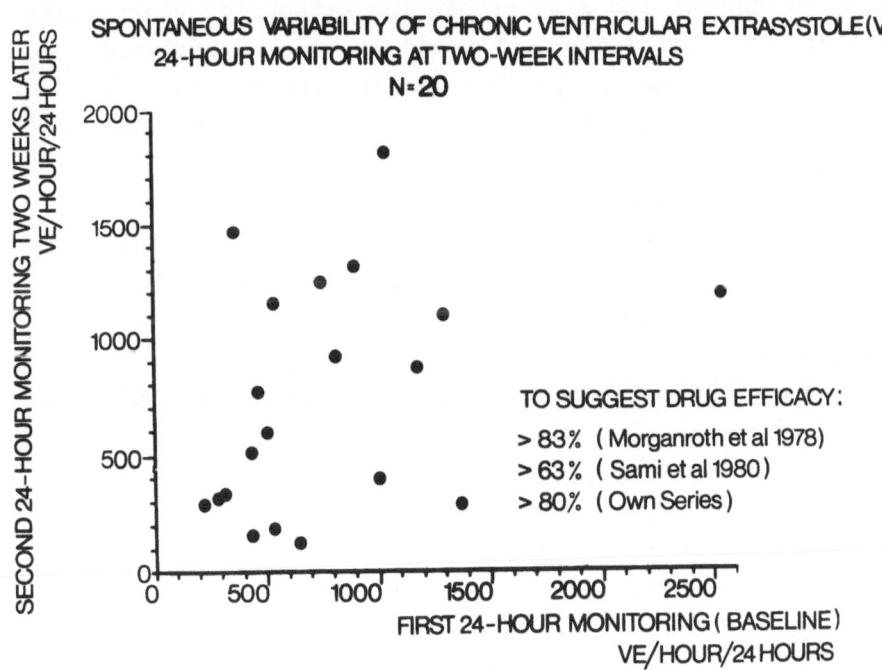

FIGURE 7. Variability of chronic ventricular extrasystole.

78

TABLE 1. Efficacy of Class I antiarrhythmic drugs against
long term mortality in hospital survivors of actue myocardial
infarction.

EFFICACY OF CLASS I ANTIARRHYTHMIC DRUGS AGAINST MORTALITY
FOUR LONG-TERM CLINICAL TRIALS AFTER MYOCARDIAL INFARCTION

AUTHORS	DRUG	DURATION MONTHS	NO. OF PATIENTS CONTROLS/TREATED	MORTALITY % CONTROLS/TREATED
RYDEN ET AL 1980	TOCAINIDE	6	56/56	8.9/8.9
BASTIAN ET AL 1980	TOCAINIDE	6	74/72	4.1/5.6
CHAMBERLAIN ET AL 1980	MEXILETINE	3-4	163/161	11.7/13.3
GENT-ROTTERDAM STUDY 1982	APRINDINE	12	152/153	12.5/ 7.8
TOTAL		3-12	445/442	10.3/10.2

DRUG TREATMENT WAS IN ALL FOUR SERIES ASSOCIATED WITH
SIGNIFICANT REDUCTION IN VENTRICULAR EXTRASYSTOLE
ASSESSED BY HOLTER MONITORING

the drug in suppressing life treatening attacks of ventricular
tachycardia or fibrillation. The problem remains unsolved
both for the asymptomatic patient and for the patient with
repeated attacks of sustained ventricular tachycardia (May et
al., 1982).

In four large long-term controlled trials with various
class I antiarrhythmic drugs in acute myocardial infarction
survivors, all drugs proved efficient in decreasing the
average frequency of ventricular extrasystoles in the treated
patient group (Table 1). However, in no group was the reduction
in ventricular extrasystole followed by a significant lowering
of sudden death mortality.

5. Control of pacemaker patients

Finally, ambulatory ECG monitoring has been used in the
control of the performance of implanted pacemakers. The need
for this type of control has so far been limited to the
pacemaker normally used now, with pacing in one chamber only,
usually in the form of non-competitive ventricular pacing

(ventricular demand pacemaker). However, with the introduction of new types of double chamber pacemakers, many of which are capable of dual chamber sensing and most of which are programmable to a broad variety of pacing modes, there is a possibility of complex pacemaker mediated arrhythmias, exacting increasing demands on ambulatory ECG monitoring. A special need for arrhythmia monitoring is required for the new types of antitachycardia pacemakers. It can only be hoped that the pacemakers may be equiped with built-in solid state ECG storage which uses the pacing electrode as a stable ECG lead (Ripart, 1982).

CONCLUSIONS

In conclusion, ambulatory monitoring is particularly useful for evaluating the role played by known or suspected cardiac arrhythmias in patient symptomatology. Ambulatory monitoring can be useful in the evaluation of the clinical significance of conduction defects or complex ventricular arrhythmias observed in the ECG-recording of the asymptomatic patient. Its role in the evaluation of risk of sudden death in the asymptomatic patient is doubtful at present. Other parameters such as ventricular failure and exercise-ECG seem more useful. Its usefulness in the control of antiarrhythmic drug therapy is hampered by the fact that ventricular extrasystoles demonstrate considerable spontaneous variability, and that drug suppression of ventricular extrasystoles does not guarantee suppression of attacks of ventricular tachycardia or fibrillation. Ambulatory monitoring will possibly play a major role in the control of more sophisticated pacemakers such as the double chamber pacemaker and the antitachycardia pacemaker. The evolution in electronics and software will make it possible to solve many of the current problems in the use of presently available recording and analysis systems such as long turn-around times and diminish the need for rigorous quality control procedures (Wenger, 1982).

REFERENCES

1. Andersen JD, Gymoese E, Arndal P et al. Problems in ambulatory monitoring. In: Trends in computer-processed electrocardiograms, 51-51 (van Bemmel JH, Willems JL, eds.).
   North-Holland Publishing Co. Amsterdam 1977.
2. Antman EM, Cohn PF. Ambulatory electrocardiographic monitoring. In: Diagnostic methods in clinical cardiology,
   pp. 29-50. (Cohn PF, Wynne J, eds.). Little, Brown & Co,
   Boston 1982.
3. Bragg-Remschel DA, Anderson CM, Winkle RA. Frequency
   response characteristics of ambulatory ECG monitoring
   systems and their implications for ST segmant analysis.
   Am Heart J 1982;103:20-31.
4. Jensen G, Sigurd B, Meibom J et al. Adams-Stokes syndrome
   caused by paroxysmal third-degree atrio-ventricular
   block. Brit Heart J 1973;35/5:516-520.
5. Jensen G, Sigurd B, Sandøe E. Adams-Stokes seizures due
   to ventricular tachydysrhythmias in patients with heart
   block: prevalence and problems of management. Chest
   1975;67/1:43-48.
6. Johansson BW. Evaluation of alteration of consciousness
   and palpitations. In: Ambulatory electrocardiographic
   recording, p. 321-330. (Wenger NK, Mock MB, Ringquist I,
   eds.). Year Book Medical publishers, Chicago 1982.
7. Josephson ME. Holter monitoring. Uses and misuses. Hospital
   Practise, May 1981, 67-81.
8. Lown B, Podrid PJ, DeSilva RA et al. Sudden cardiac
   death-management of the patient at risk. Curr Probl
   Cardiol 1980;4:7-.
9. Moss AJ, Davis HP, DeCamilla J et al. Ventricular ectopic
   beats and their relation to sudden and nonsudden cardiac
   death after myocardial infarction. Circulation 1979;60:
   998-1003.
10. Møller M. Ventricular arrhythmias following myocardial
    infarction. Odense University Press 1981.
11. Rehnquist N. Ventricular arrhythmias after acute myo-
    cardial infarction. Prognostic weight and natural history.
    Eur J Cardiol 1978;7/2:169-187.
12. Ripart A, Jacobson P. Memory technology and implantable
    Holter systems. In: The third decade of cardiac pacing.
    (Barold SS, Mugica J, eds.). Futura Publishing Co., New
    York 1982.
13. Rubermann W, Weinblatt E, Goldberg JD et al. Ventricular
    premature beats and mortality after myocardial infarction.
    N Engl J Med 1977;297:750-757.
14. Rubermann W, Weinblatt E, Goldberg JD et al. Sudden death
    after myocardial infraction: Runs of ventricular premature
    beats and R on T as high risk factors. Am J Cardiol
    1980;45:444.
15. Sandøe E, Sigurd B, Jensen G et al. Cardiac syncopes in
    patients with sinus rhythm. Singapore Med J 1973;14/3:
    312-315.
16. Sandøe E. Andersen ED, Andersen JD et al. Clinical effi-
    ciency and side-effects of new antiarrhythmic drugs. In:
    Proc. 9th world congr. cardiol, Moscow 1982. Plenum Press
    1983.

17. Schultze RA, Strauss HW, Pitt B. Sudden death following myocardial infarction: Relation to ventricular premature contractions in the late hospital phase and left ventricular ejection fraction. Am J Med 1977;62:192.
18. Waldo AL, Arciniegas JG, Klein H. Surgical treatment of life-threatening ventricular arrhythmias: The role of intraoperative mapping and consideration of presently available surgical techniques. Progr Cardiovasc Dis 1981;23:247-264.
19. Wenger NK, Mock MB, Ringquist I. Ambulatory ECG recording: clinical perspectives. In: Ambulatory electrocardiographic recording, pp. 425-440. (Wenger NK, Mock MB, Ringquist I, eds.). Year Book Medical publishers, Chicago 1982.
20. Wiener I. Pacing techniques in the treatment of tachycardias. Ann Int Med 1980;93:326-329.
21. Winkle RA. Ambulatory electrocardiography and the diagnosis, evaluation, and treatment of chronic ventricular arrhythmias. Prog Cardiovasc Dis 1980;23:99.

COMPUTERIZED ARRHYTHMIA ANALYSIS OF THE HOLTER RECORDINGS.

Ph. Coumel, J.F. Leclercq and P. Attuel.

Hôpital Lariboisière,
2, rue Amboise-Paré,
75010 - Paris, France.

ABSTRACT.

Computerized analysis of the Holter recordings (ATREC system) identifies only the QRS complexes, thus introducing a limitation in the diagnosis. The formulation of the results cannot use the classical terminology of ECG diagnosis. Despite this limitation, the possibilities of the analysis are large. The computer classifies the QRS complexes as either narrow or wide. The QRSs are analyzed for prematurity, regularity, bradycardia, pauses, transient or continuous tachycardia, and fibrillation. The premature beats are classed by their coupling interval, their distribution in bi- or trigeminy, doublets, or salvos, and the number per hour. The system gives a trend of the mean, and the 16-beat minimum and maximum heart rate. The aim of the computerized analysis is not only to detect the arrhythmias, but also to approach their mechanism, their relationships with the autonomic nervous system and to evaluate the therapeutic results.

INTRODUCTION.

A thorough analysis of the electrocardiogram, taking into account the P and QRS waves is the condition for establishing a classical ECG diagnosis and such an approach is indeed possible, though difficult, using computerized techniques. It has not been developed in the setting of the Holter monitoring not only for technical reasons (difficulty of an accurate P wave detection on ambulatory tracings, requiring an accelerated analysis of 24-hour tracings), but also because it is not really the philosophy of the ambulatory monitoring. Rather, what is expected from the Holter tapes in terms of diagnosis is to make possible the comparison between the clinical symptoms and the patient's ECG, or to detect ECG abnormalities in the absence of complaint, and to allow a quantitative approach of the arrhythmias. The classical ECG diagnosis remains the province of the physician, but the computerized analysis not only permits to save time by focusing the attention on the important parts of the tracings, but is also the first step for a comprehensive approach of the arrhythmia mechanisms and their relationships with the autonomic nervous system. As the two later applications become more and more important, they will necessitate the development of systems far more sophisticated than the presently available programs.

HOLTER TAPE ANALYSIS.

Hardware.

The ATREC system (Analyse des Troubles du Rythme de l'ElectroCardiogramme) evaluates 24-hour ECG tape recordings at 60 times real time. Any play-back unit may be used to provide the processing unit with the analog signal. The processing unit has an analog preprocessing module which suppresses T waves, P waves and power line frequencies with a 3 to 30 Hz band pass filter and a 50 Hz notch filter. The module detects the occurrence of a QRS, measures the length of the RR interval, the QRS width and polarity. The module automatically adjusts its sensitivity and eliminates a number of artefacts. The unit has been extensively tested and rarely misses or falsely indicates the presence of a QRS [Attuel et al., 1981].

The signals are fed to a Mitra model 15/35 minicomputer with a 16 k memory, of which 4 k are used for the program, and the rest of the memory stores the trend data. The computer classification is displayed on a Textronix model 4060 video screen and can be copied with a Tektronix hard copy unit.

Classification and presentation of results.

The computer classification is displayed on various panels. Some of them essentially deal with a qualitative evaluation, others with precise quantitations in terms of numbers, trends of rate, and histograms. The tables cover various period durations which are selectable from 3 to 24 hours, and each period is divided into 144 steps (according to the screen width) so that the corresponding intervals range from 75 to 600 sec. Comparing the various tables provides much information but no ECG diagnosis. The synthesis of this information should be done by the physician who is supposed to know precisely the definition of the terms used : they were chosen to avoid as much as possible any confusion with the ECG definitions of arrhythmias. Then the diagnosis proposed by the physician is controlled by direct tracing examination. Various examples of this mode of reasoning are given in the following figures.

THE DIAGNOSTIC PROCEDURE.

The problem of the artifacts.

Figure 1 represents a 3-hour analysis from 14 to 17h., so that each of the 144 steps corresponds to 75 sec. To compress the diagram, bars are placed above and below reference lines so that one line indicates 2 types of events. The events classified in the upper section deal with artifacts ("DEFAUTS CAPTEUR"), QRS width, regularity, bradycardia and tachycardia. In the example chosen, a few isolated pauses (defined as an RR interval longer

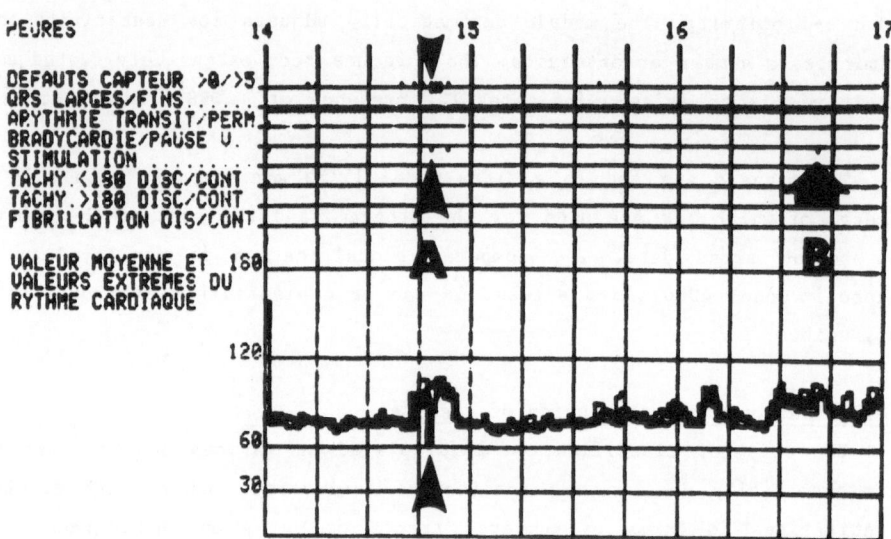

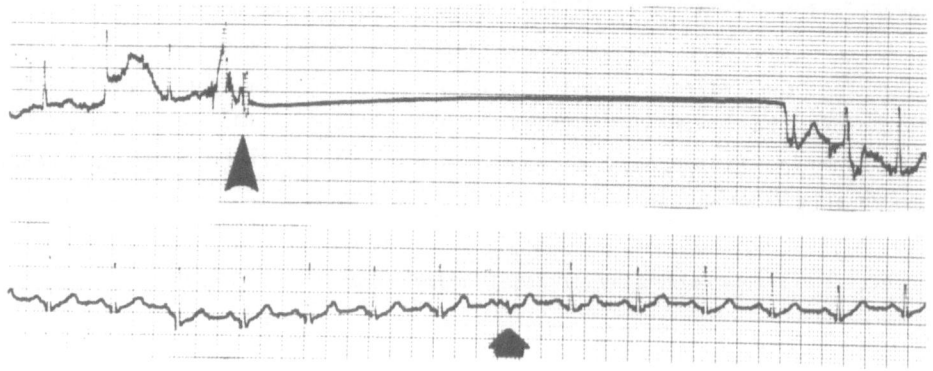

Fig. 1 Detection of pauses and the problem of the artifacts.(see text)

than 2.1 sec or 180% of the mean cycle length) are detected in the fourth line from the top, and heralded by small bars below the line. A bradycardia (mean heart rate < 40/min) would have been signaled with bars above the line. Then the problem is to authentify the reality of the pauses.

In A, shortly after 14h.45, the "pause" is detected in conjunction with the indication of the presence of many artifacts (more than 5/min in this 75 sec. period), and actually the corresponding tracing (upper strip) shows that this pseudo-pause is due to the amplifier saturation. But in B, between 16h.30 and 16h.45, by no means was it possible to suspect the quality of the tracing as no artifact was detected : the analog preprocessing module had been misled by a sudden and dramatic decrease of the QRS amplitude probably related to a fusion beat.

The ventricular response to atrial arrhythmias.

Figure 2 represents a two-and-a-half-hour analysis in a patient who from 13h.00 to 15h.00 suffers from short and intermittent attacks of atrial fibrillation and flutter (bottom strips), and develops at 15h.00 (arrows) a sustained atrial flutter with more or less irregular ventricular response. The latter is easily detected on the trends of cardiac frequency : in the lower part of the diagram, the mean heart rate (middle curve) dramatically increases, and it is encompassed by the minimal and maximal heart rates, calculated from 16 consecutive RR intervals in each considered period of 75 sec. Comparing with the 2 preceding hours makes clear that the greatly increased range reflects the variability of the ventricular response. This is further confirmed in the sixth line from top in the upper part of the diagram : a single bar is below the line, most of them are above and indicate (TACHY <180 DISC/CONT) an almost permanent but non-sustained tachycardia at more than 120 but less than 180 beats/min. The QRSs are indicated as narrow in the second line from the top, but the third line is in fact the important item : it deals with the irregularity of the ventricular beating.

In the item "ARYTHMIE TRANSIT/PERM" (irregular rhythm, transient or permanent), the objective is to separate sinus arrhythmia from atrial flutter and atrial fibrillation. This is done using the following algorithms. If the variation in 4 successive RR intervals is less than 1/16 of the mean RR interval, or the last 4 standard errors of the RR interval have the same sign, or if there is bi- or trigeminy, an order flag is placed and retained for 12 beats. If the standard error is more than 1/4 of the mean RR interval, and the order flag is absent, an irregular rhythm is recorded. It is permanent or transient if it occupies more than or less than 80% of the interval. The detection of an irregularity so defined disables the classing of narrow (supraventricular) extrasystoles.

This item is shown as reliable in the last 30 min period during which the ventricular response to the atrial flutter is not constantly irregular, and in any case the presence of the rhythm disturbance is obvious from the

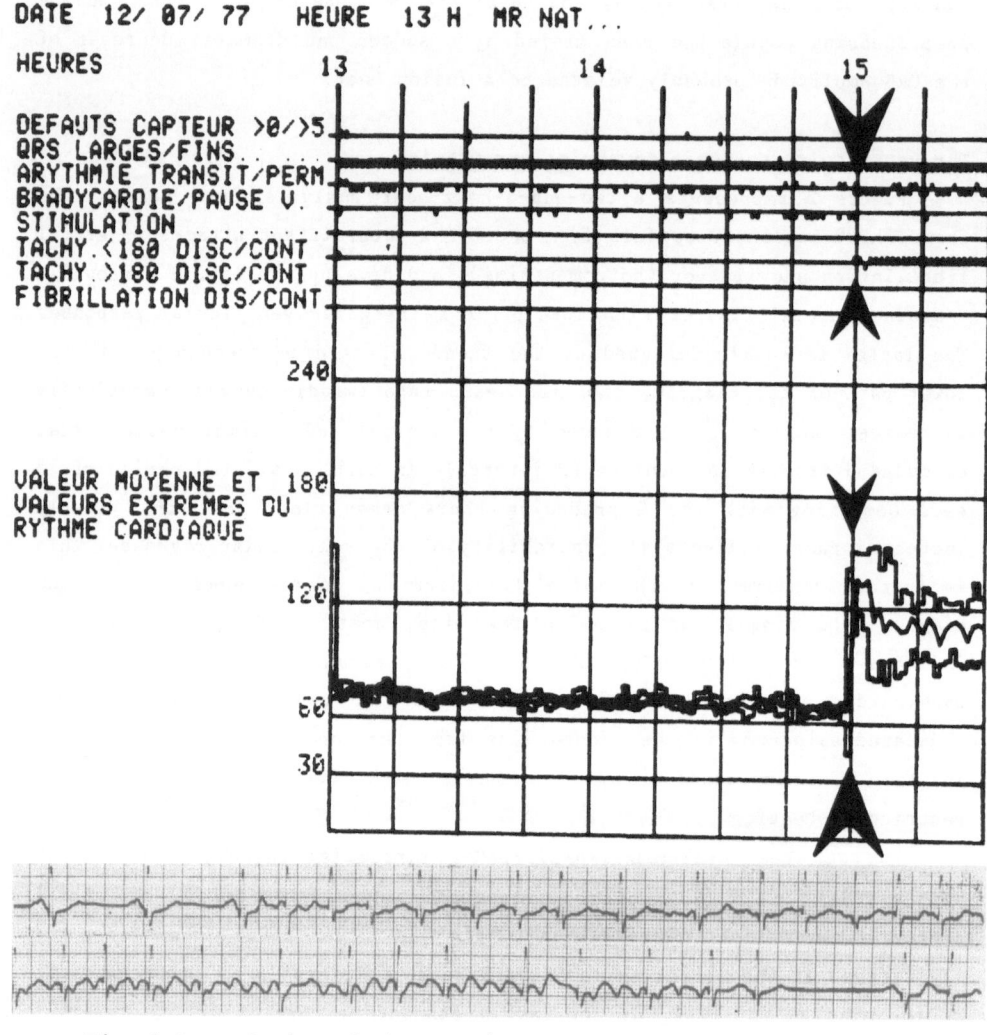

Fig. 2 Irregularity of the ventricular response during atrial arrhythmias (see text).

heart rate trends. On the contrary, during the first 2 hours, the runs of atrial fibrillation are far too short to be detectable from the heart rate, so that the indication of an irregularity is of great diagnostic importance, and easily verified on the tracings. In addition, isolated pauses, secondary to the self-termination of the short attacks, are frequently detected.

The diagnosis of ventricular tachycardia.

For the clinician, the diagnosis of ventricular tachycardia is essentially based on the presence of a rapid heart action in coincidence with enlarged QRS complexes, even if these criteria may miss the diagnosis of supraventricular tachycardia associated with a functional bundle branch block. The computer will express the conjunction of these 2 items without formulating the diagnosis of ventricular tachycardia, as in the example of figure 3, in which two episodes of this arrhythmia are recorded. The scale of analysis is 6 hours in this tracing, so that each step covers a 150 sec. duration in real time. The second line of the upper section ("QRS LARGES/FINS") shows shortly after 14h.00 and 17h.00 the replacement of narrow QRSs (small bars below the line) by enlarged QRSs (bars placed above the line). The indication of a tachycardia at a rate greater than 180/min is given concomitantly in the seventh line, as well as in the heart rate trend. The indication is also given that the tachycardia is not perfectly regular and not constantly sustained, a feature which was actually true in this patient, particularly when the ventricular tachycardia was progressively slowed by the antiarrhythmic therapy (see the bottom strip). This pattern is rather frequent in ventricular tachycardias, but usually missed by the clinician's eye when the heart rate is very rapid.

In the same way, the closer examination of the trend heart rate shows in the very few minutes preceding the onset of the tachycardia the progressive but rapid acceleration of the sinus rate, which actually reaches 107/min (see the upper strip) and constitutes a clear indication for an increased sympathetic drive as a determinant of the ventricular tachycardia.

The second section ("EXTRASYSTOLES LARGES") details events associated with wide premature beats. A beat is premature if it has a coupling interval of less than 90% of the preceding 16-beat mean RR interval and it is large if its width is greater than 150% of the preceding 16-beat average. "NOMBREUSES >1 / >6" : a bar is placed above the line if the number of extrasystoles is between 1 and 6 per minute, and below the line if there are more. "COUPLAGE MOYEN / COURT" : a bar is placed below the

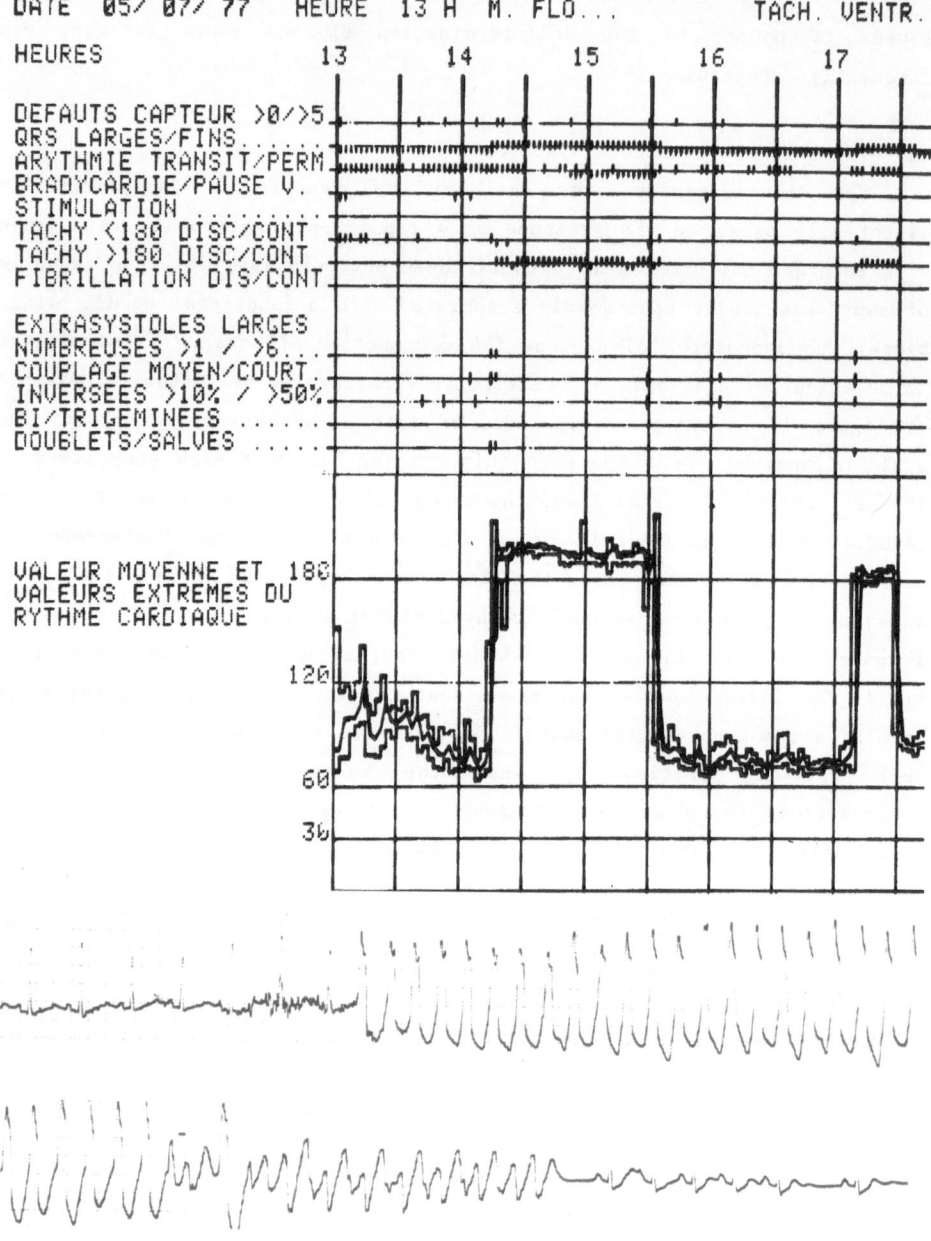

Fig. 3 Recurrent attacks of paroxysmal ventricular tachycardia.

line if the coupling interval is less than 180 ms + [mean RR interval] / 5, and above the line if it is between this value and 220 + [mean RR interval] / 5. "INVERSEES >10% / >50%" : this event records the polarity of wide extra beats with respect to the normal beats. "BI / TRIGEMINEES" : a bar is placed above the line if bigeminy occurs for 12 beats or more, and below if trigeminy is present for 15 beats or more. "DOUBLETS / SALVES" : a bar is placed above the line for 2 wide beats in a row, and below the line for 3 to 10 in a row. The same kind of analysis applies to beats which are both premature (by at least 20%) and of the same width as the basic QRSs (supraventricular extrasystoles). In the present case it should be noted that only a very few ventricular premature beats were present, so that the ventricular tachycardia was only announced by the sinus tachycardia : only the first ten beats of the arrhythmia are in fact considered (wrongly) as ventricular extrasystoles.

Detailed analysis of the ventricular extrasystoles.

This aspect of the computerized analysis of the Holter tapes has been extensively exploited, and figure 4 exemplifies what can be done in this field. The 3-hour analysis was done in a patient having mainly isolated premature beats during the first hour (bottom strip no. 1), doublets during the second hour (strip no. 2) and salvos of 3 beats during the last hour (strip no. 3). This distribution is important to consider, and is clearly indicated in the upper section of the diagram. Contrarywise, it is by no means apparent in the trend of heart rate, as well as in the step by step analysis (vertical bars) of the extrasystole frequency per minute. The numbered quantification verifies that the total number of premature beats is stable at about 2000/hour during the three 1-hour periods, but the numbers are quite different for the doublets and the salvos. Finally, another expression of the quantification appears in the RR interval histograms. Three populations (expressed in number of beats per hour) are visible : they refer to the RR interval preceding narrow (open area) or enlarged QRSs (solid areas), with 2 subsets in the latter population including an either long (isolated or first extrasystole) or short (second or third extrasystole) coupling interval.

90

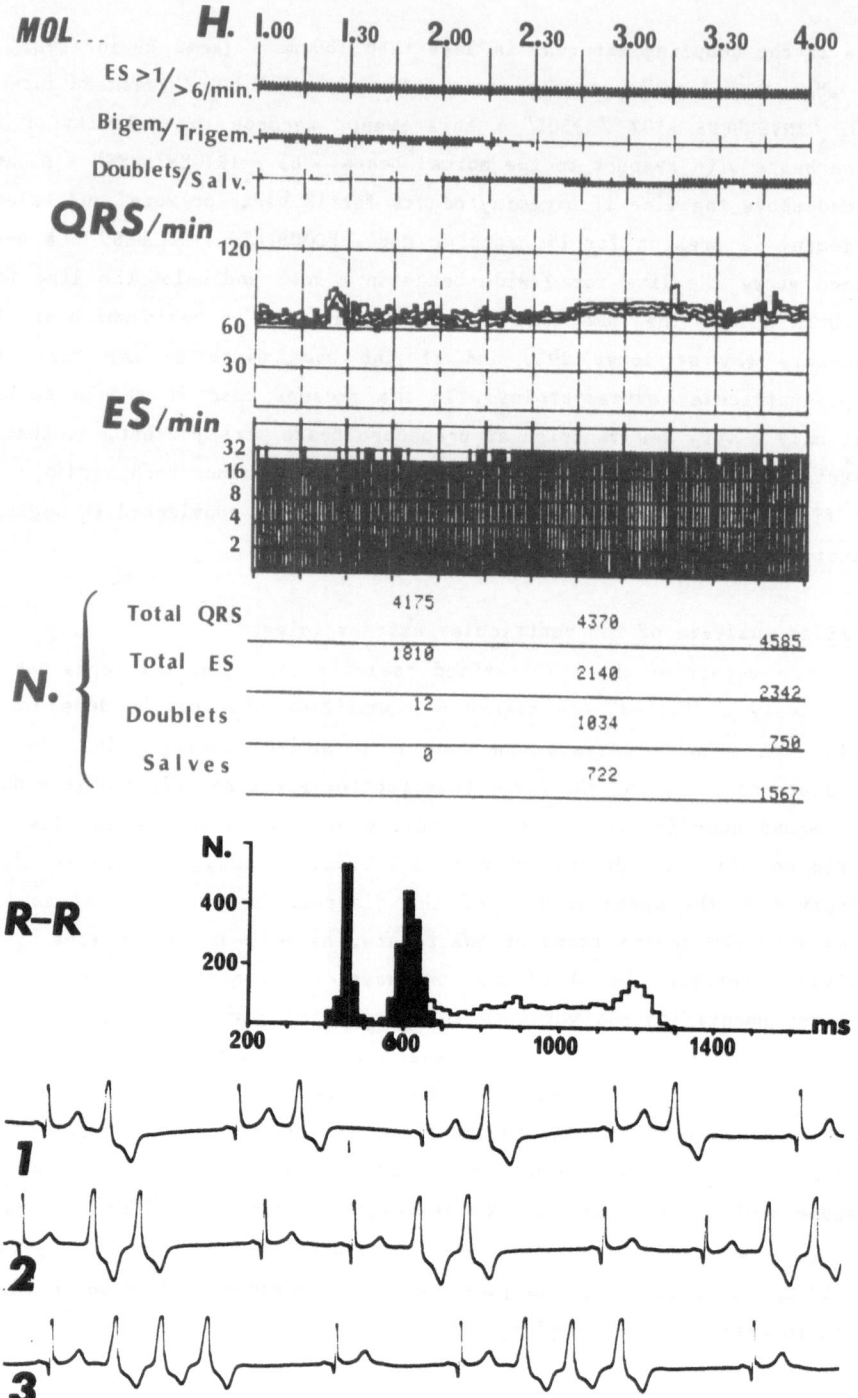

Fig. 4 Distribution and computer analysis of the ventricular extrasystoles

APPROACHING THE ARRHYTHMIA MECHANISM. FUTURE TRENDS OF COMPUTER ANALYSIS.

The computerized analysis of Holter recordings has limited ambitions in terms of ECG diagnosis. Of course it is quite conceivable to improve such an approach by taking into account the P waves thanks to an oesophageal lead. Still, in our routine experience, it is quite rare to have diagnostic problems with Holter tapes, mainly because of the context. For instance, the diagnosis of a 1/1 monomorphic tachycardia with wide QRSs may be indeed difficult in a single surface tracing lasting a few seconds, but practically it is rare not to have in a several hour recording isolated premature beats or a transient AV dissociation or block which constitute the clue of the right diagnosis. We do not think that the future trends of computerized analysis should be mainly directed towards the improvement of the electrocardiographic diagnosis.

The Holter recordings give the opportunity to place the arrhythmias in the context of the patient's normal activity. By so doing, in most paroxysmal arrhythmias, it allows to evidence the triggering mechanism of the rhythm disturbance. Atrial or ventricular premature beats, junctional escape beats usually start the paroxysmal junctional tachycardias and may become the right therapeutic target when drugs are unable to block the reentrant circuit, a situation which is frequent. A prolonged pause secondary to the spontaneous termination of a tachycardia does not have the same significance as a transient, nocturnal sino-atrial block. A number of such examples could be given.

The relationships between the arrhythmias and the autonomic nervous system have a great clinical significance which is usually underestimated. The sinus rate is the best marker we have to evaluate the level of the vago-sympathetic balance throughout the 24-hour period, and most arrhythmias do have to do with the vagal and the sympathetic drives. The same ECG aspect of a paroxysmal atrial fibrillation has a completely different significance if it happens in the context of a sinus tachycardia or bradycardia [Coumel et al., 1982a]. In figure 2 for instance it is not by chance that the sustained atrial flutter starts at 15h.00, i.e. during the digestive period, and is preceded during 2 hours by a progressive slowing of the sinus rate which indicates an increased vagal drive. On the contrary in figure 3, the ventricular tachycardia starts as a consequence of the sudden increase of the sympathetic drive : this had the practical consequence of a beta-blocking therapy in this patient.

Taking into account the sinus frequency is not only important for major but also for minor arrhythmias [Coumel et al., 1982b]. The significance of the ventricular extrasystoles is quite different as they appear or disappear in the context of a sinus bradycardia or tachycardia. But the relationship with the autonomic nervous system is not always the only important parameter, and the distinction should be made between the catecholamine-related and the rate-dependent electrophysiological phenomena [Coumel, 1982].In order to do so,we are currently developing new programs of analysis allowing to explore the tracings on a beat-by-beat basis.

Quantifying the phenomena has a limited value if the numbers are not interpreted comprehensively. This partly explains for instance why the prognostic significance of the ventricular arrhythmias in coronary heart disease is such a controversial issue in epidemiological studies [Coumel et al., 1983]. The same applies to purely quantitative, statistical studies on drugs' effectiveness [Coumel, 1983]. But it does not mean that the computerized analysis is useless in essence. On the contrary, we find of primary importance to develop the more and more sophisticated programs which are necessary for a comprehensive, electrophysiological approach in the routine of the ambulatory monitoring.

REFERENCES

Attuel, P., Rosengarten, M.D., Leclercq, J.F., Milosevic, D., Mugica, J. and Coumel, Ph, 1981. Computer quantitated evaluation of cardiac arrhythmias. Pace, 4, 23-35.

Coumel, Ph. 1982. Heart rate trend analysis : patterns and clinical significance. In "Long term ambulatory electrocardiography" (Ed. J. Roelandt and P.G. Hugenholtz). (Martinus Nijhoff, Tha Hague). pp. 51-61.

Coumel, Ph., Attuel, P., Leclercq, J.F., and Friocourt P. 1982a. Arythmies auriculaires d'origine vagale ou catécholergique. Effets comparés du traitement bêta-bloqueur et phénomène d'échappement. Arch. Mal. Coeur, 75, 373-388.

Coumel, Ph., Rosengarten, M.D, Leclercq, J.F., and Attuel, P. 1982b. Role of sympathetic nervous system in non-ischaemic ventricular arrhythmias. Brit. Heart J., 47, 137-143.

Coumel, Ph. 1983. Editorial. Ambulatory electrocardiographic monitoring and the management of arrhythmias. Precision versus inflexibility. Br. Heart J., 49, 201-204.

Coumel, Ph., Leclercq, J.F., Maisonblanche, P., 1983. Analysis of Holter tapes after myocardial infarction : are we looking for the right things ? In "The first year after a myocardial infarction" (Ed. H.E. Kulbertus and H.J.J. Wellens). In press.

CLINICAL SIGNIFICANCE OF VENTRICULAR PREMATURE BEATS

C.Contini, G.Bongiorni, G.Kraft, G.Mazzocca, M.Baratto, D.Levorato, M.Pauletti.

CNR Clinical Physiology Institute, Via P.Savi 8, 56100 Pisa

ABSTRACT
The Authors make some considerations about the clinical significance of ventricular arrhythmias and their relationship to contractile myocardial impairment. The presence of ventricular arrhythmias with depression of myocardial contractility even in a localised area can be the first sign of cardiomyopathy.The population of postinfarction patients may show a similar behaviour in the presence of a worsening of ischemic cardiopathy. Isolated arrhythmic events, even at higher degree of risk (Lown classes 4 and 5) do not necessarily imply a real worsening of the basic disease.

Many papers have been written in the last years about this topic, but a definite answer to the clinician's questions has not yet been given. Dynamic electrocardiographic recording provides a great amount of useful clinical information, but interpretation of its significance remains disputable.

There is the risk that results of Holter monitoring may actually "produce" patients, while a negative recording may hide a pathological picture.

On the other hand arrhythmias may be the first sign of disease or represent an evolutive stage of a known illness. Many characteristics of ventricular arrhythmias have been studied, particularly in post-infarction patients and in coronary heart disease without myocardial infarction; nevertheless, also in different types of heart disease, some relation can be found between ventricular arrhythmias and myocardial efficiency.

Single parameters of ventricular arrhythmias should be

examined for a complete definition of their clinical significance.

1. PRESENCE AND INCIDENCE OF VENTRICULAR ARRHYTHMIAS.

The first parameter analysed has been the presence of VA and their incidence. Holter monitoring shows ventricular arrhythmias in most cardiac patients, but presence of VA in normal subjects has also been found. The two situations differ in the incidence of VA, since in cardiac patients there are in general many thousands of VA, while in normal subjects they are always less than one hundred.

This is what usually happens although occasionally the rule can be reversed due to repetitive electrophysiological mechanisms in normal subjects or to the presence in cardiac patients of few arrhythmic events resulting in unexpected death.

Therefore presence and incidence of VA cannot provide useful clinical information unless these data are integrated by other parameters. Also evaluation of antiarrhythmic drug therapy on the only basis of quantitative decrease of arrhythmic events is not at all satisfactory: it is necessary to take into account the characteristics of residual arrhythmias.

Multiformity.

It is a very important parameter (3rd class of Lown) which has been overlooked in the classifications employed so far; its clinical significance is now being revalued, as sign of asymmetrical refractoriness and of an electrophysiological situation capable of triggering more severe arrhythmias, up to ventricular fibrillation.

This impression is confirmed by our data which include a wide range of heart diseases, from cardiomyopathies to sclerodermic cardiopathy, acquired valvular disease and postinfarction patients. This finding in cardiac patients allows to diagnose a widespread myocardial involvement which may also be shown with other techniques as diffuse contractile impairment.

Ripetitivity.

It has always been considered as a threatening aspect, particularly if besides pairs, runs of three or more beats of ventricular tachycardia are present. Ominous significance is increased if pairs occur in bigeminy or if bursts are formed by multifocal premature beats with variable coupling intervals. Besides indicating high risk of severe arrhythmias, ripetitivity may be a sign of worsening of preexistent heart disease.

Prematurity.

R on T phenomenon has always been considered the most threatening character (class 5 of Lown). However, the observation of this phenomenon in normal subjects, although has in occasional finding, has certainly decreased its unfavourable prognostic significance. R on T, like the other aforementioned parameters, should not be interpreted apart from other information. Besides foretelling more severe or fatal arrhythmias, it may be a worsening index of preexistent disease and requires selected drug treatment in cardiac patients.

In conclusion arrhythmias have a twofold clinical significance:

in the diagnostic phase, when arrhythmias may be the only demonstrable abnormality, and in the follow-up phase, when their presence may be a sign of worsening of the disease. Nevertheless this approach is not feasible if arrhythmic events are looked at as isolated phenomena rather than connected with recent onset of contractile impairment or with further deterioration of myocardial function.

In other words, a patient with significant ventricular arrhythmias and contractile impairment, should be considered a candidate to congestive cardiomyopathy; on the other hand, when a patient who has suffered myocardial infarction has arrhythmias and poor contractility in a segment other than the infarcted area, it means that a deterioration of the preexistent ischemic heart disease has occurred.

DISCUSSION

Chairman: A.L'Abbate

2.1 - Ambulatory monitoring of arrhythmias

L'ABBATE: Doctor Sandoe, do you think the indication for using Holter tapes has changed in the last ten years. I mean, are they the same reasons you would have given ten years ago?

SANDOE: I think it really has changed very much, because it is incredible what has been used, to select the patient at risk of sudden death. We will hear about it in a later talk today. You could tell me how many times are performed coronary artery disease in the asymptomatic patients? I think it would be quite a lot, wouldn't it?

L'ABBATE: I wouldn't know the answer to that. I'd like to have your personal views about the role of instrumentation. Which level of automation are you thinking of as far as the ideal system of ambulatory monitoring?

SANDOE: The ideal is very easy to speak about. That should be a solid state system where you have an on-line analysis of the ECG, but I think that's quite a time ahead. What I have tried to do was to give a presentation of what we can use, the present status of the systems for ambulatory monitoring.

CONTINI: Do you use the Holter monitoring for setting up the programmable parameters of the physiological pacing?

SANDOE: We will use it in the future, but now we have only a limited number of double-chamber pacemackers in our Institute. But I think the more we will have of these the more we would like to control them. The big problem is how many of them will get pacemaker aided re-entry tachycardia? For that, I think it would be very good to have some period of control.

BIAGINI: I would like to know some more about the relationship between arrhythmyas and ischemia. You have shown some slides where there was ST elevation and ventricular tachycardia.

SANDOE: I think that might be an interesting research project. If you say it from a practical point of view, then I think it would be the exception that you find ischemia before arrhythmias. That's just my personal impression, but I think there should be some research projects about that.

BIAGINI: My impression is that we are understimating the ischemia in episodes of arrhythmias because we are using a wrong lead or a few leads or the sensitivity of the available system to detect ST-T changes is inadequate.

SANDOE: We should really have at least three or four leads.

BALASUBRAMANIAN: I think we've been looking at incidence of arrhythmias and sudden death, and have failed in that so far. Some recent results seem to prove that sudden death in block patients is quite closely related to the change in variability of heart-rate and if we go and look at heart rates more closely and try to locate it, it might be a new avenue to find an answer.

SANDOE: I think that Holter monitoring plays an important role in this kind of correlation study.

BIAGINI: Dr. Coumel, I enjoyed your presentation especially for the philosophy that you give to the analysis of Holter monitoring. I would like to make only one comment about the patient with sudden death that you have shown. You have shown an increase in the heart rate to about 95 beets/min. but perhaps we also have to look at ischemic changes. I think this is another example of the correlation between ischemia and arrhythmias.

COUMEL: You're perfectly right. I did not have enough time to call your attention to this problem, but it is a fact that in this particular case, it was difficult to decide whether the very determinant is the arrhythmias or the ST depression. This had cardiac insufficiency and in this particular case both are very indicated. The only point is that from the clinical point of view he had no pain at all. But it's not a sufficient reason, I agree with you.

BIAGINI: In fact cardiac pain is present only in about 20-30 percent of the ischemic episodes.

MANCIA: Did you say that by beta-blocking agents you reduced the verall heart-rate variability?

COUMEL: Yes.

MANCIA: But isn't this in contrast with the fact that the vagal mediation has a great influence in the heart rate variability? I think this is well established. The reason I'm asking is that we also studied heart-rate variability by several beta-blocking agents and we found, for example that we had to go to long term variability observation to see a reduction with the beta blocking agents.

COUMEL: It's also a very complicated matter, I agree with you. Particularly, I would say that classically the vagal activity is supposed to provoke the very short term, the beat to beat variations of the heart rate.

And if you examine the beat to beat variations of the patient on beta blocking treatment you see no large variations compared to the basic tracings. You see, indeed, some variations, because after all the best way to depress the vagal tone is to depress the sympathetic tone, so you see some very short term, beat to beat variations.

Those links of the system are always working together, and the very results of beta blocking treatment is above all to modify the long term variations of the heart rate. You perfectly know that you have normally an S-shaped curve of the 24 hour rate, and the main effect of beta blocking treatment is that you make it flat. But if you compare variuos beta blockers, with various intrinsic beta blockant effect, you stabilize your 24 hour rate at different levels according to the importance of beta blocking effect. We must never think only in term of vagal tonic action of blockade or sympathetic action of blockade, because the two links of the system are always working together.

WALSH: Early in your presentation you seemed to stress certain patterns in the change of R to R interval as predictive of a fibrillation, that is to say an acceleration of heart rate versus a deceleration. I wondered if you had considered the possibility of studyng a simple pattern recognition scheme on the changes of R to R versus time able to predict incidents.

COUMEL: It depends on which scale you are working with. For example in the vagal induced arrhythmias, you have the general trend of decreasing heart-rate, but in the very few beats preceding the fibrillation, you have a further increase of the R - R intervals. So you have both a mean-term and a very short term influence of the vegal-drive, and this applies to sympathetic induced fibrillation.

WALSH: What I'm suggesting is that this pattern might have a very characteristic shape which might be predictive for you.

ZEELENBERG: More comments to the previous question. We calculate an index of R-R dispersion which is very similar to standard deviation of the R-R interval, and at some point we started to put this out towards the user of the computer system and then we noticed that several times at quite some time preceding atrial fibrillation, there was a sort of step response in the dispersion. It went up from a very low level to a very high level.

TOPIC: 2.2

Ambulatory monitoirng of ischemic patients

AMBULATORY ST SEGMENT MONITORING- PAST AND FUTURE

BY

Dr. V.Bala Subramanian, MD,FACC
Brunel University, Uxbridge, Middx, UK

SUMMARY

Monitoring the ST segment of the electrocardiogram has become technically accurate with the introduction of frequency modulated recorders. The extended lower frequency enables accurate registration of ST segment changes without distortion. The recorders, however are fragile and failure rate is high. The clinical role of ambulatory ST segment monitoring is not in predicting coronary artery disease, but in identifying variant forms of angina either occuring alone or in combination with classical angina, estimating efficacy of treatment or its withdrawal and defining heart rate variations. The technique must be used in conjunction with other non-invasive methods of diagnosis such as exercise testing and if used in isolation may not yield its full potential.

INTRODUCTION

It has been previously assumed that direct recording tape recorders such as the Oxford Medilog Mark I, normally used for documenting arrhythmias can be used for ST segment recording. These recorders and the replay system have a poor and inadequate low frequency response and suffer from phase shift problems. Use of such recorders could lead to unpredictable and unquantifiable artefacts which could be erroneously interpreted as normal or representing ischaemic changes in the electrocardiogram. In a previous communication, the limitations of the Oxford Medilog Mark I recorder for ST segment recording and the superiority of frequency modulated recorders were clearly demonstrated (Bala Subramanian et al 1980). In validation experiments, a real time FM recorder was found to yield recordings closest to control values and the Oxford Medilog Mark II FM recorder produced adequate results. Using the latter recorders we have obtained 1200 tapes in patients with suspected ischaemic heart disease. The experience with this system and the possible directions for future research are reviewed.

RECORDER

The Oxford Medilog Mark II FM recorder is a small and contoured machine using cassette tape and 9 volt alkaline battery to obtain 24 hours of two channels of ECG continuosbly. One channel is used for flutter compensation and another for recording timing signals. Events can be marked by the patient on another channel. The tapes are played back at 60 times recording speed into the analytical system through a demodulating playback system - Oxford Medilog PB4.

The recorder commercially supplied by the company is not adequate for satisfactory recordings. Common problems were the poor quality of cables and the electrode wires easily pulled off from the cables. It is recommended that the following modifications are carried out before using the recorder and follow the procedures to obtain good recordings.

1. A cable similar to the one used in Avionics tape recorders is connected and the cable length cut to approximately 6 to 9 inches.

2. Electrode wires with a locking device is used to prevent them being pulled out.

3. The end connectors of the electrode wires should be as flat as possible.

4. The electrode wires must be checked for internal fracture before every recording and the wire should be discarded at the first evidence of internal fracture.

5. All tapes, even the new ones must be demagnetised by a bulk eraser before use to avoid loss of clock signals.

6. The recording and playback heads must be regularly cleaned with isopropyl alcohol.

7. The heads must be regularly demagnetised.

8. A 25% spare must be kept to replace defective recorders.

ELECTRODE APPLICATION

The following steps are recommended

1. The hair over the chest is shaved if necessary.

2. The electrode sites are carefuly chosen. The ideal sites are manubrium sterni, 6th rib on the right and left side. In women with large breasts the electrodes must be applied below the breasts and a brassiere worn. The electrodes should be applied over the bones and not on interspaces or major muscle masses.

3. The electrode sites are briskly rubbed with isopropyl alcohol till erythema is produced.

4. The sites are stained with a felt marker.

5. The marked sites are abraded by a battery operated burr until only the epidermis is removed. Blood should not be drawn as it increases the skin impedance.

6. The elctrodes are applied taking care not to press the centre which would result in the electolyte jelly weeping into the adhesive area.

7. The electrodes and the wires are fixed by adhesive strips.

8. The recorder is worn around the neck on a cloth pouch and the entire system stabilised by giving the patient an elastic vest.

CALIBRATION

It is essential to record square wave calibrations at the beginning and end of a recording session and these must last at least for 5 minutes.

ANALYSIS

Some workers have used "eyeballing" to identify ST segment changes. This could be grossly inaccurate. The ST segment and heart rate must be written out as an analogue trend using a trending system. If facilities are available, digital methods of analysis are accurate and yield objective data free from observer variations and subjective bias. They also reduce the technician time required for data analysis and allow the data to be stored and retrieved rapidly.

ARTEFACTS

The commonest artefacts encountersed are those due to inadequare eletrode site preparation, choosing poor quality electrodes and cable movement. Internal fracture of electrode wires can give rise to high frequency artefacts. Battery depletion can occasionally distorts the ECG to resemble ST segment elevation. Mismatched recording and playback heads can produce severe flutter of the base line. Inadequate flutter compensation of the playback system can lead to thick base lines. Careful attention to details enumerated above should eliminate most of these and enable satisfactory recordings in at least 90% of patients. Two channel recordings are recommended as at least one channel will be available if another fails.

CLINICAL ROLE

There is considerable controversy about the diagnostic role of ambulatory ST segment monitoring. Some physicians consider all vague undiagnosed chest pains as Prinzmetal's angina and expect the technique to be useful. Others try to interpret the recordings in isolation and find the false positive ST segment changes disconcerting. In my experience, the technique has very little role in the diagnosis of chronic stable angina as an uncontrolled investigation cannot be expected to displace techniques such as exercise testing. Ambulatory ST segment monitoring is invaluable in the following clinical situations and research applications.

1. Diagnosis and follow-up of patients with vasospastic angina.

2. Defining effects and duration of action of anti-anginal drugs.

3. Defining effects of sudden withdrawal of these drugs.

4. Identifying effects of heart rate on ST segment canges.

5. Identifying tachycardia or undue bradycardia induced by drug therapy.

6. Study of heart rate variability.

CONCERTED ACTION

The FM recorders available are technically adequate, but are not robust and reliable for routine clinical use. New recorders must be investigated to define their performence to record ST segment changes. Effort must be made to develop methods of analysis which permit rapid and accurate analysis and archival storage. The new generation of digital recorders need to be evaluated for their suitability. The available electrodes are still unsatisfactory and efforts must be made to develop good quality electrodes.

REFERENCES

1. Bala Subramanian V, Lahiri A, Raftery EB etal (1980) Br. Heart J. 44,419

SIGNIFICANCE OF ELECTROCARDIOGRAPHIC CHANGES
IN ACUTE TRANSIENT MYOCARDIAL ISCHEMIA

A. Biagini, C. Carpeggiani, M.G. Mazzei, Testa R., A. L'Abbate.

C.N.R. Institute of Clinical Physiology and

Istituto Patologia Medica,

University of Pisa, Pisa, ITALY.

INTRODUCTION

The significance of different electrocardiographic alterations in relation to myocardial ischemia, derives normally from studies performed in animals, where it is possible, during the experimental setting, to correlate directly the entity of ischemia with the observed electrocardiographic variations. The information obtained in this way has been used in the clinical setting and also has been compared with the data obtained from the follow up of these patients and eventually from autoptic examinations. Moreover in recent years techniques have become available which allow to study more accurately and precisely, in patients and in animals, the distribution of myocardial blood flow, the myocardial contractility and the anatomy of the coronary vascular bed. More recently the possibility to monitorize the electrocardiogram of ambulatory patients for long periods of time has given rise to new questions that in part are still open to discussion. Object of this report will be to review the data in the literature on the correlation of the different electrocardiographic changes to acute transient myocardial ischemia, in patients and animals with particular reference to the data obtained in ambulatory patients.

EXPERIMENTAL DATA

The use of the microspheres techniques to study the regional distribution of myocardial blood flow, has allowed to obtain most of the actual knowledge on physiology and pathophysiology of the myocardial circulation, and has also allowed to define more precisely the significance of different electrocardiographic alterations. It is now well known that the myocardial blood flow is uniformly distributed in the left ventricle with a slight prevalence to the subendocardial layers being the normal ratio ENDO/EPI equal to 1-1.2 (Buckberg et al., 1972; L'Abbate et al., 1980; Geary et al., 1981).

An alteration of the normal hemodynamic situation as caused by the presence of a critical coronary stenosis or by an abnormal increase in the left ventricular pressure, causes a redistribution of flow with the development of ischemia always in the subendocardial layers (L'Abbate et al., 1980), but never in the subepicardial layers alone. Therefore if myocardial ischemia develops this is either localized to the inner part of the ventricular wall or it involves transmurally the whole myocardial wall; the second condition occurs usually by an occlusion of one of the large epicardial coronary artery in absence of collaterals.

Therefore it is important to stress that in the animal model it is impossible to produce a myocardial ischemia localized only to the subepicardium. We will now briefly discuss the different changes observed during experimentally induced ischemia on the surface electrocardiogram.

Transmural myocardial ischemia

(Normally produced by the transient occlusion of a major epicardial coronary vessel).

A few seconds after the appearance of the vessel occlusion, peacked T waves were followed by clear ST segment elevation which rapidly subside after the release of the ischemia. It is important to note that the alteration of the T wave can be the only apparent phenomenon, also if a great territory is involved by the ischemia and for a long period. Often are present in conjunction with the ST-T changes also variation of the QRS amplitude, in absence of any increase of the myocardial volume, which can be the only apparent ECG changes even during long periods of time (the origin and the specificity of this electrocardiographic alteration is still debated). The transient appearance of pathological Q waves is seldom observed usually during the episodes of longer duration.

Subendocardial myocardial ischemia.

This is usually produced by a reduction of the coronary flow and/or by an increase in the ventricular pressure. The electrocardiographic changes observed during this pathological condition are difficult to study in animal. Due to the surgical manipulation of the chest wall and of the pericardium, already in basal condition, when no myocardial ischemia is present, in the surface electrocardiogram are apparent changes of the ST segment and of the T wave which mask the changes due to the subendocardial ischemia.

CLINICAL DATA

The actual knowledge of the significance of the different electro-cardiographic changes in patients during myocardial ischemia derives greatly from the widespread diffusion of techniques that allow to study directly in humans the regional changes of myocardial blood flow (coronary arteriography or myocardial scintigraphy) or to monitorize for long periods of time the myocardial contractility (echocardiography, blood pool gating ect.).

Transmural ischemia

The complete occlusion of one of the major epicardial coronary artery in absence of collaterals as during Prinzmetal angina causes acute trans-mural myocardial ischemia. The intensive study of patients with Prinzmetal angina has given most of the information that we now have on the significance of the different electrocardiographic changes that can be observed during acute transmural myocardial ischemia.

1. ST segment elevation: angiographic studies have documented the occurrence of a complete occlusion of one of the major coronary vessels supplying the myocardial zone corresponding to the ST changes on the surface electrocardiogram (Maseri et al., 1977; Bertrand et al., 1977; Maseri et al., 1978). Transmural reversible deficit of perfusion has been described during scintigraphic studies (Maseri et al., 1976).

   Regional transient loss of contractility has been described during echocardiographic study (Distante et al., 1983) or during blood pool gated scintigraphy (Parodi et al., 1982), while massive global ventricular impairment has been documented by hemodynamic studies (Maseri et al., 1975).

   Most of these experiences have been repeated in our istitute also during Holter monitoring, therefore the occurrence of a clear ST segment elevation is now considered indicative of acute transmural myocardial ischemia.

2. Pseudonormalisation of a negative T wave (PNTW). The angiographic (Biagini et al., 1982), scintigraphic (Parodi et al., 1981) and hemodynamic (Chierchia et al., 1980) patterns observed during PNTW are identical to the episodes characterized by ST segment elevation, therefore in our experience the pathophysiological significance of those 2 different electrocardiographic changes has to be considered equal.

3. Peacking T wave. Hemodynamic data (Chierchia et al., 1980) have shown ventricular impairment similar to those observed during ST segment elevation, but at the present time there are non enough available data to consider the peacking of T wave always indicative of transmural ischemia. We believe that only in patients who show also, episodes of ST segment elevation this particular sign can be considered indicative of ischemia, also if we are aware of the fact that the origin of this change can be different.

   On the other hand we have to consider that in animal model periods of transmural ischemia may cause only a peacking T wave since the ST segment elevation is quite a late phenomenon. Furthermore patients with episodes of ST segment elevation on Holter monitoring show normally also many episodes of peacking T wave always of shorter duration and sometimes with typical chest pain, indicating the possible ischemic origin of this electrocardiographic sign (Biagini et al., 1982).

4. U waves conversion. Complete occlusion of the left anterior descending artery with a massive reduction of regional uptake has been documented (Matsuguch et al., 1982), in conjunction with a peaking T wave. It is our impression that at the present time this particular electrocardiographic change needs more exhaustive studies to identify its real pathophysiological significance.

5. QRS amplitude variation. Changes in QRS amplitude in absence of clear ST-T variations have been described in patients with Prinzmetal angina (Biagini et al., 1982), but we attribute very poor specificity to this particular sign.

6. No apparent electrocardiographic changes. The use of techniques that directly or indirectly measure the myocardial ischemia has given the impression that transient episodes of myocardial ischemia may present no apparent electrocardiographic changes. This particular finding of clear practical importance needs first of all to be clearly demonstrated and than quantitated before giving an estimation of the phenomenon.

Subendocardial ischemia. The incomplete occlusion of one of the major coronary vessel or its complete occlusion in presence of collateral circulation, or the increasing of the oxygen demand in presence of a fixed reduced coronary reserve causes subendocardial ischemia.

The electrocardiographic signs that can be appreciated during this particular situation are the following.

1. ST segment depression. Angiographic studies (Maseri et al., 1977; Biagini et al., 1982) have shown a variety of different anatomic patterns associated to this electrocardiographic sign: incomplete vasospasm of a major epicardial vessel or incomplete occlusion in presence of collateral circulation, or fixed coronary stenosis.

Scintigraphic studies (Parodi et al., 1981) have shown a diffuse fainty reduction of uptake in the inner layers of the myocardium with not precise limits. Often a direct correlation between the region of reduced uptake and the sites of the electrocardiographic changes is not observed. Hemodynamic studies (Chierchia et al., 1981) have shown ventricular impairment of various degree. We believe that this variety of angiographic, scintigraphic and hemodynamic patterns are due to the different regional involvement of the myocardium during episodes of subendocardial ischemia and to the not perfect correlation between the extent of the electrocardiographic sign of subendocardial ischemia on the electrocardiogram and the real extent of the ischemia.

2. Negative T wave. This particular electrocardiographic sign is usually observed after an episode of transmural myocardial ischemia indicating the permanance of the ischemia in the subendocardium for a longer period of time. We believe that this isolated electrocardiographic change is difficult to appreciate, while it is frequent in association of episodes of ST segment elevation or depression.

3. No apparent electrocardiographic changes. It is possible to postulate that episodes of transient subendocardial ischemia can present any apparent electrocardiographic changes also if at the present we do not have available data to confirm this hypothesis.

AMBULATORY MONITORING

The capability of Holter monitoring system to evaluate the ST-T changes typical of myocardial ischemia, has been questioned by many Authors who believed that the low frequencies which described the ST-segment and the T wave should not be appreciated by this technique (Bragg-Remschel et al., 1982). Therefore the ambulatory monitoring system has been employed mainly to study patients with arrhythmic problems.

The practical demonstration the electrocardiographic changes recorded during ambulatory monitoring are comparable to those obtained by standard electrocardiographic devices (Stern et al., 1975; Biagini et al., 1980), has convinced most of the cardiologists to use this technique to study their anginal patients. Furthermore the contemporaney use of the Holter in conjunction of different techniques like angiography (Biagini et al., 1982) has clearly demonstrated that this technique is capable to appreciate the electrocardiographic changes due to myocardial ischemia. Therefore most of the knowledge on the significance of the different electrocardiographic changes obtained in animals and in humans by traditional electrocardiography has been transferred to the Holter technique.

Nevertheless it has to be keep in mind that the technical characteristics of the Holter system are not completely similar to that of a traditional electrocardiographic devices and that due to the tremendous amount of information obtained during 24 hours of recording (about 100.000 cardiac cycles), the analysis of the Holter tapes requires the use of algorithms which at the present are not completely reliable especially in the measure of the ST-T changes.

A particular aspect that we would like to stress is that in clinical practice only 2 leads are recorded and often only 1 lead is analyzed, while acute transient myocardial ischemia usually involves only regionally the myocardium and often could be appreciated only by the electrode directly exploring the ischemic zone (Biagini et al., 1982). Therefore we suggest to record the electrocardiographic signals from 2 different myocardial regions (as the anterior and the inferior), unless a priori the region that will become ischemic would be previously known.

It should also be emphasized that the correlations described between myocardial ischemia and the various electrocardiographic changes, were always obtained in patients, while very little is known on their significance in a normal population. Therefore it should be incorrect to consider of the same value electrocardiographic changes recorded in a patient in whom different and more specific techniques have documented transient myocardial ischemia and in a person considered to be normal; because the origin of the same phenomenon could be different.

In conclusion it is our belief that the Holter monitoring is a useful technique to monitorize patients known or strongly suspected to present ischemic problems. Most of the information obtained with standard electro cardiography on the pathophysiological significance of the different electrocardiographic changes during myocardial ischemia can be used also to intepret data obtained with Holter monitoring. Only the simultaneous use of different techniques in conjunction with the electrocardiogram, whatever obtained, can give precise informations on their pathophysiological significance.

REFERENCES

Bertrand, M.E., Laisue, C., Lefebvre, J.M., Carre, A., Warembourg, H. and Leikieffre J. 1977. Le spasme des arteres coronaires. Arch. Mal. Coeur., 70, 1233.

Biagini, A., L'Abbate, A., Mazzei, M.G., Carpeggiani, C., Testa, R., Antonelli, R., Michelassi, C., Benassi, A. and Maseri, A. 1980. Inaffidabilità del monitoraggio elettrocardiografico in Unità di Cura Coronarica per il riconoscimento di episodi di ischemia miocardica. Giorn. It. Cardiol., 10, 1449.

Biagini, A., Mazzei, M.G., Carpeggiani, C., Testa, R., Antonelli, R., Michelassi, C., L'Abbate, A. and Maseri A. 1982. Vasospastic ischemic mechanism of frequent asymptomatic transient ST-T changes during continuous electrocardiographic monitoring in selected unstable angina patients. Am. Heart. J., 103, 13.

Biagini, A., Michelassi, C., Mazzei, M.G., Carpeggiani, C., Testa, R., Benassi, A., Varanini, C.M., Riva, A., Marchesi, C. and L'Abbate, A., 1982. Electrocardiographic changes during Prinzmetal angina: QRS versus ST segment variation. IEEE Computer Society Press, Silver Spring, Maryland, p. 237.

Biagini, A., Testa, R., Carpeggiani, C., Mazzei, M.G., Emdin, M., Michelassi, C. and L'Abbate, A. 1982. Contributo dell'elettrocardiografia dinamica alla conoscenza della cardiopatia ischemica silente. In: "La Cardiopatia Ischemica Silente", Prati P.L., edr. p. 81.

Bragg-Remschel, D.A., Anderson, C.H. and Winkle, R.A. 1982. Frequency response characteristics of ambulatory ECG monitoring system and their implications for ST segment analysis. Am. Heart J., 103: 20.

Buckberg, G.D., Fixler, D.E., Archie, J.P. and Hoffman, J.I.E. 1972. Experimental subendocardial ischemia in dogs with normal coronary arteries. Circ. Res., 30, 67.

Chierchia, S., Brunelli, C., Simonetti, I., Lazzari, M. and Maseri A. 1980. Sequence of events in angina at rest: primary reduction in coronary flow. Circulation, 61, 759.

Chierchia, S., Lazzari, M., Simonetti, I. and Maseri A. 1980 Hemodynamic monitoring in angina at rest. Herz, 5, 188.

Distante, A., Rovai, D., Picano, E., Moscarelli, E., Palombo, C., Morales, M.A., Michelassi, C. and L'Abbate, A. 1983. Transient changes in left ventricular mechanics during attacks of Prinzmetl angina: an M-Mode echocardiographic study. Am. Heart J. (in press).

Geary, G.G., Smith, G.T., Mc Namara, J.J. 1981. Defining the anatomic perfusion bed of an occluded coronary artery and the region at risk to infarction. A comparative study in the baboon, pig and dog. Am. J. Cardiol., 47, 1240.

L'Abbate, A., Marzilli, M., Ballestra A.M., Camici, P., Trivella, M.G., Pelosi, G. and Klassen, G.A. 1980. Opposite transmural gradients of coronary resistance and extravascular pressure in the working dog's heart. Cardiov. Res., 14, 21.

Maseri, A., L'Abbate, A., Pesola, A., Ballestra, A.M., Marzilli, M., Severi, S., Maltinti, G., De Nes, M., Parodi, O. and Biagini A. 1977. Coronary vasospasm in angina pectoris. Lancet, 1, 713.

Maseri, A., Mimmo, R., Chierchia, S., Marchesi, C., Pesola, A. and L'Abbate, A. 1975. Coronary artery spasm as a cause of acute myocardial ischemia in man. Chest, 68, 625.

Maseri, A., Parodi, O., Severi S. and Pesola, A. 1976. Transient transmural reduction of myocardial blood flow demonstrated by thallium-201 scintigraphy as a cause of variant angina. Circulation, 56, 280.

Matsuguch, T., Koiwaya, Y., Nakasaki, O., Orita, Y., and Nakamura, M. 1982. Negative U wave and peaked T wave without ST changes during spontaneous and ergonovine-induced vasospastic angina. Am. J. Heart, 6, 918.

Parodi, O., Marzullo, P., Galli, M., Bencivelli, W., Agostini, F. and L'Abbate, A. 1982. Different pattern of contractility and perfusion in resting angina with ST segment elevation and depression. Am. J. Cardiol., 49, 1016.

Parodi, O., Uthurralt, N., Severi, S., Bencivelli W., Michelassi, C. and Maseri, A. 1981. Transient reduction of regional myocardial perfusion during angina at rest with ST segment depression or normalization of negative T waves. Circulation, 63, 1238.

Stern, S., Tzivoni, D. and Stern, Z. 1975. Diagnostic accuracy of ambulatory ECG monitoring in ischemic heart disease. Circulation, 52, 1045.

ACKNOWLEDGMENTS

The authors gratefully acknowledge the cooperation of Miss Emanuela Campani, Miss Daniela Banti and Mrs Hilda Biagini de Ruyter, for assistance in manuscript preparation.

PREVALENCE AND MAGNITUDE OF ST SEGMENT AND T WAVE ABNORMALITIES IN HEALTHY ADULT SUBJECTS DURING CONTINUOUS AMBULATORY ELECTROCARDIOGRAPHY

P. BJERREGAARD

University Department of Cardiology
Aarhus Kommunehospital
8000 Aarhus C, Denmark

From studies with ordinary ECG recording technique and multiple leads ST-T changes have been observed in relation to change in posture (Lachman et al. 1965), emotional strain (Sigler 1961), vagotonia (Iglesias et al. 1969), inhalation of tobacco smoke (Graybiel et al. 1936) and several other situations encountered by most subjects during an ordinary 24 hour period (Marriott 1959, Marriott 1967). Some of these changes have been observed in precordial leads and must therefore occasionally show up during ambulatory ECG recording, where the most frequently used leads are "V_5-like" with the exploring positive electrode at the V_5 position and the negative electrode at various locations, but mostly at the manubrium sterni (lead CM_5) or at the level of the fifth intercostal space in the right anterior axillary line (lead CC_5).

ST SEGMENT DEPRESSION

Only very few studies of the ambulatory ECG in healthy adult subjects have focused on the ST-T changes possibly because of the question of the validity of ST segment depression reproduced by earlier instruments for ambulatory electrocardiography (Hinkle et al. 1967). Most later models for ambulatory ECG recording are, however, acceptable for grossly reproducing ST-T changes, but some may overestimate the magnitude of ST segment depression. Djiane et al. (1977) found J point depression with ascending ST segment ("junctional changes") especially during periods of sinus tachycardia in 70% of the subjects in their study, and such changes are probably a consequence of the limited frequency response of the equipment used. Some of these changes may, however, represent the physiological ST changes with increase in heart rate reported by Sjöstrand (1950). In the study by Tzivoni and Stern (1973) especially designed for an investigation of the electrocardiographic pattern during sleep in healthy subjects and in patients with ischemic heart disease the ST segment remained isoelectric both day and night in all the healthy subjects, and the height of the T waves showed only minimal changes. It is unfortunate, that the study does not provide information about the sex of the subjects studied, because the most conspicuous results from other studies involving both males and females have been the great difference between the proportion of males with ST depression compared to females.

TABLE 1   ST segment depression in the ambulatory ECG

AUTHOR AND YEAR OF PUBLICATION	POPULATION STUDIED			LEAD	ST DEPRESSION of $\geq$ 1 mm % of Subjects
	No	Sex	Age Years		
Engel & Burckhardt 1975	35	Male & Female	24 ± 4	CM_5	9
Djiane et al. 1977	50	Male & Female	22 - 57	CM_5	4
Tzivoni & Stern 1973	39	?	Mean 38	$V_1 (\blacksquare)$ - $V_5 (+)$	None
Armstrong et al. 1982	50	Male	35 - 49	CC_5 & CH_6	30
Bjerregaard 1982	125	Male	40 - 59	CM_5	1
Bjerregaard 1982	57	Female	40 - 59	CM_5	18

In the study by Engel and Burckhardt (1975) 4% of the males and 15% of the females had significant ST depression, and in the study by Djiane et al. (1977) the corresponding figure for males was 3% and for females 8%, but the actual number of subjects with ST depression was very low in these studies. In a somewhat larger group of subjects studied by Bjerregaard (1982) these differences were, however, even more evident (1% for males and 18% for females). The same difference in behavior

of the ST segment in males and in females has been observed in
response to exercise (Cumming et al. 1973), but not explained
satisfactoryly.

In some contradiction to previous studies are the results
recently published by Armstrong et al. (1982) from a study of
ST-T changes in 50 normal men ranging in age from 35 to 49
years (mean 44.6). During scanning of 24 hour ECG recordings
they found 1.0 mm or greater of horizontal or downsloping ST
segment depression persisting 80 ms after the J point of the
QRS complex in a total of 15 subjects or 30%. In contrast to
other studies of ST segment abnormalities in healthy subjects
they used, however, 2 leads (CC_5 and CH_6) instead of one (normally CM_5). The clinical importance of ST segment abnormalities
reported in patients with angina pectoris (Stern et al., 1975;
Biagini et al., 1982; Johnson et al., 1982) suggests, that the
high percentage for such abnormalities found by Armstrong et
al. (1982) in normal men is very unusual and possibly due to
the special lead systems used or a high incidence of latent coronary artery disease in the subjects studied.

T WAVE INVERSION

A negative T wave would in light of the previously mentioned large number of causes for T wave changes by most investigators be considered a non-specific finding in an ambulatory ECG, but the findings by Tzivoni et al. (1978) seem to
indicate, that such an assumption may not be correct. In a
study of 48 patients with precordial pain findings in the ambulatory ECG were correlated with findings on coronary arteriography, and in 5 patients with deeply inverted T waves as a
transient phenomenon, severe coronary artery disease was demonstrated in all of them. The T wave changes observed in the study by Engel and Burckhardt (1975) were not described in detail,
but Bjerregaard (1982) found "major" T wave changes in only 2
out of 182 subjects, both males. Again in contrast to other
studies Armstrong et al. (1982) found labile T wave inversions
of up to 3.0 mm in depth lasting 20 seconds to 20 minutes in 18
out of 35 (51%) of the subjects without ST segment depression.

TABLE 2   Negative T waves in the ambulatory ECG

AUTHOR AND YEAR OF PUBLICATION	POPULATION STUDIED			LEAD	NEGATIVE T WAVE %
	No	Sex	Age Years		
Engel & Burck-hardt 1975	35	Male & Female	24 ± 4	CM_5	11
Djiane et al. 1977	50	Male & Female	22 - 57	CM_5	0
Armstrong et al. 1982	50	Male	35 - 49	CC_5 & CH_6	36
Bjerregaard 1982	125	Male	40 - 59	CM_5	5
Bjerregaard 1982	57	Female	40 - 59	CM_5	7

Available data have in this way demonstrated the occurrence of "significant" ST-T changes in the ambulatory ECG in
apparently healthy adult subjects. Studies in patients with
chest pain have shown, however, that such changes may be of
both prognostic and diagnostic importance. Further studies with
various leads and instruments of high performance able to quantitate ST-T changes in an accurate way are therefore urgently
needed in order to establish "normal" limits for ST-T changes
in the ambulatory ECG.

REFERENCES

Armstrong, W.F., Jordan J.W., Morris, S.N. and McHenry, P.L.
1982. Prevalence and magnitude of S-T segment and T wave
abnormalities in normal men during continuous ambulatory
electrocardiography. Am J Cardiol 49, 1638-42
Biagini, A., Mazzei, M.G., Carpeggiani, C., Testa, R., Antonelli, R., Michelassi, C., L'Abbate, A. and Maseri, A. Vasospastic ischemic mechanism of frequent asymptomatic transient ST-T changes during continuous electrocardiographic
monitoring in selected unstable angina pectoris. Am Heart
J 1982;103,13-19
Bjerregaard, P. 1982. ST-T changes in the ambulatory ECG on
healthy adult subjects. Proceeding: IXth World congress of
Cardiology. Moscow. Vol.II,0133
Cumming, G.R., Dufresne, C., Kich, L. and Samm, J. 1973. Exercise electrocardiogram pattern in normal women. Br Heart J
35,1055-9

118

Djiane, P., Egre, A., Bory, M., Savin, B. and Serradimigni, A. 1977. L'enregistrement électrocardiographique continu chez 50 sujets normaux. In: Puel P, ed. Troubles du rythme et electrostimulation. Toulouse: Societé de la Nouvelle Imprimerie Fournié. 161-7

Engel, U.R. and Burckhardt, D. 1975. Haüfigkeit und art von herzrhythmusstörungen wowie Ekg.-veränderungen bei jugendlichen herzgesunden probanden. Schweiz Wochenschr 105, 1467-9

Graybiel, A., Starr, R.S. and White, P.D. 1936. Electrocardiographic changes following the inhalation of tobacco smoke. Am Heart J 12,89-99

Hinkle, L.E., Carver, S.T., Meyer, J. and Stevens, M. 1967. Tape recordings of the ECG of active men. Limitations and advantages of the Holter-Avionics instruments. Circulation 36,752-65

Iglesias, R., Echenique, R. and Conzales, G. 1969. T-wave inversion of the ECG of healthy individuals with vagotonia. Aerospace Med 40(3),318-20

Johnson, S.M., Mauritson, D.R., Winniford, M.D., Willerson, J.T., Firth, B.G., Cary, J.R. and Hillis, D. 1982. Continuous electrocardiographic monitoring in patients with unstable angina pectoris: Identification of high-risk subgroup with severe coronary disease, variant angina, and/or impaired early prognosis. Am Heart J 103,4-12

Lachman, A.B., Semler, H.J. and Gustafson, R.H. 1965. Postural ST-T wave changes in the radioelectrocardiogram simulating myocardial ischemia. Circulation 31,557-63

Marriott, H.J.L. 1960. Coronary mimicry: Normal variants, and physiologic, pharmacologic and pathologic influences that simulate coronary patterns in the electrocardiogram. Ann Intern Med 52,411-27

Marriott, H.J.L. 1967. Normal electrocardiographic variants simulating ischemic heart disease. JAMA 199(5),103

Sigler, L.H. 1961. Abnormalities in the electrocardiogram induced by emotional strain. Am J Cardiol 8,807-14

Sjöstrand, T. 1950. The relationship between the heart frequency and S-T level of the electrocardiogram. Acta Med Scand 138(fasc III),201-10

Stern, S., Tzivoni, D. and Stern, Z. 1975. Diagnostic accuracy of ambulatory ECG monitoring in ischemic heart disease. Circulation 52,1045-49

Tzivoni, D. and Stern, S. 1973. Electrocardiographic pattern during sleep in healthy subjects and in patients with ischemic heart disease. J Electrocardiol 6(3), 225-9

Tzivoni, D., Wolf, E., Stern, Z., Orkan, E. and Stern, S. 1978 Ambulatory ECG monitoring and bicycle ergometry: correlation with findings on coronary arteriography. Eur J Cardiol 8/1,19-26.

DISCUSSION

Chairman: A.L'Abbate

2.2 - Ambulatory monitoring of ischemic patients.

CLEMENT: I have 2 questions for Dr. Balasubramanian. The first question is: a few years ago the people of the Rotterdam group convinced us, or did not convince us, I do not know, that we should use for ST-segment study the ortogonal leads, and that specificity and sensitivity would be better than with the regular EKG. My question is: is it technically feasible or not? The second question is a technical one: we had been using for years the Medilog Mark One System and four years ago we got convinced that we should move to the FM Modulator Mark 2 system. So we replaced our Oxford Medilog Mark 1 by Mark 2. And on that day all our troubles started: particularly an enormous recording of noise, and we got regular visits of the Oxford people changing electrodes, cables, plugs, we were about to change technician - we have not done it. But in fact they never got it fixed and they are trying now to replace the Medilong 2 with the MR14, I believe, but I'm not familiar with it, and I would like to know really, from an expert, what to do to get this thing fixed.

BALASUBRAMANIAN: For the 1st question about the ortogonal leads, it's technically very difficult to use ortogonal leads in a Holter monitoring system. And now the evidence is gradually mounting that a combination of CM5, CC5 and CS5 gives a 93% specificity in ST-T testing. So this combination for Holter monitoring probably might be technically adequate to produce a good specificity. We have been plagued at the beginning by these problems with the Oxford Medilog Mark 2. I think the recorders have recently improved. Of our 1st generation recorders, we had 17 recorders, we had none working. All 17 were in the workshop at some stage going up or down. The moment we buy a recorder from Oxford Medilog, we don't use it as they supply it to us. It undergoes an internal modification by us, which I have tried to convince Oxford to use, but they've never been convinced by us. We cut the recording lead short to 9 cms, the cable is cut to 9 cms and secondly, the battery contacts are changed. And, number three, we don't use the electrodes they recommend, we use the electrodes which we have found to be satisfactory. The entire record procedure is changed. The recorders are not worn around the waist, they are worn around the chest. And most of the noise has now been identified due to 2 problems: one is the lack of pressure compensation in the replay deck: and second is the mismatch between replay head and the recording head. What we do normally is have 2 or 3 replay decks without noise problem, we try to play back on other deck and find that the noise can be considerably reduced if the head-match can be obtained between replay and recording head. But they are very critical records: they have a good performance but poor reliability.

MANCIA: You showed us a very nice record of changes in ST segments. I think the other speakers, however, had put into focus another quite important aspect, that, maybe, these changes are not enough to give a good diagnosis of ischemic attack. You have no specific changes that may be associated with ischemia, you may have ischemia with no changes in ST segments, you may have false positive, particulartly in women.

BALASUBRAMANIAN: Yes I'm glad you brought this point up. I don't think that ambulatory monitoirng of ST segment is a viable diagnostic technique when looked in isolation. It is like the blind man looking at the elephant. You must compare it and add the information you get with other variables. When you look at it in isolation, because of the uncomtrolled native of data which comes out, because of the problems which must be faced with the equipment we are using, the predictive accuracy, So it could be very nicely used to locate changes, like what I have done on for therapy, for diagnosing ST segment elevation or a combination of this and proven ischemia. But if you want to use it for diagnosis, there are better methods available. So in my opinion the technique is good for some things but not for everything.

WALSH: I have a question for Dr. Hinsen. I'm very intrigued by your approach of using multiple leads placed in close proximity to the heart, where the ST elevation occurs. This is a very attractive idea, but what I'm wondering is, did you compare this lead system to a randomly placed signal or dual lead system or to the standard 12 leads ECG, for specificity or sensitivity analysis?

HINSEN: We have several lead systems, up to 100 or 200 leads systems, but this is of course impracticable for Holter monitoring. We have considered several optimum types of these total electrode systems, and we are now comparing, all the results to all the other available clinical results. At the end of the year, we are planning to announce the first results at the Computers in Cardiology meeting in Aachen.

BIAGINI: I would like just to make a comment about the specificity of recording the Electrocardiogram for ST segment changes analysis. I agree with Dr. Balasubramanian. But also one more thing is important, is to say which kind of lead we are monitoring, because most of the time we don't know where the patient will have an ischemia attack. In our experience, about 42% of the episodes of the ST segment changes will be lost monitoring only anterior lead. And most systems use anterior lead only. I think we need at least 2 leads systems.

BALASUBRAMANIAN: I think that's a well taken point. Even though I have shown only one channel of electrocardiogram in all my tracings, we have recorded 2 channels (CM5 and CC5) in all our recordings. And again I'm enphasising the point that you can't interpret ambulatory monotoring in isolation. All our recordings are done the day after an exercise test recording, so we know precisely the site where the changes are occuring, and we are going to monitor the same thing. One of the advantages of the Oxford Medilog Mark 2 system is its slimmess, at times we put 4 recorders in tandem and we have recorded 18 simultaneous leads, and the patients have no inconvenience. So it's quite possible to correlate 18 simultaneous recordings.

COUMEL: I have two questions for the speakers: one is very short, and one is, maybe, very large. The short one is, do you have any minimal standard duration for istance, for Prinzimetal anginal attacks? I mean that rather often we see very typical changes but during a very few seconds, does it matter, is it of diagnostic importance? And my second question is: did you pay attention and, you certainly paid attention, to the relationship between, for istance, prinzimetal angina and autonomic nervous system? This is a very complicated affair, but do you have any precise idea on this controversial point and could you schematize, what are the currently available opinions?

BALASUBRAMANIAN: I thought that as far as chronic stable angina is concerned the position is much more clear. We hardly ever get ST segment depression which does not last at least for a minute, before the changes become normal. We did find patients who became normal within 10 beats after an episode occurred, and we also found that patients could became remarkably ST segment elevated within another 10 beats, and some of the episodes lasted between 20-30 seconds only, and some could last 20 minutes or so. So we think that even if episodes shorter than 20 seconds could mean coronary artery spasm, manifesting in changes on the electrocardiogram. As far the autonomic changes are concerned, I could only refer to literature. A lot of people have tried to treat them with beta blocking drugs, with no success, and a lot of people have tried to treat them with alpha blocking drugs with no success, and people have tried to stimulate myocardial ischemia with ST segment elevation by injecting various sympathomimetic and parasymoathetic drugs without success. And people have tried to inject various things to produce spasm without much success. So I think the state of the art is really not known.

BIAGINI: I would like to say that by using different techniques, such as echography, (as performed by the group of Dr. Distante at our Institute) you can see very short periods of improvement of the left ventricular wall that last seconds, as Dr. Balasubramanian said before, and so you have changes of a few seconds, let's say 20 seconds, 50 seconds or 1 minute, that are preceded by changes in the thickness and in the contractility of the left wall. So it depends maybe on the technique you used.

MANCIA: I can add a comment to the second question: although I fully agree that the mechanism of the Prinzimetal angina are unknowr I think there could be suggestions that there are some reflexes involved during the Prinzimetal angina, and with regards to this I was surprised to see that in one of your episodes you showed, you had an increased heart rate during the Prinzimetal angina episode. I remenber the paper by Guazzi and co-workers, whom I think were the first in the field, at the beginning of the seventies. They monitored blood-pressure and heart rate continuously during several episodes of Prinzimetal angina and found, I believe bradicardia in almost all the episodes.

BIAGINI: Perhaps the vertical line that was on the slide was a bit confusing. The line was drawn at the beginning of the electrocardiographic changes, and at that time the heart rate was increased. But if you look at the first changes in the contractility and relaxation, which are much before the changes in the electrocardiogram, you see that at that time you have no heart rate changes. The electrocardiogram in fact shows changes with delay, as it is possible to document by experimental studies, closing the coronary artery. There our experience is not in contrast with that of Guazzi.

MANCIA: Can I ask a question to Dr. Bjeregaard. How can you be sure that these people, aged 40-59, were healthy?
The reason of the question is that I think that the signs you have shown

are probably not enough to exclude the existence of coronary heart disease. Particularly I am refering to the ST changes you have shown.

BJEREGAARD: That's right. ST segment depression, in fact may be due to ischemia. I don't know. Especially now we know that 75% of ischemic attacks are without pain. So maybe a follow up on this would show that it has prognostic importance to find ST segment depression in healthy people.

VAN BEMMEL: I have a few comments and questions. I think that a concerted action is fairly worthwhile, Dr. Marchesi, since already quite a lot of problems are coming up, the first question will be for you: did you have any idea that in your review of those instruments you showed us this morning, that there were such horrible instruments, connected with such famous names? I thought we had already solved this problem 15-20 years ago. Maybe you can comment on that, and if there are any other instruments of that type. I have a question also for Dr. Hinsen: did you use your eight electrodes primarily to increase diagnostic sensitivity and specificity, or did you in the end only improve your signal to noise ratio, since your different electrodes are located in the same area and I just wondered if you could not cope with the problem when using just one or two pairs CC5, CM5, CS5, instead of having 8 electrodes in the same area?

HINSEN: We want to manage both the problems you spoke of. We improve our signal to noise ratio averaging over the special area. Moreover by increasing the signal-noise ratio, we get better primary information about the ischemic process. Because we do not know the border zone of the ischemic side, and where the electrodes will go when they shift. So if we have only one electrode in the centre; it may be that the ischemic zone is shifted, and we have such shifts during exercise. So we get wrong results. We think that the more electrodes you take, the better will be the specificity and sensitivity, and the signal to noise ratio.

VAN BEMMEL: Certain electrode position, not related to the type of ischemia or the location of ischemia are more sensitive· and more specific for ST depression, which you have not compared.

HINSEN: We are now looking for the best set of electrodes.

VAN BEMMEL: It has been asked to you already, Dr. Bjerregaard but I should like to ask you the same question in a different way: didn't you just prove by your study that there is a difference in prior probabilities in selecting certain leads in different sexes, since it is known that certain leads are more sensitive to detect certain abnormalities in women or in men?

BJERREGAARD: Maybe.

MARCHESI: The former question of Dr. Van Bemmel about the quality of instrumentation is an important one. Let me take only a few points. First we have considerable problems of information regarding the medical end user. Let's just take the question of magnetic recording. Early recorders were using direct recording method. When FM recorders have been introduced, all users wanted the new type of recorder, without knowing, perhaps, that they could be worse, in absence of a more sophisticated speed control device. This problem of dissemination of technical knowledge applies of course to other aspects of the instrumentation. Secondly we have problems coming from limited production, which doesn't allow standardization, so affording cost and quality of the instrumentation. This is also a crucial problem, because I think it is motivated by the absence of standardization of the medical procedures of analysis of Holter recordings. Finally a third point, linked also to the previous observation, is that no standard for performance evaluation has been accepted by manufacturers, so it's almost impossible to compare the quality of the different instruments available. I believe that these are major points to be considered in a concerted action.

TOPIC: 2.3

Ambulatory monitoring of hypertensive patients

CLINICAL VALUE OF NON-INVASIVE AMBULATORY
BLOOD PRESSURE MEASUREMENTS AND COMPARISON
WITH OTHER METHODS.

D.L. Clement, M. Bobelyn, L. Packet, G.O. Van
Maele

Department of Cardiology, University Hospital, 185
De Pintelaan, B-9000 Gent, Belgium

ABSTRACT

For years, the diagnosis of arterial hypertension has been largely
based on the level of blood pressure measured in the doctor's office.
Studies with either continuous or semi-continuous blood pressure recordings have shown that variability of blood pressure is so large that
casual pressure only is a tiny part of the spectrum of the blood pressure profile. Ambulatory blood pressure recordings are very helpful
in this respect ; most of the information can be obtained by non-invasive means. Besides a more correct diagnosis of the hypertensive disease as made in normal life, ambulatory blood pressure recordings permit a better definition of the effect of hypotensive drugs on blood
pressure and its variations.

INTRODUCTION

There is a growing interest in continuous or semi-continuous recordings of arterial blood pressure (Clement, 1979 ; Stott et al.,
1981). From the early days of this experience the argument has been
alife whether invasive or non-invasive recordings should be preferred
and whether recordings should be made ambulatory or rather in better
controled and standardized conditions.

Invasive versus non-invasive recordings

The invasive methods provide the clinician with intra-arterial
recordings, avoiding several of the well-known errors in measurements
of indirect blood pressure recording techniques. Also data are given
on a beat-to-beat basis for a 24,48 or even 72 hours period without
active participation of the patients who are allowed to move freely
during their normal daily activities.

The non-invasive ambulatory methods provide the clinican with
information derived from the Korotkoff sounds, recorded in normal daily
life without (Del mar Avionics systems) or with little (Remler systems)
participation of the patients. Because of their non-invasive character, recordings can be repeated many times without any significant risk
to the patients.

Even accepting the higher degree of accuracy of intra-arterial readings, there is a definite trend in several institutions to use for their clinical and even scientific work, the non-invasive techniques. First, they do inform about Korotkoff sounds, which is the parameter used for years in the definition of blood pressure and also the parameter used to determine prognosis of hypertension (Kannel, 1974) as well as efficacy of treatment (Veterans Administration studies, 1974, HFDP study 1979, Australian Study, 1980). Second, they provide with the answer to the most important part of the question being posed which is : what is the blood pressure outside of the clinic in the normal surroundings of the patients ; that information is given in the format of a curve or of an histogram (Van Maele and Clement, 1981) very much like the invasive recordings ; moreover, recent data that will be discussed in this issue, have shown that beat-to-beat analysis of the blood pressure curve is no longer necessary to define the major components of the blood pressure profile (Di Rienzo et al., Abstract, 1982). Third, even with a low rate of complications in experienced hands, invasive recordings are hard to accept in patients that are largely asymptomatic and show mild to moderate hypertension as it is the case in the vast majority of the patients. It becomes even more difficult to accept when normotensive or normal subjects have to be studied and when repeated recordings are necessary such as for ex. as in drug studies.

In light of these arguments, it was decided that for the questions to be answered, the non-invasive techniques were more appropriate and that the invasive recordings should be restricted to a limited number of specific or exceptional conditions.

Validation of non-invasive ambulatory techniques

To record blood pressure and heart rate in the patients' normal environment, the portometer (Remler M 2000) was used. This apparatus was developed by Hinman and associates (1962) ; it has been extensively tested and widely used by Sokolow and coworkers (Kain et al., 1964 ; Sokolow et al., 1966 ; Sokolow et al., 1973 ; Perloff et al., 1981).

In 50 patients, reliability of this technique was checked by comparing the data recorded on tape and those simultaneously defined by sphygmomanometer (fig. 1). There is a very close correlation be-

tween both these measurements, both for systolic and for diastolic values ($r^2 = 0.99$, p <0.001) confirming earlier findings (Cowan et al.,
1979 ; Bachmann and Bäuerlein, 1981) ; only at higher levels of pressure, small differences are documented.

Some of the technical difficulties encountered with the Remler

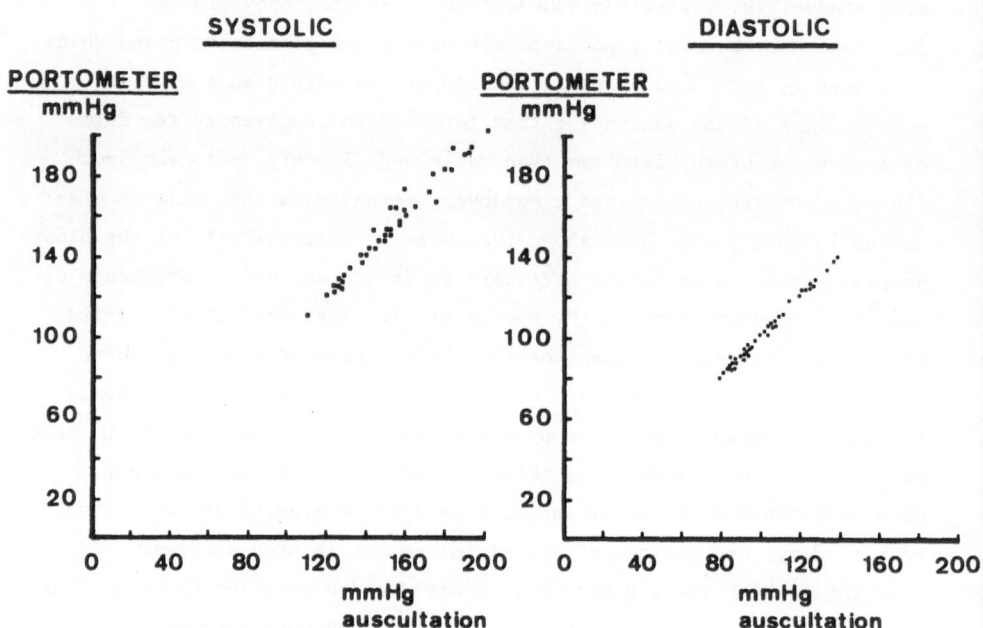

Fig. 1

Correlation between portometer and sphygmomanometer recordings.

apparatus are largely corrected with newer instruments (Flanders
Technology, 1983).

Applications of the technique
1. Definition of blood pressure and evaluation of prognosis.

It has since long been shown both by invasive and non-invasive techniques, that large differences exist between office readings of blood pressure and ambulatory recordings (Perloff et al., 1981). In most of these studies only the means obtained with both techniques are compared and the differences listed ; it is in most cases impossible to find out whether the office readings are part of the spectrum of blood pressures recorded by ambulatory monitoring and if so, where they are localized on the histogram. Therefore, in 29 patients, office readings were compared to the data obtained in the same patients, by two different non-invasive techniques, including first a portometer recording, performed during 12 hours with a measurement every 30 minutes. Second, a three hours recording of blood pressure, in the supine position, using either Arteriosonde or Dinamap, with a measurement every five minutes. In fact, this second technique was included to investigate the relationship between histograms derived from ambulatory devices and those coming from recordings made in quiet relaxed conditions. In favour of the latter techniques, is the fact that these recordings are easier, cheaper and that the conditions can better be standardized. Against this is the questionable relationship of such a curve to the ambulatory recordings made in normal life.

As could be expected, office readings were significantly ($p < 0.01$) higher than the mean of the values obtained by portometer (169/103 versus 146/94 mmHg) ; surprisingly, the latter were only slightly higher than the arteriosonde readings (139/89 mmHg, $p < 0.01$). Individually, office readings were higher than portometer readings in 85 % of the cases and higher than Arteriosonde readings in 100 % of the cases ; portometer readings were higher than Arteriosonde in 80 % of the cases (fig. 2).

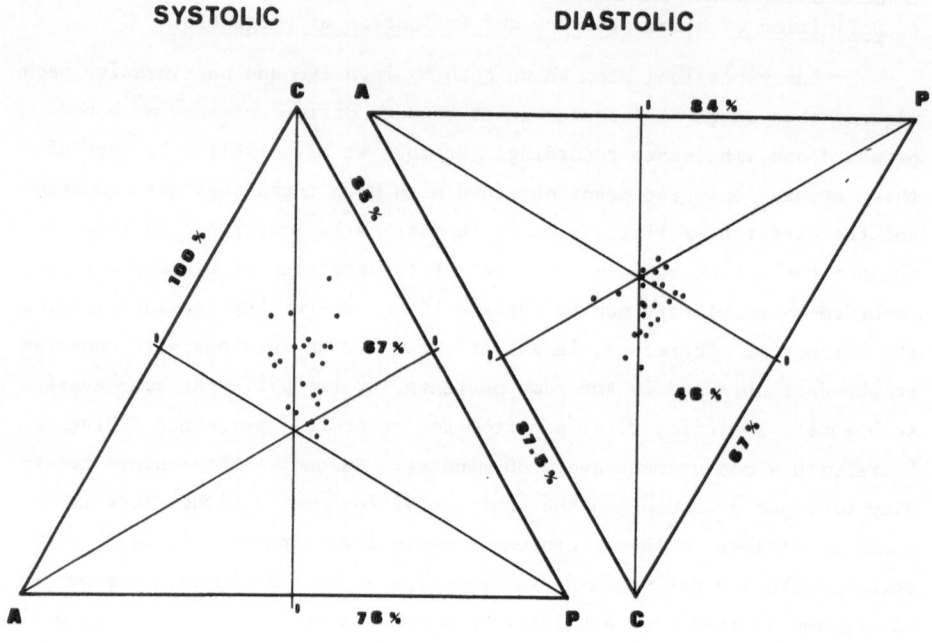

SYSTOLIC   DIASTOLIC

Fig. 2

Comparison of casual blood pressure (C) to Arteriosonde (or Dinamap) recordings (A) or portometer recordings (P). A point is situated at the
zero line when both techniques yield the same result ; the data for every
comparison are given on each side of the triangle ; the numbers indicate
how many times (in percentage) one technique gives higher results than
the other.

Notice that blood pressure which was always higher than 140/90 mmHg
in the office, was lower than this value in respectively 30 % (portometer)
and 46 % of the cases (Arteriosonde).

Although there is a positive and significant (p < 0.001) correlation
between the office readings and the non-invasive recordings in group, which
is better for systolic than for diastolic values, the individual figures
of either portometer or Arteriosonde cannot be predicted from the office
readings alone.

When the histograms coming from both the methods are compared, a surprisingly large degree of overlapping is found both for systolic as for diastolic blood pressure.

That the casual blood pressure is by far not ideal to identify the patients' blood pressure is illustrated by its localization on the histograms where it can be found around the 85° percentile.

These data illustrate again the large differences existing between office readings and ambulatory recordings of blood pressure ; the most unexpected finding was the very close relationship between ambulatory recordings and those performed during three hours, in relaxed conditions but with a larger number of measurements. It can be speculated that, to plot the histogram, one needs a large enough number of points regardless of whether these have been recorded over 12 hours or 3 hours, regardless of whether recordings were made ambulatory or in the supine position.

As far as prognosis is concerned, ambulatory recordings do help largely in better defining the complication rate of the hypertensive disease. Best documented data in that respect come from the group of Dr Sokolow who has accumulated information starting from the sixties. They first compared prevalence of vascular complications in the optic fundi, electrocardiogram and roentgenogram of the chest in a sample of 675 untreated hypertensive patients. It was clearly shown that for the same level of blood pressure, prevalence of complications was lower in those patients with a lower ambulatory blood pressure (Perloff et al., 1981) ; this was particularly true for the lower levels of pressure and was less pronounced at higher blood pressure. The same group has now very nice prospective documentation on this point confirming that ambulatory recordings do permit a sharp discrimination in patient presenting with the same office pressure (Cowan et al., 1981). The latter does by no means contradict the results of the Framingham studies but show that association of office readings and ambulatory readings do perform better in estimating prognosis.

2. <u>Study of effect of blood pressure lowering drugs</u>.

Ambulatory methods are most useful to assess on objective basis the effect of antihypertensive drugs. Data can be expressed in several ways which are totally beyond the possibilities of office readings. Data of individual patients can be given as means $\pm$ S.D. ; intraindividual figures can be analyzed with paired comparison ; data can be repre-

sented as curves in function of time which can illustrate the duration
of the hypotensive effects ; also, data can be given as histograms which
are interesting as they inform what part of the curve is influenced by the
drug under study.

The differences between office readings and ambulatory blood pressure are observed during treatment as frequently as in the control conditions ; everyone has encountered the case of a patient with persistent
high blood pressure despite high doses of drugs, experiencing many side
effects. Frequently these patients show much lower values in ambulatory
recordings and do, in fact, require much lower doses of the hypotensive
drugs to effectively control their blood pressure.

3. Study of blood pressure variability.

Although there is no clear evidence that variability has any relation to prognosis, still it is from a scientific point of view most in-
triguing to know why and how blood pressure varies so much. Ambulatory
recordings of blood pressure and heart rate can provide us with that
information. The most regular way is to define blood pressure variability as the standard deviation of the mean of all individual blood pressure readings. As this value is positively correlated to the level of
pressure (Clement et al., 1979), most investigators prefer to use the
coefficient of variation (Mancia et al., 1983).

Main criticism against using the standard deviation or the variation
coefficient, is that this value is also influenced by non stationarity
of blood pressure. Still, by far, most investigators continue to use
this parameter because of its simplicity and lack of acceptable alternative solutions.

It has been a challenge for several years to unravel the mechanism of blood pressure variability. It has been a common belief that
variations are largely due to variations in the activity of the sympathetic system ; still there is a large body of evidence showing that
beta adrenoceptor blockade is unable to diminish blood pressure variations regardless of which beta adrenoceptor blocking agent is being
used and whether intraarterial (Heyndrickx et al., 1979 ; Mann et al.,
1979 ; Watson et al., 1979 a) or non-invasive (Clement, 1977 ; Clement
et al., 1977 ; Clement et al., 1983) recordings are performed. Similarly, blockade of peripheral (Clement, 1979) or central alpha adre-
noceptors (Clement et al., 1983) is unable to significantly influence

the amplitude of the variations ; this correlates with a lack of correlation with sympathetic function tests (Watson et al., 1979b ; Clement
et al., 1979). The question on what mechanism blood pressure variability depends remains a challenging point for all investigators working
in this field.

REFERENCES

Bachmann, K. and Bäuerlein, G. 1981. Ambulatory monitoring of arterial
    blood pressure. Comparison between blood pressure measurements
    obtained with the Remler M-2000 portable recorder and by radio-
    telemetry under laboratory conditions and during everyday activities.
    Biotelemetry Patient Monitg., 8, 47-55.
Clement, D.L. 1977. Blood pressure variability in hospitalized patients.
    Acta Clin. Belg., 32, 163-167.
Clement, D.L., Bogaert, M.G. and Pannier, R. 1977. Effect of beta-
    adrenergic blockade on blood pressure variation in patients with
    moderate hypertension. Europ. J. Clin. Pharmacol., 11, 325-327.
Clement, D.L., Mussche, M.M., Vanhoutte, G. and Pannier, R. 1979. Is
    blood pressure variability related to activity of the sympathetic
    system ? Clinical Science, 57, 217-219s.
Clement, D.L. 1979. Blood Pressure Variability, MTP Press.
Clement, D.L. 1979. Effect of sympathetic nervous activity on blood
    pressure variability. In : Blood Pressure Variability, MTP Press,
    43-48.
Clement, D.L., Cardon, E., Castro, M., De Pue, N., Packet, L. and Van
    Maele, G.O. 1983. Effect of metoprolol and of guanfacine on am-
    bulatory blood pressure and its variations. Brit. J. Clin. Phar-
    macol. In press.
Cowan, R.M., Sokolow, M. and Perloff, D. 1979. Methodological considera-
    tion in determining the accuracy of an indirect blood pressure re-
    corder in : ISAM. Ed. F.D. Stott, E.B. Raftery, L. Gould, 241-
    245.
Heyndrickx, G.R., Nellens, P. and Clement, D.L. 1979. Autonomic nervous
    control of blood pressure variability in conscious dogs.
    In : Blood Pressure Variability, Ed. D.L. Clement, MTP Press,
    49-54.
Hinman, A.T., Engel, B.T., Bickford, A.F. 1962. Portable blood pressure
    recorder : accuracy and preliminary use in evaluating intradaily
    variations in pressure. Am. Heart J., 63, 663.
Hypertension Detection and Follow-Up Program Cooperative Study (HFDP) :
    five year findings of the hypertension detection and follow-up
    program. I. Reduction in mortality of persons with high blood
    pressure, including mild hypertension. 1979. JAMA, 242, 2562-71.
Kain, H., Hinman, A.T., Sokolow, M. 1964. Arterial blood pres-
    sure measurements with a portable recorder in hypertensive
    patients : I. Variability and correlation with "casual" pres-
    sures. Circulation, 30, 882.
Kannel, W.B. 1974. Role of blood pressure in cardiovascular morbi-
    ditiy and mortality. Prog. Cardiovasc. Dis., 17, 5.

Mancia, G. 1983. Blood pressure variability at normal and high blood pressure. Chest, 83, supplement february, 317-319.

Mann, S., Millar Craig, M.W., Altman, D.G., Melville, D.I. and Raftery, E.B. 1979. The effects of metoprolol on ambulatory blood pressure. Clinical Science, 57, 375-377s.

Perloff, D. and Sokolow, M. 1978. The representative blood pressure : usefulness of office, basal, home, and ambulatory readings. Cardiovascular Medicine, 3, 655-668.

Perloff, D., Sokolow, M. and Cowan, R. 1981. Clinical relevance of ambulatory blood pressure measurements. Biotelemetry Patient Monitg., 8, 67-80.

Sokolow, M., Werdegar, D., Kain, H.K. et al. 1966. Relationship between level of blood pressure measured casually and by portable recorders and severity of complications in essential hypertension. Circulation, 34, 279.

Sokolow, M., Perloff, D., Cowan, R. 1973. The value of portably recorded blood pressures in the initiation of treatment of moderate hypertension. Clin. Sci. Mol. Med., 45, 195s.

Stott, F.D., Raftery, E.G., Clement, D.L. and Wright S.L. (Editors) 1982. ISAM Gent, Academic Press.

The Australian therapeutic trial in mild hypertension. Report by the management Committee. 1980. Lancet, i, 1261-7.

Van Maele, G.O. and Clement, D.L. 1981. Methods of processing semi-continuous blood pressure recordings. Proceedings of 2nd Gent Workshop on Blood Pressure Variability. Academic Press. Ed. Clement D.L., Stott, F.D., Wright, S.L., Raftery, E.B., 607-619.

Van Maele, G.O. and Clement, D.L. 1982, How shall we define blood pressure variability ? In : Proceedings of the 2e International Symposium on Blood Pressure Variability, 608-611.

Veterans Cooperative Study Group on Antihypertensive Agents : Effects of treatment on morbidity in hypertension : results in patients with diastolic blood pressures averaging 115 through 129 mmHg. 1967. JAMA, 202, 1028.

Watson, R.D.S., Stallard, T.J. and Littler, W.A. 1979a. Influence of once-daily administration of beta-adrenoceptor antagonists on arterial pressure and its variability. Lancet, 1, 1210-1213.

Watson, R.D.S., Stallard, T.J. and Littler, W.A. 1979b. Factors determining the variability of arterial pressure in hypertension. Clinical Science, 57, 283-285s.

CONTINUOUS BLOOD PRESSURE MONITORING IN THE CLINICAL EVALUATION OF HYPERTENSIVE PATIENTS AND IN THE STUDY OF NEURAL CARDIOVASCULA CONTROL

G.Mancia, A.Ferrari, G.Bertinieri, M.Di Rienzo*, G. Gras-si, G.Parati and G.Pomidossi.

Istituto di Clinica Medica IV, Università di Milano and Centro di Fisiologia Clinica e Ipertensione, Ospedale Maggiore, Milano, Italy.

*From Centro di Bioingegneria, Politecnico e Fondazione Don Gnocchi, Milano, Italy.

ABSTRACT

Towards the end of the sixties Pickering and his Oxford group (1,2) deviced a method that allowed blood pressure to be measured intra-arterially in ambulant subjects with limited interference with their ambulation and to some extent with their life-patter. Beside being repeatedly referred to in this workshop, the Oxford method is too well known to necessitate a detailed description. Suffice it to say that its design effectively minimizes the incovenience and risk inherent to the invasiveness of the procedure, and that its technical features usually allow a blood pressure signal of adequate quality to be recorded (3). By means of some precautions the recording can be carried out under condition of stable 0 signal and equal sensitivity throughout the range of existing blood pressures.

We have adopted the Oxford method since 1977 and have so far completed few hundred 24 hour blood pressure recordings in normotensive subjects and in subjects with untreated or treated hypertension of essential or secondary nature. Although this large experience has allowed us to gather information on several pathophysiological and clinical aspects of conditions of deranges blood pressure, we will limit ourselves to three topics only: 1)effects of bahaviours on blood pressure, 2) blood pressure variability and 3) clinical applications of continuous blood pressure recording.

Behaviours and blood pressure

Continuous blood pressure recording represents the
ideal approach to clarify the effects of different behaviours on blood pressure, and this is indeed the field
on which most information has been collected during the
early years of the Oxford method (2, 4-7). Thanks to the
original studies of the Oxford group, and to other studies
performed later, we know that behaviours can strikingly
alter blood pressure in either hypotensive and hypertensive directions.

Behaviours that produce hypotension have their most
classical example in sleep during which blood pressure is
markedly lowered with respect to the values occurring
during wakefulness (4,8). Figure 1, which is taken from
one of our studies (9), shows mean arterial pressure values
recorded during 2 hours of the morning, 2 hours of the
afternoon, 2 hours of the evening, and 2 hours of night
sleep in a group of normotensive subjects, and in 2 groups
of essential hypertensive subjects of moderate and severe
degree respectively. Within each group blood pressure was
similar during the different day times and showed a marked
reduction during sleep. Interestingly, the magnitude of
the reduction was similar among the 3 groups which also
shared similar day time heart rate values and sleep-induced
bradycardias.

On the contrary side the spectrum behaviours that increase blood pressure have their most classical examples
in exercise and emotions. We have addressed our attention
to an emotional condition that has a special clinical relevance, i.e. that evoked in the patient during cuff blood
pressure assessments by the physician (10). To this aim
ambulant inpatients on 24 hour intra-arterial blood pres-

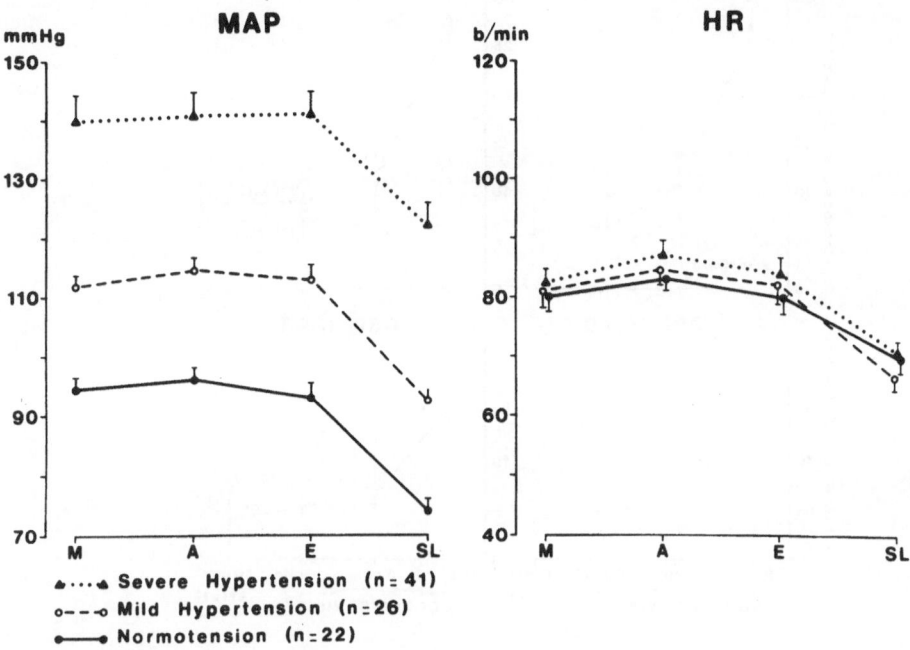

Figure 1. Mean arterial pressure (MAP) and heart rate (HR)
values recorded during a 2 hour period of the morning (M),
a 2 hour period of the afternoon (A), a 2 hour period of
the evening (E) and a 2 hour period of sleep (SL) selected
from midnight to 4 a.m. Data represent average values from
a group of normotensive subjects and 2 groups of subjects
with mild and severe essential hypertension. MAP and HR were
calculated by a computer in the manner described in the text.

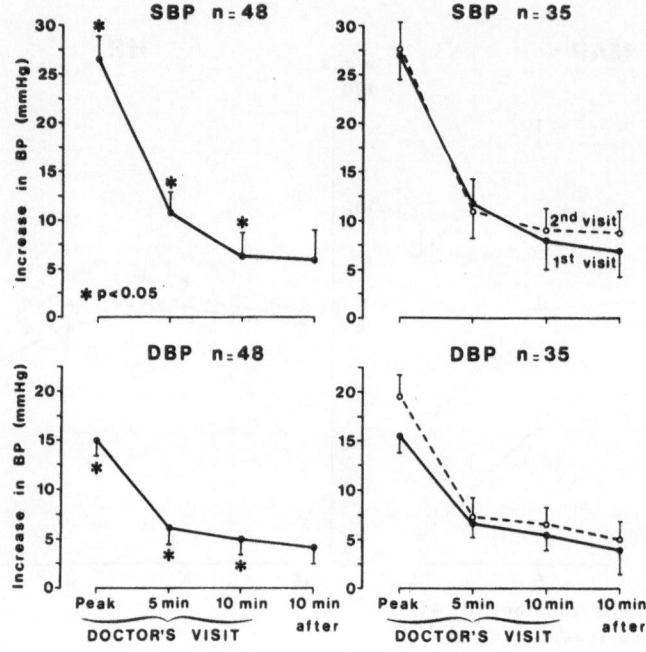

Figure 2. Changes in systolic (SBP) and diastolic (DBP) blood pressure occurring during the 10 minute visit of the physician in charge of performing cuff blood pressure assessments. The left panels show average data from 48 subjects who underwent one visit, whereas the right panels show average data from 35 subjects in which two visits by the same physician were made. All data have been calculated in comparison to a reference value taken 4 minutes prior to the physician's arrival. Peak responses mean the maximal blood pressure changes that occurred 1 to 4 minutes after the doctor's arrival. Asterisk refers to the statistical significance of the differences with the reference value before the physician's arrival.

sure monitoring were subjected to a morning visit by a
hospital doctor unfamiliar to them who performed 3 or 4
cuff inflations within a 10 or 15 minute time. After
completion of the 24 hours the doctor's visit was identified on the replayed tape and its blood pressure and
heart rate values were analyzed in comparison to the values
observed during the periods preceding and following the
visit. The doctor's arrival caused an immediate rise in
blood pressure which brought systolic and diastolic values
respectively 26.7 ± 2.3 mmHg and 14.9 ± 1.6 mmHg above the
values measured before the doctor's arrival. These pressure
rises (whose emotional nature was confirmed by the con-
comitant marked tachycardia) were reached within 1 to 4
minutes after which blood pressure declined so that at
the 10th minute of the doctor's visit systolic and diastolic blood pressure exceeded the pre-visit by 6.3 ± 2.6
mmHg only. These differences, which were statistically
significant, persisted at the 15th minute of the visit,
and disappeared slowly after the doctor's departure (Figure
2, left panel).

These findings exemplify how much blood pressure can
be altered by behavioural influences. They also demonstrate that some of these influences probably lead to overestimation of patients' blood pressure, and that this over
estimation is large if blood pressure measurements are
made too early in the course of the doctor's visit. This
may interfere with the diagnosis of the existance and the
severity of hypertension, and thus with the decision
process concerning the rationale of treatment.

It should be emphasized that additional features appear
to make the above mentioned "overestimation error" a
serious one to consider. In our experience the blood pressure rise observed during a second visit by the same doctor

was similar to that observed during the first visit, suggesting that attenuation and extinction of the error
may not be quick to be achieved (Figure 2, right panel).
Furthermore, the large interindividual variability that
characterized the magnitude of the maximal blood pressure
rise (4-75 mmHg range for systolic and 1-36 mmHg range
for diastolic pressure) eluded any attempt of correlation
with patients' data such as age, sex, basal blood pressure and blood pressure short- and long-term variability
(see below). Even the correlation between the doctor-in-
duced blood pressure and heart rate rises was surprisingly poor (r=0.37). Thus we face not only a large but also
a variable and unpredictable error (11). Presumably this
error is responsible for the large and variable difference
that has been shown to exist between casual and continuously monitored day or 24 hour blood pressure (12,13). In
agreement with our results Floras et al (12) have failed
to predict the magnitude of this difference on the basis
of patients' day blood pressure, blood pressure variability
or blood pressure responses to stress.

A final comment concern the possibility that behaviours
may differently affect blood pressure in normotensive and
hypertensive people. It has been suggested that exercise
and emotions may increase blood pressure and/or heart rate
more in hypertensives, affording a criterion on which to
identify hypertension-prone subjects and to improve hypertension diagnosis (14). We (9,10) have never found substantial differences in the behaviourally-induced changes
in blood pressure and heart rate between normotensive and
hypertensive subjects (see effects of sleep and emotions),
and neither have others (12). The possibility of greater
(and more prolonged) blood pressure rises during emotions
in more restricted subgroups of hypertensives, for example

the young borderline hypertensives, cannot be ruled out, however (15).

Blood pressure variability

Intra-arterial blood pressure recording in ambulant subjects has offered a quantitative approach to an old observation concerning blood pressure, i.e. its spontaneous variability (1). In our studies (9,16) a computer sampled the blood pressure signal every 60 msec, calculated average mean arterial pressure values every 3 seconds, and used these data to provide means and standard deviations for each half hour of the 24 hour recording. Half hour standard deviations were then averaged to obtain a standard deviation that reflected the tendency of blood pressure to vary within half hours. Half hour means were also averaged to obtain a standard deviation that reflected also the blood pressure tendency to vary among half hours. These two standard deviations were considered to express short- and long-term blood pressure variabilities. Of course these terms are conventional as long-term variabilities should be defined as those within weeks, months or years. These variabilities are not measurable, however, and ours have at least the advantage of attempting a separation between more prolonged and short (including moment-to-moment) blood pressure variations.

A crucial question concerning blood pressure variability is that of its origin and mechanisms. Although humoral (17) and mechanical (i.e. respiration) factors may be responsible for a certain amount of blood pressure variability, there is no doubt that the major fraction of this phenomenon is accounted for by neural modulation of cardiovascular functions via the autonomic nerves. In this respect

we have found in 89 subjects that half hour mean arterial
pressure variabilities are positively related to half
hour heart rate variabilities (calculated from average
3 second values, see above), and that this is the case
also for half hour mean arterial pressure and heart rate
means (Figure 3). Similar positive relationships have been
observed in animals (19,20). These findings might originate
from a dependance of short-term blood pressure variations
on cardiac events, i.e. on changes in stroke volume induced by heart rate alterations. However, because in cats
abolition of heart rate changes by atropine does not reduce
blood pressure variability, a second explanation is more
likely. Blood pressure and heart rate variabilities are independent phenomena originating from a common source. This
source is likely to be a central influence which affects
in the same direction cardiac and vascular targets. This
explanation implies a primary role of central factors in
24 hour cardiovascular modulation.

Two further questions concerning blood pressure variability are: 1) its dependance on arterial baroreceptor reflexes and 2) its alterations in arterial hypertension.
Figure 4 shows that short- and long-term mean arterial
pressure variabilities have a weak negative correlation
with the sensitivity of the baroreflexes as measured by
the phenylephrine method.   This suggests that the buf-
fering action of baroreflexes so clearly demonstrated in
animals (20,21) is operative also in man. It also suggests,
however, that this action is not a major one and that differences in blood pressure variabilities commonly observed
among subjects can only minimally be ascribed to baroreflexes. The lack of significant negative correlations
between blood pressure variabilities and baroreflex sensitivity as measured by the alternative trinitroglycerine

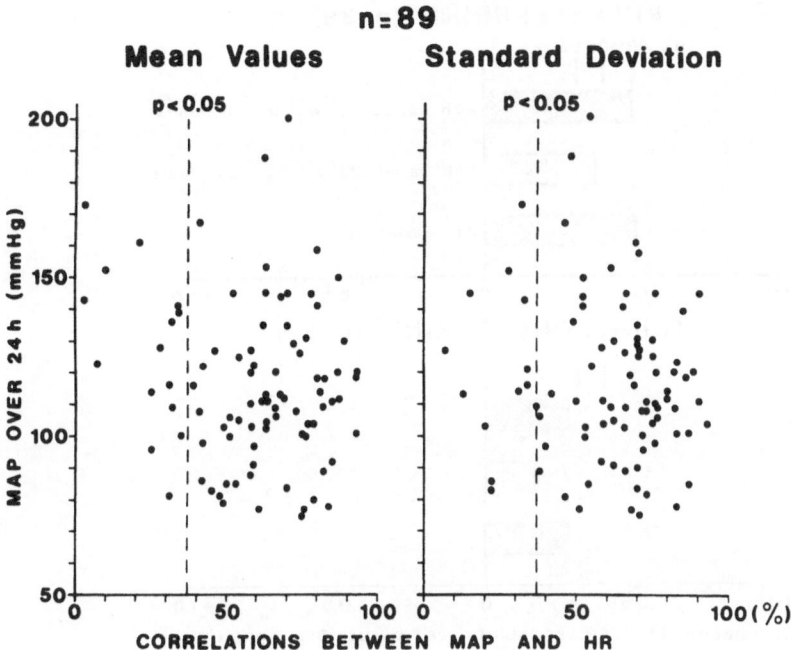

<u>Figure 3</u>. Correlations between mean arterial pressure (MAP) and heart rate (HR) means (left panel) and between MAP and HR variabilities (right panel) in 89 subjects. Original data on which correlations were calculated are half hour averages and standard deviations. Each point refers to one subject. Notice that correlations were always in the positive side, in most cases achieving the level of statistical significance (p < 0.05, dashed line). Also notice that this was the case both for subjects with lower and for those with higher 24 hour MAP. Correlation indices were calculated by the non-parametric test of Smirnov (22).

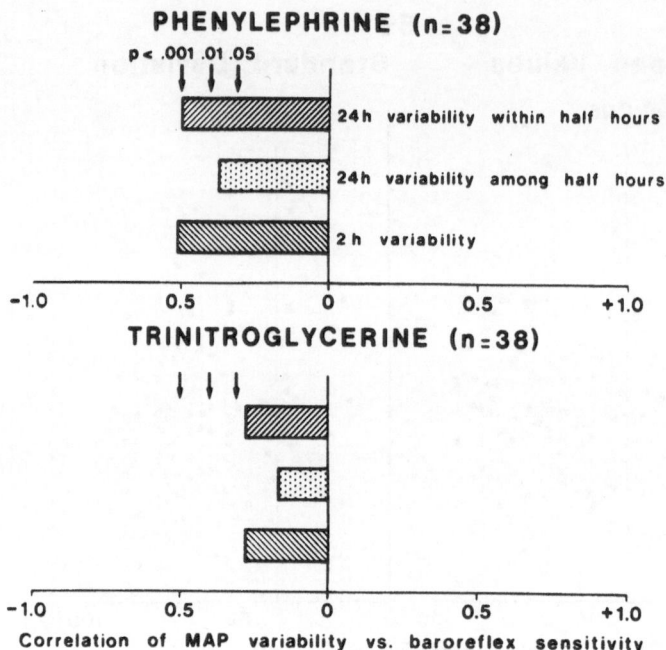

Figure 4. Correlations between short-term (within half
hours) and long-term (among half hours) MAP variabilities
and sensitivity of the arterial baroreflexes as measured
by the phenylephrine (upper panel) and the trinitroglycerine
method (lower panel) in 38 subjects. Correlations are also
shown for the 2 hour periods in which the baroreflexes were
tested. Notice that correlations were on the negative side,
achieving statistical significance only in the case of the
phenylephrine method.

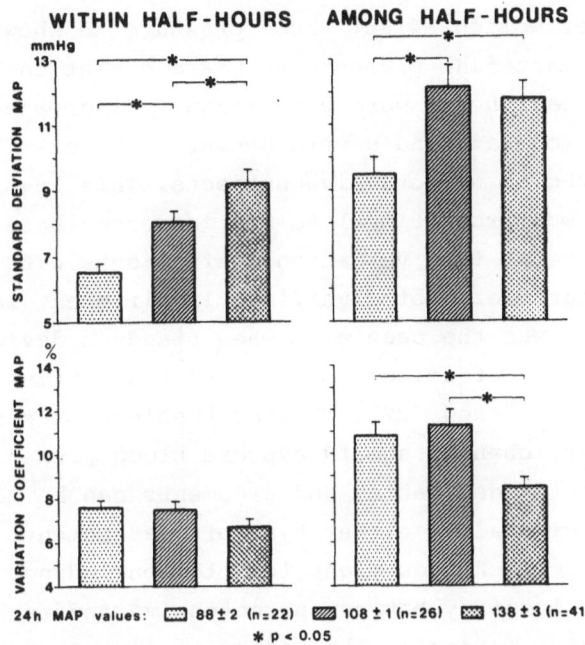

Figure 5. Short- (within half hours) and long-term (among half hours) MAP variabilities in the 3 groups of subjects of Figure 1. Data are shown as absolute variabilities (standard deviations, upper panels) and percent variabilities (variation coefficients, lower panels). Patients' age was matched in the 3 groups.

method sounds confirmatory of this suggestion.

How   hypertension affect blood pressure is shown
in Figure 5. Mean arterial pressure standard deviations
within and among half hours were significantly increased
in subjects with moderate and severe essential hypertension as compared to normotensive subjects. This increase, however, was proportional to the increased baseline blood pressure so that variation coefficients within
and among half hours were not significantly different in
the 3 groups. This was the case also when standard deviations and variation coefficients of day and night times
were separately considered (22). Whether absolute or percent blood pressure changes should express blood pressure variabilities is debatable, and arguments can be advanced in favour or against either type of measurement.
Preference to percent changes might lead to concluding
for a fundamental identity between normotensive and essential hypertensive subjects with regard to neural modulation of the circulatory system. This conclusion appears
to be strengthened by the observation that normotensive
and essential hypertensive subjects do not differ in terms
of absolute and percent long- and short-term heart rate
variabilities (Figure 6).

Clinical applications

We believe that continuous blood pressure recording
is a valuable tool for studying human cardiovascular regulation in normal and abnormal conditions, and for critically advancing clinical research in hypertension (11,23),
but do not believe it has and will ever have a large
practical application.

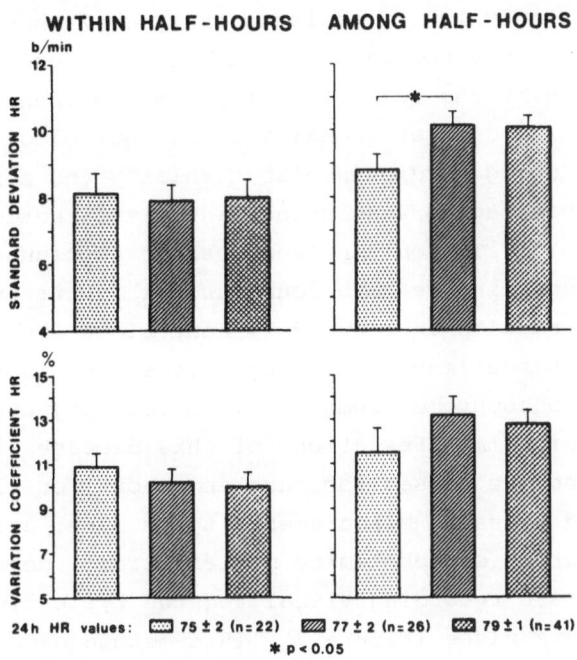

Figure 6. Short-(within half hours) and long-term (among half hours) HR variabilities in the 3 groups of subjects of Figure 1 and 5. Data are shown in the same manner as those of Figure 5.

Present clinical application is limited by the lack
of reference data on which to evaluate daily or 24 hour
average values obtained through the continuous recording.
It is also limited by the lack of undisputable evidence
on the greater value of average daily or 24 hour blood
pressure in predicting cardiovascular morbidity and mortality, although encouraging suggestions in this direction
have emerged (12,13). The only present use of continuous
blood pressure recording we have found useful (apart from
anecdoctical information on reduced 24 hour blood pressures in labeled borderline or mild hypertensives) is for
the diagnosis of pheochromocytoma (24). In few subjects
in which the clinical manifestations of this disease con-
sisted of hypertensive crises too rare and short for allowing cuff blood pressure measurements to be made, and
for inducing clearcut catecholamine modifications, continuous blood pressure recording visualized the typically
huge blood pressure rises (Figure 7). This method also
allowed to exclude the existance of a pheochromocytoma in
few cases in which short-lived palpitations and other
symptoms had raised the suspicion of this disease.

Further application of continuous blood pressure recording will of course be persistently hindered by its
invasiveness. In this respect we share the opinion that
non-invasive automatic blood pressure monitoring might
represent a more promising solution. We wish to underscore,
however, that this approach faces problems that are still
unsolved. These problems do not include the fact that
over the 24 hours non-invasive devices provide only few
hundred blood pressure values (a tiny fraction of the
thousand values occurring during this interval), because
intermittent blood pressure sampling, even when spaced
by 30 or 60 minutes, guarantee an accurate average 24

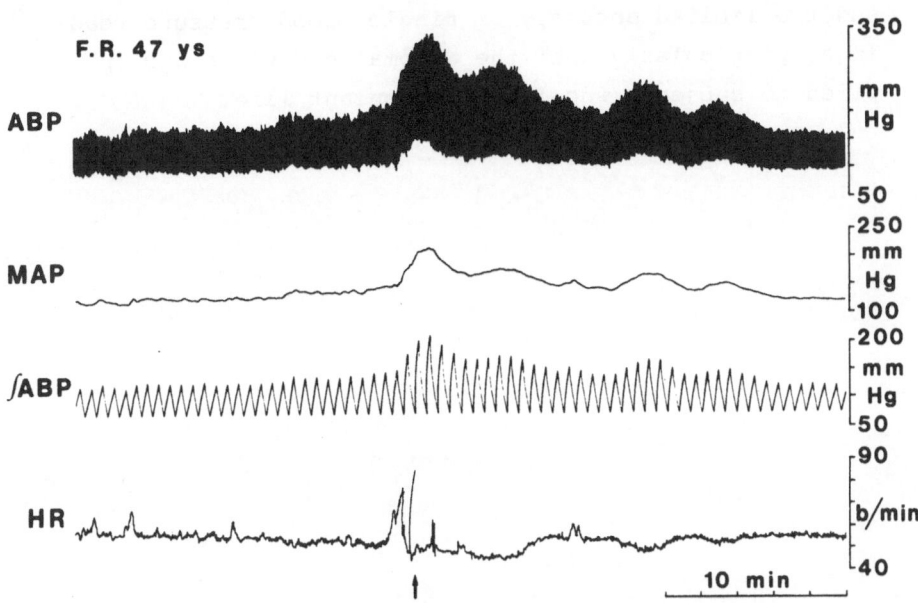

Figure 7. Example of an hypertensive crisis recorded in a patient with pheochromocytoma. Data were obtained by connection of the Oxford recorder with a Grass polygraph via an ordinary tape recorder. This allowed to visualize pulsatile blood pressure (ABP), mean arterial pressure (MAP), ABP integrated at regular time intervals ($\int$ ABP) and heart rate (HR). The arrow indicates the beginning of the crisis and signalled by the patient. Notice that during the crisis systolic blood pressure exceeded 350 mmHg, while heart rate was reduced after an initial rise.

hour value (25). They include, however, the artifacts
and the limited accuracy of single blood pressure readings, particularly when the automatic devices are applied to subjects who live an ambulant life.

References

1. Pickering GW. High Blood Pressure. JA Churchill, Ltd, London, 1968.
2. Bevan AT, Honour AJ, Stott FM. Direct arterial blood pressure recording in unrestricted man. Clin Sci 36, 329-344, 1969.
3. Stott FD, Teny VG, Honour AJ. Factors determining the design and construction of a portable pressure transducer system. Postgrad Med J 52 (suppl 7) 97-99, 1976.
4. Littler WA, Honour AJ, Carter RD, Sleight P. Sleep and blood pressure. Br Med J 3, 346-348, 1975.
5. Littler WA, Honour AJ, Sleight P, Stott FD. Continuous recording of direct arterial pressure and electrocardiogram in unrestricted man. Br Med J 3, 76-78, 1977.
6. Raftery EB. Hypertension day by day. The Practitioner 223, 166-175, 1979.
7. Littler WA, Honour AJ, Sleight P. Direct arterial pressure, pulse rate and electrocardiogram during micturition and defecation in unrestricted man. Am Heart J 88, 205-210, 1974.
8. Mancia G, Zanchetti A. Cardiovascular regulation during sleep. In Physiology of Sleep, edited by J Orem, New York, Academic Press, pp 1-55, 1981.
9. Mancia G, Ferrari A, Gregorini L, Parati G, Pomidossi G, Bertinieri G, Grassi G, Di Rienzo M, Pedotti A, Zanchetti A. Blood pressure and heart rate variabilities in normotensive and hypertensive human beings. Circ Res, in press.
10. Mancia G, Bertinieri G, Grassi G, Parati G, Pomidossi G, Ferrari A, Gregorini L, Zanchetti A. Measurement of blood pressure by the doctor: effects on the blood pressure and heart rate of the patient. Lancet, in press.

11. Mancia G. Methods for assessing blood pressure values in humans. Hypertension, in press.

12. Floras JS, Assan MD, Sever PS, Jones JV, Osikowska B, Sleight P. Cuff and ambulatory blood pressure in subjects with essential hypertension. Lancet 2, 107-109, 1981.

13. Sokolow M, Wertegard D, Kain HK, Hinman AT. Relationship between level of blood pressure measured casually and by portable recorders and severity of complications in essential hypertension. Circulation 34, 279-298, 1966.

14. Loriman AR, MacFarlane PW, Provan G, Duffy T, Lawrie TDV. Blood pressure and catecholamine responses to "stress" in normotensive and hypertensive subjects. Cardiovasc Res 5, 169-   , 1971.

15. Falkner B, Onesti G, Angelakos ET, Fernandes M, Langman C. Cardiovascular response to mental stress in normal adolescents with hypertensive parents. Hypertension 1, 23-30, 1979.

16. Mancia G, Ferrari A, Gregorini L, Parati G, Pomidossi G, Bertinieri G, Grassi G, Zanchetti A. Blood pressure variability in man: its relation to high blood pressure, age and baroreflex sensitivity. Clin Sci 50, 401s-404s, 1980.

17. Watson RDS, Stallard TJ, Littler WA. Factors determining the variability of arterial pressure in hypertension. Clin Sci 57 (suppl 5), 283s-295s, 1979.

18. Smirnov NV. Table for estimating the goodness of fit of empirical distributions. Ann Math Statistics 19, 279-281, 1948.

19. Anderson DE, Yingling JE, Sagawa K. Minute-to-minute covariations in cardiovascular activity of conscious dogs. Am J Physiol 236, H434-H439, 1979.

20. Ramirez AJ, Bertinieri G, Belli L, Cavallazzi A, Di Rienzo M, Pedotti A, Mancia G. Reflex control of blood pressure and heart rate by arterial baroreceptors and cardiopulmonary receptors in the unanesthetized cat. Submitted for publication.

21. Cowley AW, Liard JF, Guyton AC. Role of the baroreceptor reflex in daily control of arterial blood pressure and other variables in dogs. Circ Res 32, 564-576, 1973.

22. Mancia G. Blood pressure variability at normal and high blood pressure. Chest 83, 317S-320S, 1983.

23. Mancia G, Zanchetti A. Continuous arterial blood pressure recording in human hypertension: A methodological approach. Atherosclerosis Reviews, vol 7: Measurement and control of cardiovascular risk factors, edited by R Hegyeli, Raven Press, New York, pp 247-254, 1980.

24. Mancia G, Ferrari A, Gregorini L, Parati G, Pomidossi G, Zanchetti A. Prolonged intra-arterial blood pressure recording in the diagnosis of pheochromocytoma. Lancet 2, 1193-1194, 1979.

25. Di Rienzo M, Grassi G, Pedotti A, Mancia G. Continuous vs intermittent blood pressure measurements in estimating 24 hour average blood pressure. Hypertension 5, 264-269, 1983.

COMBINED ECG AND INTRA-ARTERIAL BLOOD PRESSURE ANALYSIS
FOR THE BEAT TO BEAT EVALUATION OF THE
SYSTOLIC TIME INTERVALS IN AMBULATORY PATIENTS

C.Palombo*, C.Marchesi*, A.Macerata*,
S.Giaconi**, A.Montereggi***,
M.Raciti**, A.Benassi*, D.Levorato*, S.Ghione*

*C.N.R. Clinical Physiology Institute
**A.R.MED. Associazione per la Ricerca Medica
***Medical Student, University of Pisa
via Savi, 8 - 56100 Pisa, Italia

ABSTRACT

The Oxford intraarterial blood pressure monitoring has been extensively used, up to now, for pathophysiological and pharmacological studies in arterial hypertension. However, all currently available methods for data analysis have been restrained to the extraction of data on blood pressure and heart rate. In order to try to explain the possibility of obtaining also a beat-to-beat evaluation of cardiac function in unrestricted patients, we developed an original computerized method for the determination of systolic time intervals by means of the combined analysis of blood pressure and electrocardiogram continuously recorded.
Preliminary results will be reported which show that intraarterial digitized systolic time intervals are able to reflect at least to some extent the known physiological changes expected after a wide spectrum of physical and pharmacological tests. However, further studies will be needed for the full validation of the preejection time by our technique.

INTRODUCTION

The arterial pressure monitoring in unrestricted patients has been up to now extensively utilized for continuous evaluation of blood pressure (BP), heart rate (HR) and indexes of their variability.

This approach has widely extended our knowledge about BP profile and variability in normal and hypertensive patients (Millar Craig et al.,1978a; Millar Craig et al., 1978b; Floras et al.,1978; Mancia et al.,1980; Pessina et al.,1982).

However, the simultaneous availability of ECG and BP signals offers, at least theoretically, also the possibility of obtaining in unrestricted patients a beat to beat evaluation of systolic time intervals (STIs), which are well known indexes of cardiac performance. In fact, the STIs have been shown to reflect hemodynamic events, and have become a well-established tool for assessing left ventricular function and its response to physiological and pharmacological interventions (Lewis et al.,1977; Weissler,1977; Steriotis et al.,1979; Ahmed et al.,1972; Levi et al.,1982). Furthermore, a technique has been validated for assessing STIs without the phonocardiogram (PCG) (Spodick et al.,1976), and a few papers have been published on their monitoring and automatical analysis (Haffty et al.,1977; Gribbin et al.,1979).

This study reports the preliminary results of a technique for continuous monitoring of STIs in ambulant patients by the combined analysis of ECG and BP. Data will be reported obtained in patients during hemodynamic changes either spontaneous or induced by physiological and pharmacological interventions; moreover the data obtained by the intraarterial monitoring have been compared with the conventional STIs recorded simultaneously.

MATERIALS AND METHODS

1.Patients selection and experimental protocol

Five hospitalized patients (4 females, 1 male) with borderline to moderate hypertension (I-II W.H.O. stage), with age ranging from 35 to 58 years, underwent a 24-hours intraarterial monitoring of BP and ECG using the well known Selyg-Oxford technique, described elsewhere (Millar Craig et al., 1978a).

Each patient did a dynamic (bycicle ergometer) and an isometric (handgrip) exercise during the recording.

Furthermore, in order to induce consistent hemodynamic modifications reflected in changes in STIs, acute administrations (usually i.v.) of drugs known to affect left ventricular preload, afterload and/or contractility were also accomplished. Drugs administred, usually by stepwise incremental infusion (in one case only, for the calcium-antagonist nifedipine, the sublingual route was utilized), were beta-receptors agonists or antagonists, calcium- antagonists, angiotensin II, atropine, sodium nitroprusside, ergonovine maleate. Fourteen pharmacological tests were performed in the 5 patients studied.

During these tests, STIs were also obtained by external carotid pulse (ECP) and phonocardiogram (PCG) at each stage of infusions, with the purpose of comparing the intraarterial parameters to the conventional

156

non-invasive ones.

2.Computerized analysis of signals

The ECG and the BP signals were digitized and analyzed according to the steps indicated in Fig. 1.

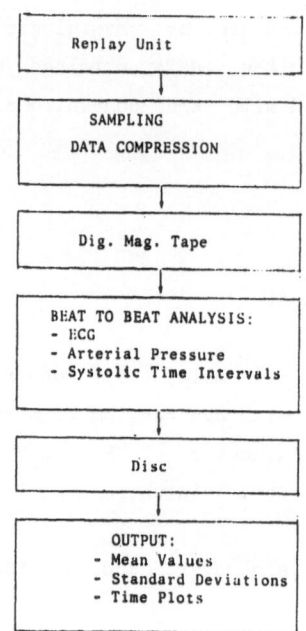

Fig. 1 – Block diagram which shows the main steps of the computerized analysis of the signals obtained by the combined ECG–BP monitoring. See text for further details.

In brief, the signal reproduced by the Replay Unit were sampled and compressed in such a way that a 24 hours recording for two channels was stored in a 24 hundred feet digital tape with a density of 800 bytes per inch. The sampling rate was 100 samples per second, both for ECG and BP. The time course of the overall process was 24 min., corresponding to 60 times the real time of recording. After sampling, the beat-to-beat analysis of ECG and BP was started and, by combining these two parameters, a continuous evaluation of STIs was also obtained. The information, stored on a disc, was available for presentation as absolute beat-to-beat values, mean values, standard deviations, time plots. The "time-window" for averaging the values of the parameters analyzed could be selected by the operator from 15 seconds to many hours. Ninty minutes were needed for this part of the analysis.

As regards the STIs derived by the arterial pressure curve, the left ventricular ejection time (LVET) was measured from the brachial upstroke to the dichrotic notch, and the pre-ejection period (PEP) from the Q-wave of the ECG to the upstroke of the brachial pressure curve (Fig.2). This approach for the PEP without the PCG values relies on the assumption that the transmission time of the arterial pulse wave (PTT) does not consistently change during a wide variety of cardiocirculatory conditions (Spodick et al.,1976).

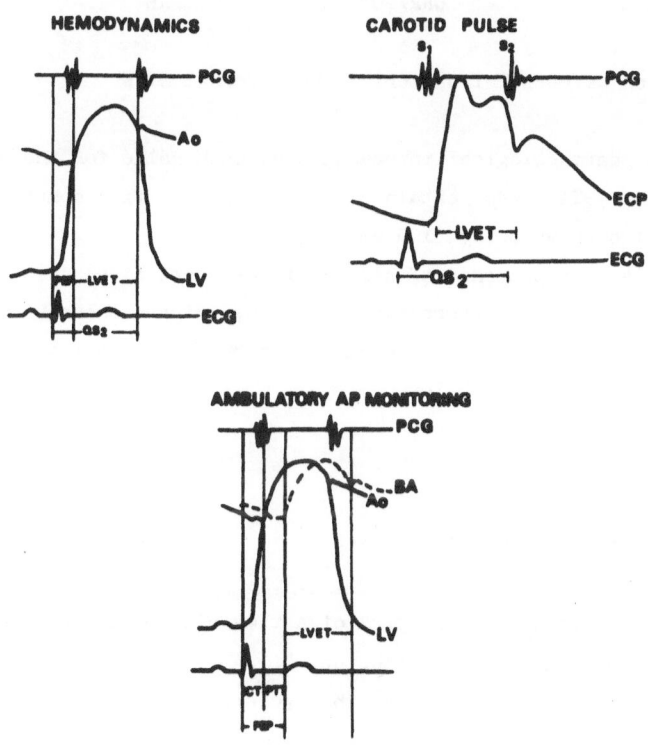

Fig. 2 - Diagrams showing the methods for computation of STIs by central hemodynamics (top, left), by ECP, PCG and ECG (top, right) and by ambulatory arterial pressure (AP) monitoring, with the catheter inserted in the brachial artery (BA) (bottom).

In the catheterization laboratory the true PEP, corresponding to the isovolumetric contraction time (ICT), is obtained. Also the external carotid pulse, combined with PCG and ECG, gives a measurement of PEP unaffected by the PTT (Lewis et al.,1977; Weissler,1977).

On the contrary, combining the peripheral arterial monitoring and the ECG, the measurement of PEP from Q-wave to the brachial upstroke always consistently overstimates the preejection time, which also includes -through this technique- the PTT.

Ao= aortic root LV= left ventricle

From the direct parameters, the corresponding one adjusted for heart rate (LVETC, PEPC) were also derived, according to the following equations:

$$LVETC = \frac{LVET}{\sqrt{RR/1000}} \quad ; \quad PEPC = \frac{PEP}{RR} \times 1000$$

3.Comparison between intraarterial and external STIs

During the pharmacological interventions, each value for the conventional, non-invasive STIs was obtained by averaging five consecutive cycles recorded at high velocity (100 mm/sec.).

Finally, the presence of a significant correlation was investigated, by means of the linear regression analysis, between these values and the corresponding mean values -averaged over 30 sec.- simultaneously obtained by the intraarterial technique.

RESULTS

1.Physiological interventions

In the Fig.3 an example of a time-plot obtained from a part of a 24-hours recording has been reported.

It is evident that during the bycicle stress test the intraarterial STIs have the expected pattern, represented by a decrease in the PEP and an increase in LVET, more pronounced after normalization for the increase in HR (LVETC).

The Fig.4 shows for the same recording the data represented as mean values over 30 seconds with their corresponding standard deviations.

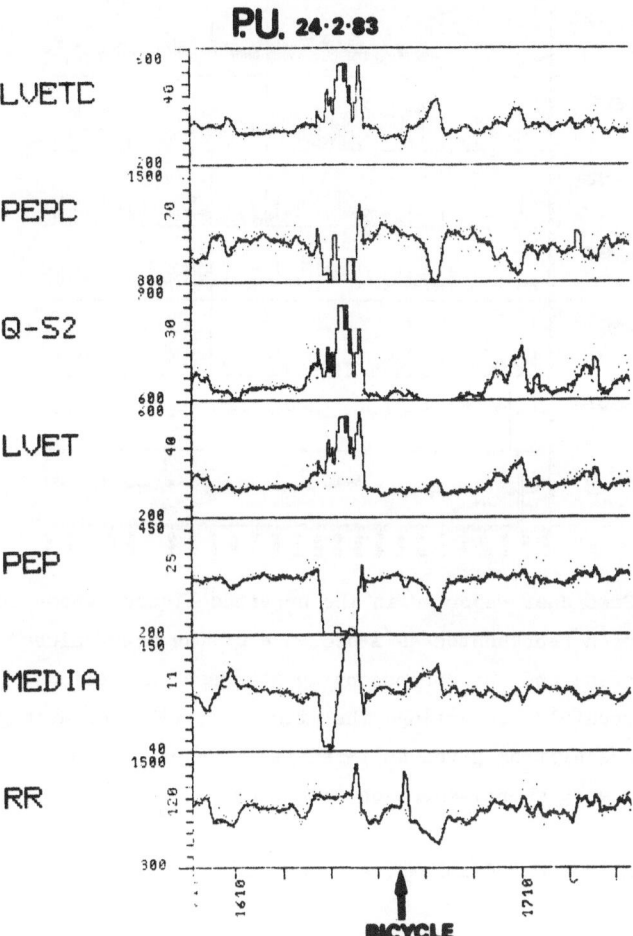

Fig. 3 — Time-plot (part of the 24-hours recording) obtained after digitization of the ECG and BP signals. From the top to the bottom: the STIs, the mean arterial pressure (MEDIA, in mmHg) and the HR (expressed as R-R intervals) have been reported. For each parameter, the line is composed of single dots, each representings the values averaged over 15 seconds. The time is on the abscissa, where each interval corresponds to 10 min. The rough —well detectable— initial artifacts correspond to the calibration of BP. Two sharp increase of the R-R are well evident before the exercise test (bicycle), and represent two markers of events obtained switching off the ECG for a brief period.

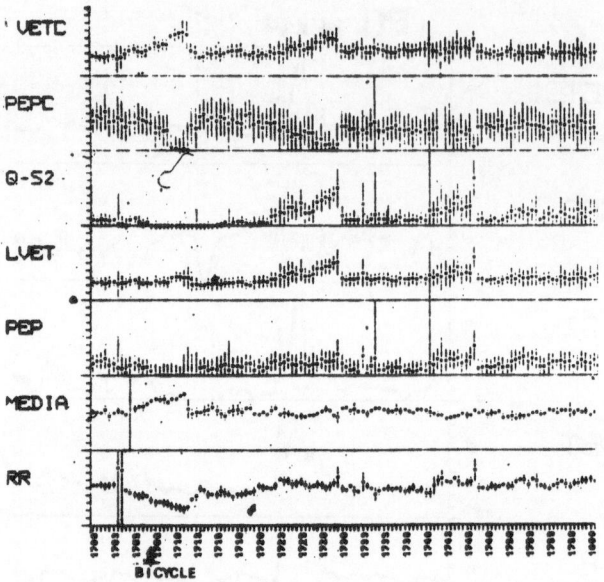

Fig. 4 – Same case reported in the previous figure, whose digitized data have been represented as a sequence of the mean values over 30 sec. (squares) and the corresponding standard deviations (vertical bars). Adequately selecting the time-intervals for averaging this kind of representation gives an immediate idea of variability for each parameter at very short, short or long term.

2.Pharmacologically-induced and spontaneous changes

The Fig.5 shows an example of utilizing the digitized intraarterial monitoring for pharmacological studies.

During the incremental infusion of angiotensin II (from 0.0015 µg/kg/min to 0.03 µg/kg/min, since record 540 to record 630), it is possible to observe a gradual but well evident increase in BP without consistent changes in HR and STIs; however, at the peak infusion rate, both BP and HR show a sudden, sharp increase, associated to a marked reduction in PEP and an increase in LVET and LVETC (three arrows). This last pattern could be suggestive of a widespread, angiotensin-induced sympathetic stimulation.

It may be interesting to note, on one hand that during this episode the patient, a young woman affected by essential borderline hypertension,

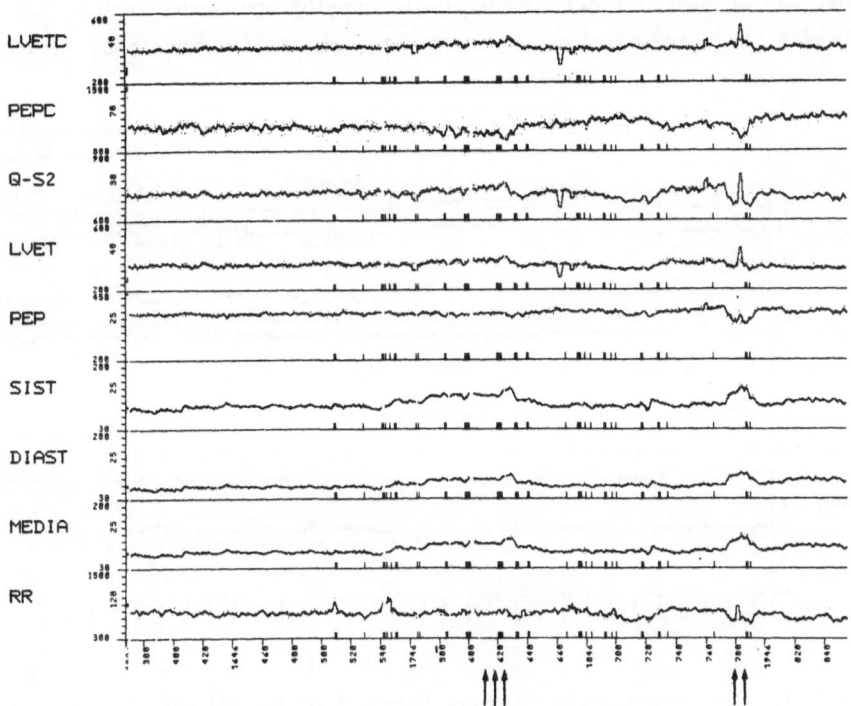

Fig. 5 - Time-plot of a part of 24-hours recording, showing the response to a stepwise infusion of angiotensin II. See text for details. It is interesting to observe that the increase in systolic, diastolic and mean BP (SIST, DIAST, MEDIA) observed on standing (two arrows), after the infusion, is associated to a marked decrease of PEP, thus indicating a widespread, sympathetic stimulation.

complained the same symptoms observed during spontaneous hypertensive paroxisms, such as facial flushing, headache, dizziness, and on the other hand that a similar pattern could be observed both during orthostatic stimulation (two arrows) and spontaneous increase of BP occurring at rest (in the evening or during the night) (Fig.6).

3.Correspondence between intraarterial digitized and external STIs

The results obtained correlating the STIs derivated by the intraarterial monitoring with those simultaneously recorded by ECP, ECG and PCG have been reported in Table I.

High correlation coefficients were observed in 4/5 patients for LVET, whereas no statistically significant correlations were obtained for PEP. However, the lack of significancy can be partially ascribed, in 3 cases, to the low number of observations.

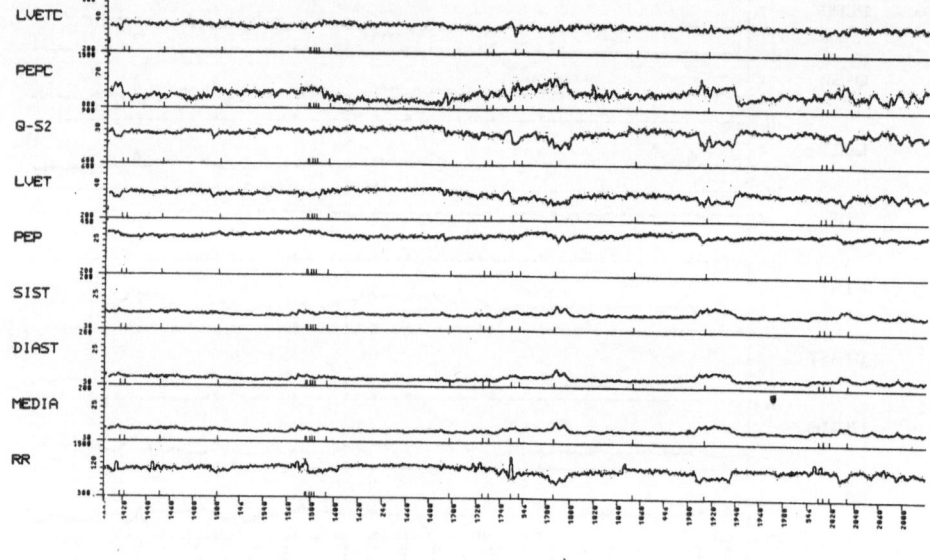

Fig. 6 - Spontaneous changes (arrows) of BP, HR and STIs observed at rest during the same recording of Fig. 5. The observed pattern is suggestive of sudden increase in sympathetic cardiac drive.

DISCUSSION

The monitoring of cardiac performance in ambulatory unrestricted patients represents an attractive goal for cardiovascular investigation. In fact , it could have a wide spectrum of applications, ranging from continuous hemodynamic evaluation of patients with fainting or transient myocardial ischaemia to the analysis of the sympathetic control of circulation; this last point appears to be specially worthwhile for the evaluation of hypertensive patients and their sympathetic system activity.

The STIs are related to the indexes of left ventricular function (Lewis et al.,1977; Weissler, 1977; Ahmed et al.,1972) and to plasma catecholamines (Levi et al.,1982) and appear to be, therefore, indicated for monitoring cardiac performance and its neural control.

The preliminary results presented in this report, obtained by an original method for continuous evaluation of STIs by the ECG and BP monitoring in unrestricted patients, showed good measurement of LVET, whose values were in the known physiological range and well correlated with the correspondent non-invasive values. On the contrary, the PEP was always overestimated (because the measurement without the PCG does not permit to eliminate the PTT, which sum to the "true" PEP) and poorly related to the external parameter.

This last fact can be due in part to the different variability, respect to the basal values, of the same parameter obtained by the two different techniques; furthermore, the external, not-continuous evaluation of STIs can not be considered a "gold standard" for the validation of a monitoring system, because of some difficulty in the assessment on the intraarterial recording of the exact time during which the external STIs are recorded. Finally,variable changes in PTT could limit an exact evaluation of PEP.

STIs: INTRAARTERIAL AMBULATORY MONITORING VS EXTERNAL CAROTID PULSE

Patient	Intercept (msec) a=	Slope (msec/msec) b=	Correlation coefficient r=	N.	p	Parameter
P.U.	−42.58	1.29	0.683	15	<0.01	
F.G.	29.16	1.15	0.718	11	<0.05	
I.C.	256.26	0.25	0.656	7	n.s.	LVET
T.M.	194.06	0.51	0.812	11	<0.01	
C.P.	889.40	−1.76	0.424	12	n.s.	
P.U.	279.50	0.45	0.435	15	n.s.	
F.G.	263.61	0.29	0.173	11	n.s.	
I.C.	255.83	0.56	0.600	7	n.s.	PEP
T.M.	299.10	0.20	0.173	11	n.s.	
C.P.	348.67	0.20	0.346	12	n.s.	

Tab. I - Linear regression analysis between intraarterial digitized STIs and the external parameters simultaneously recorded.
N= number of observation. A good agreement for LVET is evident, whereas no significant correlation was observed for PEP.

However, a good agreement was observed from a qualitative point of view both for LVET and for the PEP between the intraarterial and external technique, when the trend of the events during the interventions performed was graphically represented. It is also evident that in most occasions the STIs monitoring shows a pattern which can be well explained on physiological basis (Fig.7-9).

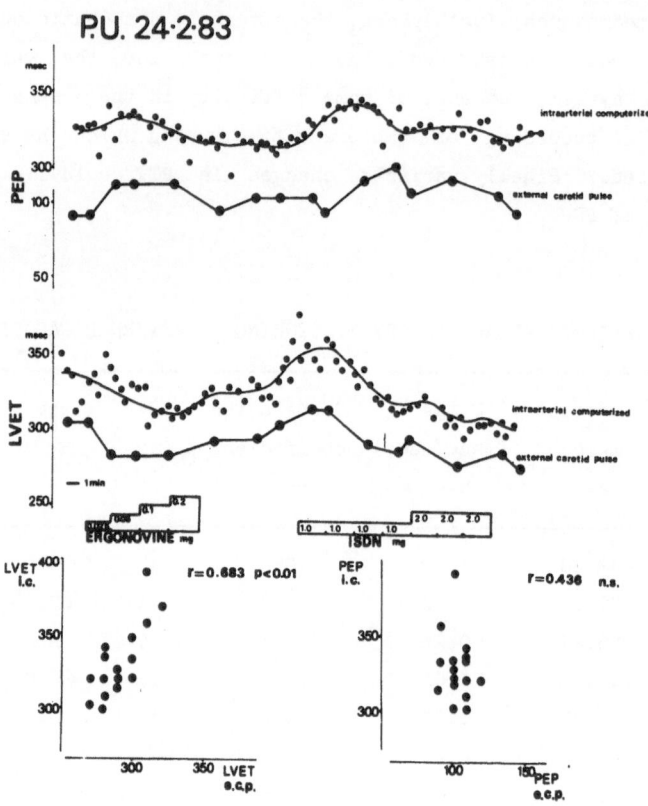

P.U. 24·2·83

Fig. 7 - The comparison between the pattern of PEP and LVET obtained by the intraarterial technique (upper curve) and the non invasive one (lower curve) during infusion of ergonovine maleate and isosorbide dinitrate (ISDN) has been represented. For each "external" data the intraarterial value —obtained by averaging all the values recorded during the corresponding 30 sec— has been reported, together with the two immediately previous and following values. This representation shows a good agreement also for PEP, although the correlation between the intraarterial values (i.c.) and the external values (e.c.p.) is not statistically significant. The more "smooth" trend of the events continuously evaluated by the intraarterial technique is also evident.

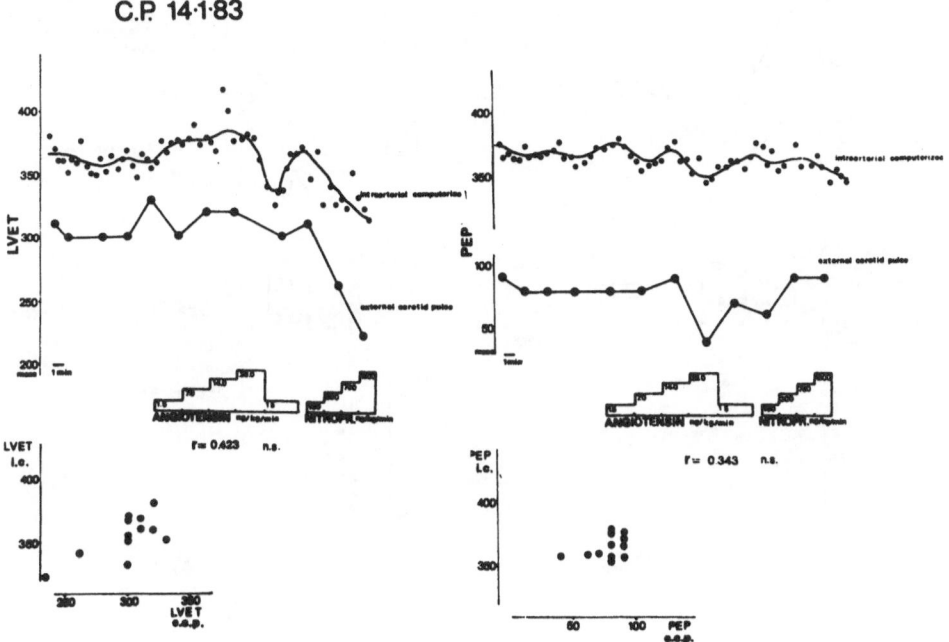

Fig. 8 - Graphic representation of the STIs during infusion of angiotensin II and nitroprusside, obtained as in the previous Figure. No significant correlations between the intraarterial and the external technique are observed in this patient. However, a substantial agreement is evident when the trends of events are compared.

In our opinion these results suggest that the ambulatory BP monitoring can be utilized for monitoring -at least in a semiqualitative way- also some indexes of cardiac performance. Further validation, however, is needed, in particular for the assessment of the constancy -at least from a practical point of view- of the PTT, because of data reported in the literature are somewhat conflicting (Spodick et al.,1976; Gribbin et al.,1979).

166

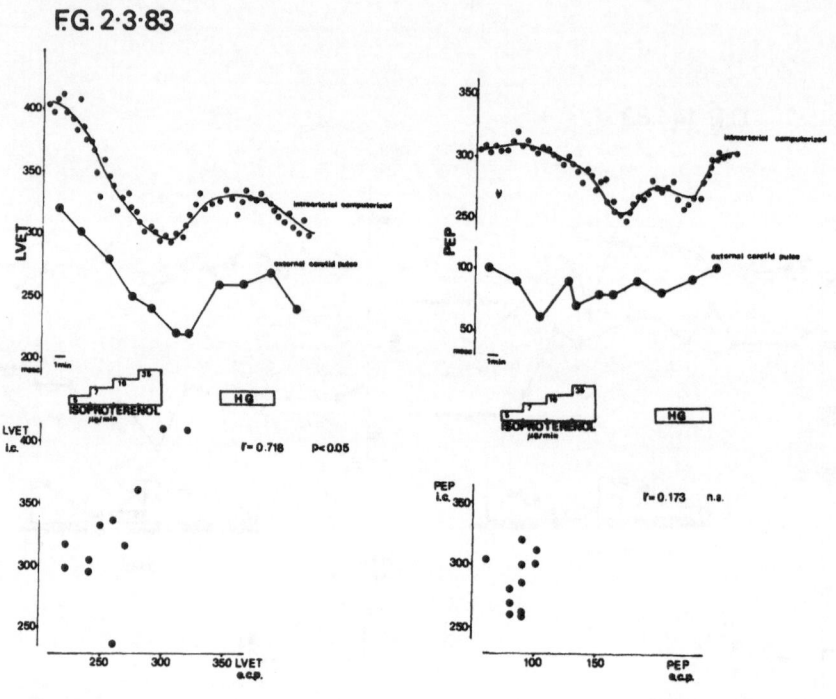

Fig. 9 – The trend of STIs during isoproterenol infusion and isometric exercise (HG) has been reported. The comparison between the two techniques gives results similar to those observed in Figg. 7 and 8.

REFERENCES

Ahmed, S.S., Levinson, G.E., Schwartz, C.J. and Ettinger, P.O. 1972. Systolic time intervals as measure of the contractile state of the left ventricular myocardium in man. Circulation, 46, 559-571.

Floras, J.S., Jones, J.V., Johnston, J.A., Brooks, D.E., Hassan, M.O. and Sleight, P. 1978. Arousal and circadian rhithm of blood pressure. Clinical Science and Molecolar Medicine , 55, 395s-397s.

Gribbin, P., Pickering, T.G. and Sleight P. 1979. Arterial distensibility in normal and hypertensive man. Clinical Science, 56, 413-417.

Haffty, B.G., Kotilainen, P.W., Kobayashi, K., Bishop, R.L. and Spodick D.H. 1977. Development of an ambulatory systolic time interval monitoring system. Journal of Clinical Engineering. July-September, 199-210.

Levi, G.F., Ratti, S., Cardore, G. and Basagni, M. 1982. On the reliability of systolic time intervals. Cardiology, 69, 157-165.

Lewis, R.P., Rittgers, S.E., Forester, W.F. and Boudoulas, H. 1977. A critical review of the systolic time intervals. Circulation, 54, 146-158.

Mancia, G., Ferrari, A., Gregorini, L., Parati, G., Pomidossi, G., Bertinieri, G., Grassi, G. and Zanchetti, A. 1980. Blood pressure variability in man: its relation to high blood pressure, age and baroreflex sensitivity. Clinical Science, 59, 401s-404s.

Millar Craig, M.W., Hawes, D. and Whittington, J. 1978a. A new system for recording ambulatory blood pressure in man. Med. Biol. Eng. Comput., 16, 727- .

Millar Craig, M.W., Hawes, D. and Whittington, J. 1978b. Circadian variation of blood pressure. Lancet, 1, 795-797.

Pessina, A.C., Palatini, P., Semplicini, A., Mormino, P., Casiglia, E., Ventura, E., Agnoletto, V., Sperti, G., Gava, H., Hlede, M. and Dal Palu, C. 1982. Ambulatory blood pressure monitoring: quantification of blood pressure variability before and after antihypertensive therapy. Int. J. Clin. Pharm. Res., 11, 211-214.

Spodick, D.H. and Quarry Lance, V. 1976. Non invasive stress testing methodology for elimination of the phonocardiogram. Circulation, 53, 673-676.

Steriotis, J., Ioannidis, P.J., Ktenas, J. and Aravanis, C. 1979. Systolic time intervals before and after the management of hypertension. In " Non invasive cardiovascular diagnosis " (Ed. E.B. Diethrich). (PSG, Publishing Company, Littleton). pp. 499-504.

Weissler, A.M. 1977. Systolic time intervals. The New England Journal of Medicine, 296, 321-324.

DISCUSSION

Chairman: G.Mancia

2.3 Ambulatory monitoring of hypertensive patients.

WALSH: I have a question for Dr. Palombo. In light of the fact that systolic time intervals are considered to be marginally good to poor predictors of such cardiac parameters as after load and pre load etc., and the fact that in the sixties and seventies many efforts to measure the pulse wave velocity with the peripheral pulse were failed by the fact of distortion of the peripheral wave. I wonder if your group has considered or is considering independent verification of the systolic time intervals by your method, with independently calculated cardiac parameters such as resistance stroke volume derived from indocynine green or therm dilution?

PALOMBO: The problem is done by the invasive nature of the evaluation. Then it could be necessary to study by left ventricular catheterization the patient during simultaneous recording of intrarterial blood-pressure. However, this is a work in progress. And at first, we prefer to evaluate our technique with a non-invasive one.

WALSH: But both techniques have questionable values in this case.

PALOMBO: I hope that the different kind of two techniques can explain the poor results obtained by us for PEP evaluation.

ZYWIETZ: I would like to comment on those blood-pressure measurements of the first two speakers, based on a study we have performed on 3000 hypertensive subjects. If you compare blood-pressure measurements you have to mantain very rigidly simultaneous measurements. We have done, for example, measurement of incidental blood pressure measurement and then at 2 minutes distance, or even less. First finding was that there is a significant decrease during this first period. This decrease depends highly on the incidental systolic blood-pressure the patient has itself. For example cases where patients have incidental blood-pressure of around 80; that means you just measure casual values if the patient sets down, immediately after that measurement. Then patients which show low systolic blood-pressure around 100-110, tend to increase slightly blood-pressure during the first minutes of rest. Other cases where you have blood-pressure, or incidental blood-pressure of 150 or 160 mm. show a drastic decrease. If you want to reduce and understand variability of those measurements, one needs to group the cases according to the systolic blood-pressure you get in your first measurement, and then you see a very systematic behaviour, strong decrease of case with high blood-pressure, and slight increase or just stable behaviour of cases with 100-120 systolic pressure. These decreases or changes in blood-pressure correlate very well with measurements we take during a standardized exercise. So, first point is: you have to mantain very rigid timing if you compare blood-pressure measurements; and second point is dependent on the starting situation of the measurements. Depending on these conditions, you can group and reduce variability.

CLEMENT: We never managed to find out any correlation of the difference between casual and continuous recordings. Whether this was due to the level of pressure that was initially recording, or to whatever stress that was being done in those patients. We have used a whole battery of what we call sympathetic stress tests. And there is no correlation among these tests whatever the way you represent data. The same result applies to the difference between casual and ambulatory recordings. And that's about all what I can say. The other aspects that I don't understand from your statement is that you could somewhere accept that people having a certain level of casual pressure, would be that lower when you record ambulatory pressure. We have never been able to find out this answer. We have people with enormously high blood-pressure, who become totally normal in normal life outside the clinic, and we have other people who have 160 and they become 140 outside the clinic.

MANCIA: We are still wondering about whether or not there is a certain sub-group of people in a certain age that might be hyper reactive and if there is some evidence suggesting this I don't know. What I can say is that our experience is like that of Dr. Clement. We are surprised by similarities of responses of people with different blood-pressure when taken in big numbers, and not by differences.

ZYWIETZ: Grouping people according to age, according to weight and so on, I belive this is a good way to get similar findings in the different groups. We have no explanation for that, but that's what we found, and the number of patients was large.

GHIONE: I would like to ask Dr. Clement a question: You compared, I understand, the blood-pressure measured during ambulatory monitoring, with pressure measured for a couple of hours in a patient staying in a quiet room and you found very similar average blood pressure. That is very striking for everybody expecting that putting somebody on a led, and leaving him without much noise around, his blood pressure should go down. How would you interpret this data?

CLEMENT: We are often looking at data, and I never would like to speculate about what you see. What we have seen is that, surprisingly, the histograms of both techniques are very close to each other. Now, you want, me to speculate. In order to define someone's blood-pressure profile it could maybe not be necessary to have enormous amounts of points. You have to define X numbers of measurements, and if those measurements are done properly in conditions which have to be defined, that you get a blood-pressure curve, which is the curve of that individual.

GHIONE: How representative are these measuremets in a quiet room for your patient?

CLEMENT: I just can not do other than show that one histogram is very close to the other one, to my great surprise.

GHIONE: So we just keep our patients in a quiet room for 2 hours and avoid ambulatory monitoring?

CLEMENT: I don't know. I'd like to have some people repeating the study and doing exactly the same thing. If they do show the same result, then it could be a very easy and cheaper and better standardized way to do it, yes, but that is all I know.

TOPIC: 2.4

Aspects of the organization of the ambulatory monitoring

MULTILEVEL ORGANIZATION OF AMBULATORY MONITORING UNITS.

C.Contini, G.Kraft, G.Mazzocca, G.Bongiorni, M.Pauletti, M.Baratto D.Levorato.

CNR Clinical Physiology Institute, Via Savi 8, 56100 Pisa.

ABSTRACT
The Authors review the various constructive philosophies employed in instrumentation for dynamic ECG recordings;these have been classified into 4 levels of complexity and cost.On the other hand clinical problems presented by cardiac patients can be classified into similar complexity levels.The best utilization of Holter analysis systems is obtained if complexity level of both instrumentation and clinical problems are taken into account.
Real time recorders are now under validation and cannot be considered in this classification, while computerized systems have found a useful application in newer physiological studies.

In the last years several constructive philosophies have been outlined in the field of instrumentation for dynamic electrocardiography,which were mainly determined by technological progress.

They have different and diversified aims,both as to costs and as to results obtainable with the analysis of 24 hour tracings.

Various levels of instrument complexity can thus be defined; choice of which level to employ must be suggested by the complexity of the individual patient's clinical problem;in consequence distribution of the equipment will be guided by the functions of the cardiologic centre to which the instruments are assigned.

The following possible levels may be listed:

1 - the first level has the least constructive complexity and

requires total involvement of the operator.

The type of analysis obtainable with such devices is entirely founded upon the operator's technical and professional ability; his task consists in reading and interpreting more or less compacted ECG tracings. In a particular type of instrument which may be placed on this level, a certain complexity of the electronics has allowed a typical tracings display, capable of stimulating in real time the human perceptive system so that it provides a highly reliable performance.

2 - The second level represents a compromise between electronic automatisms and human perceptive system. The operator may at any time chose the role of controller or of analyser.

To this section belong the high-cost dedicated devices which represents the majority of commercial systems.

3 - The third level is characterized by complete automation which is made possible only by automatic computer elaboration. Operator's intervention is limited to the final phase of the procedure, where interpretation and decision are required. There is always the possibility of optional signal control.

4 - in the fourth level I have included instruments which can make a real time analysis and acquire only abnormal events on solid state memory; elaboration is limited to abnormal events and to few other physiological parameters.Any control of system's reliability is lacking.

Once this kind of instrument classification by complexity

is accepted, and the clinical questions more frequently encountered in everyday practice are taken into account, an element which in my opinion largely contributes to the success of the method is adaptation of the expected performance of one of the listed systems to the individual clinical problem.

In this way waste of time and money will be avoided and quality of information, where necessary, will be improved. However one must keep in mind that systems without perceptive control or at least manual control in a subsequent time (point 4) still need further validation; on the contrary, in systems where this possibility is considered, it should be actually employed rather than placing total confidence in automatisms.

In order to complete the picture of relationships between instruments and clinical problems, it will be useful to attempt to classify the latter, taking into account the most frequent clinical problems in everyday practice.

1. The simplest clinical problem is to ascertain the correspondence of a given symptom to an abnormal recorded event, in other words to document symptomatic conduction or rhythm disturbances. The main drawback of such clinical situations is the sporadic and irregular occurrence of symptoms, so that a 24 hour recording seldom solves the diagnostic problem. For this purpose the most suitable recorders are the ones so called " Circadian " which may be started at the occurrence of symptoms by the patient himself and may remain applied for long periods of time, up to fifteen days. In these cases analysis is extremely simple and a single

recording lead is sufficient.

2. A more complex level of clinical problem is the documentation of the nature of chest pain in apparently healthy subjects, in whom all provocative tests yielded negative results.Reliability of 24 hour recordings for the diagnosis of ischemia and whether such a diagnosis can be made with only 2 ECG leads has been a matter of extensive discussion. Apart from this problem, I believe in these cases instruments of the second and third level and repeated recordings should be employed. The same is true for the evaluation of malignancy of ventricular arrhythmias and for the control of the efficacy of antiarrhythmic and antianginal treatment.

3. The third level shows its full potentiality when employed for accurate functional evaluation of subjects who have already been recognized as cardiac patients, and for a dynamic study of apparently normal subjects, whose normality has been assessed with other methods; it is important to remember that today's elements of physiology still derive from static observations.

4. As to the 4th level, I think it is not realistic to consider it available for the solution of clinical problems. However a validation of the recognition algorhythms is still lacking, which would allow us not to regret the lack of signal control in this kind of devices.

The adaptation of the level of the instrumentation to clinical problems allows the best use and the lowest running costs. This is adequate both for a public health service, which includes at least three levels of cardiological interventions, and to a private structure, which also comprises three levels, from Cardiology office, to private Clinic up to Institution of Clinical Research.

Finally, the application of these criteria allows a more rational distribution of loads and tasks to the various cardiological units of the health service either private or public.

An absolute validation of the performance of all types of instruments will become possible only when a database is set up which collects the majority of possible ECG alterations.

This is a complex and time-consuming work, since the range of abnormalities present in human cardiac pathology is wide enough to defy almost always the evaluating system.

CHAPTER 3

RECENT ADVANCES OF METHODS FOR THE AMBULATORY MONITORING
OF THE CARDIOVASCULAR SYSTEMS

TOPIC: 3.1

Algorithms for cardiac cycle detection

ALGORITHMIC APPROACHES TO QRS DETECTION

O. Pahlm[*], L. Sörnmo[**]

* Department of Clinical Physiology
University Hospital, Lund, Sweden

** Department of Telecommunication Theory
University of Lund, Lund, Sweden

ABSTRACT

The QRS detection algorithm is an essential part of any computer-based system for the analysis of ambulatory ECG recordings. This survey asserts that all one-channel QRS detectors, described in the literature can be considered as having the same basic structure. A discussion of some of the current detection schemes is presented in regard to this structure. Some additional features for QRS detectors are mentioned. The problem of multi-channel detection now gaining importance is also briefly treated.

INTRODUCTION

During recent years, digital QRS detectors have replaced analog ones in most ECG processing applications. The cost of microprocessors are now so low that even simple devices, such as heart rate meters, are often equipped with digital QRS detectors. The present workshop is devoted to the processing of long-term ECG recordings from ambulatory patients. Figure 1 demonstrates the signal processing steps employed in computer-based analysis of such recordings. We use the term "post processor" (step 6) for all further algorithmic or human processing of the QRS detector output. Examples include heart rate measurements, R-R interval analysis and QRS waveform classification. In all-digital systems, which perform QRS detection and post-processing in real time, steps 1 and 2 are, of course, omitted.

It is important to be aware that the various links in the signal processing chain are highly interdependent. For example, a QRS detection algorithm which has been "tuned" to a certain recording/replay system (steps 1-3) may have to be retuned if it is to be used with another system having e.g. different frequency characteristics. Furthermore, if the post-processor is a sophisticated waveform classifier, the demands on the QRS detector are quite different from those when the post-processor is simply an algorithm for R-R interval analysis. The waveform classifier can typically accept more false alarms from the QRS detector than the R-R interval analyser.

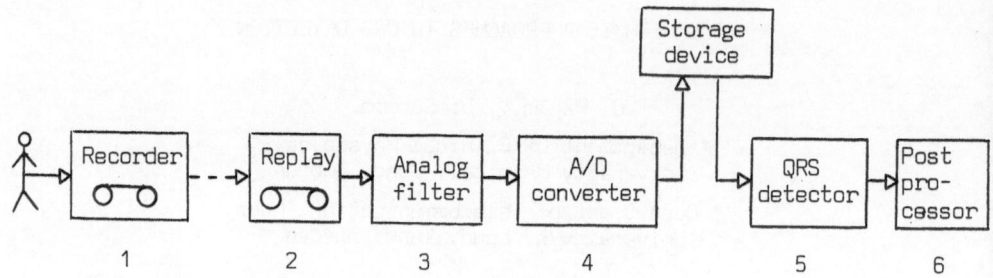

Fig. 1 Block diagram of signal processing steps in monitoring/ana-
lysis of ambulatory ECG recordings.

Conceptually the QRS detector can be divided into two entities, which
we call the pre-processor and the decision rule. These two entities are
discussed in the following sections, as well as some additional features
of QRS detection schemes. In order to further improve detector performance,
morphological information acquired in step 6 can be incorporated in the QRS
detector, see e.g. Mead et al. (1975). Since such feedback tends to be very
system-dependent, it will not be considered here. The evaluation of performance is also briefly considered.

DIGITAL PRE-PROCESSING

The purpose of the pre-processor is to enhance the QRS portion of the
digitized ECG, while suppressing noise and artefacts. Pre-processing can be
divided into linear filtering and non-linear operations. The non-linear
operations consist of e.g. rectification or squaring of the filtered signal. Not all pre-processors employ non-linear operations; the filtered signal is instead fed directly to the decision rule.

The earliest efforts made to produce a signal better conditioned for
the decision rule were to use the 1st difference of the ECG (Caceres, 1963;
Pryor et al., 1969; Holsinger et al., 1971). This further accentuates the
R-wave due to its relatively sharp peak. Since such a filter also accentuates high-frequency noise, it is not appropriate in situations with moderate signal-to-noise ratios (SNR), e.g. ambulatory monitoring. More recent detectors instead incorporate a bandpass filter in the pre-processor,
usually with a center frequency between 10 and 20 Hz, and bandwidth of 5
to 10 Hz. This choice of filter is indicated by the theory of detecting a
known signal in Gaussian noise. It is well-known that the optimum detector
includes a matched filter, which for a white noise situation has an impulse

response equal to the QRS complex, but reversed in time and shifted. In contrast to the case in communication theory, however, the form often varies with time and the noise is not stationary. The design of a BP-filter must therefore be a compromise, taking into consideration that the lower cut-off frequency should be chosen such that large-amplitude P- and T-waves are rejected while still accentuating PVCs, and, when choosing the upper cut-off frequency, that motion artefacts should be rejected but not narrow QRS complexes.

The design of a filter for QRS detection has been investigated by Thakor et al. (1980); see also the review of Brydon (1976). They conclude from a limited data base that a BP-filter with f_c = 18 Hz yields good performance. A class of digital filters has been suggested by Börjesson et al. (1982). The impulse response of each filter is defined by two integer parameters K and L:

$$h(k) = Z^{-1}\left\{(1-z^{-K})(1+z^{-1})^L\right\} \tag{1}$$

where $Z^{-1}\{\cdot\}$ is the inverse Z-transform. In the time domain, the first part $(1-z^{-K})$ forms a difference between the input signal and the delayed input (K samples), and the second part $(1+z^{-1})^L$ is a lowpass filter with decreased bandwidth for increased L. The filters in this class have linear phase, and they can be implemented by using only additions and subtractions. Sörmmo et al. (1982) found that, for the sampling rate f_s = 100 Hz, a good performance is obtained by using (K,L) = (1,2). These parameters yield a BP-filter with f_c = 20 Hz and a rather large bandwidth, see Fig. 2. Since the spectral variability of the QRS complex is large, a smaller bandwidth seems to be too restrictive. For f_s = 100 Hz the filter (K,L) = (1,1) has been employed by Nygårds and Hulting (1978) and Fancett and Wong (1980). For a higher sampling rate, i.e. f_s = 250 Hz, (K,L) = (5,4) may be an appropriate choice, also yielding a filter with f_c = 20 Hz, see Fig. 2 (Engelse and Zeelenberg, 1979). By using the above combinations of sampling rate and filter parameters, the mains frequency is cancelled. Other digital filters which have been designed with reference to matched filters are found in Dillman et al. (1978) and McClelland and Arnold (1976).

Several heuristic approaches to non-linear operations on the filtered ECG can be found in the literature, e.g. Murthy and Rangaraj (1979) and Okada (1979). A common objective of such schemes is to deduce a signal which yields a single positive peak for each QRS, and thus enables the use

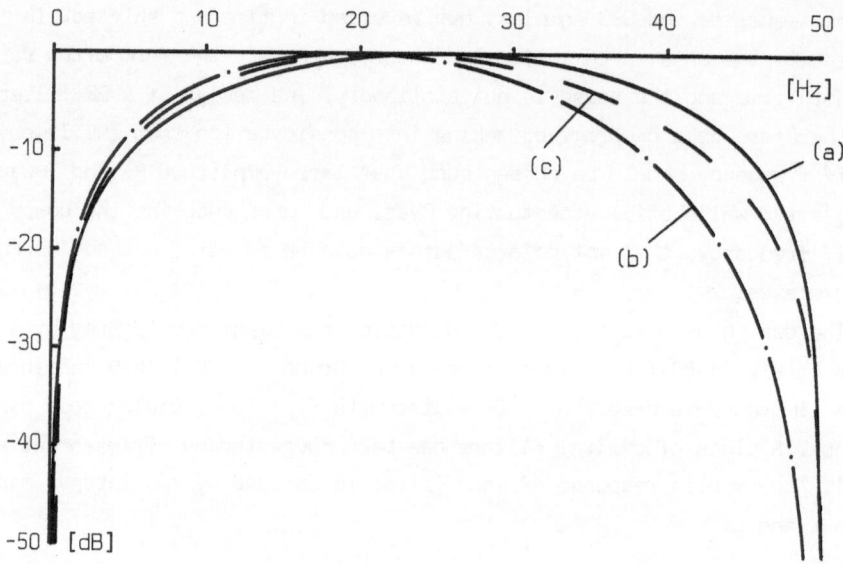

Fig. 2   Frequency characteristic for h(k) and (a) (K,L) = (1,1),
f_S = 100 Hz,   (b) (K,L) = (1,2), f_S = 100 Hz,   (c) (K,L) = (5,4),
f_S = 250 Hz.

of a one-sided amplitude threshold. Murthy and Rangaraj (1979) accomplish
this by weighting each sample in the squared, 1st-differenced ECG by a triangular window. In order to reduce the large ripple that can occur in the
weighted signal, it is subjected to heavy smoothing. Although the above
non-linear schemes may perform satisfactorily, it is not clear from a theoretical point of view why these schemes should be employed.

By applying techniques known from optimal estimation to a stochastic
model for the ECG, the resulting detector includes a non-linear operation
on the filtered ECG (Börjesson et al., 1982). Essentially that scheme forms
a function of the rectified, maximal amplitude difference between two samples separated by a certain distance. Due to the computational requirements,
an approximation of that scheme is introduced, which relies only on the
peaks in the filtered signal; for details see Sörnmo (1982).

DECISION RULE

In order to determine if a QRS complex has occurred or not, a decision
rule is applied to the output of the pre-processor. The rule, which often
takes the form of an amplitude threshold, may be fixed or incorporate some
kind of adaptivity. Although there are recent proponents for using a fixed

threshold (Bolton and Coleman, 1981), adaptive thresholds are now by far
the most commonly applied. This is due to the fact that in ambulatory ECG
recordings, the QRS amplitude can change drastically during the recording.
In order to detect low-amplitude QRSs with a fixed threshold, one is inevitably forced to accept several false alarms. Besides comparison of the
amplitude to a threshold, some detectors also embody the width of the waveform as a basis for decision.

Even if the whole recording usually is available to the detector (i.e.
from a computer disc), most workers treat the signal in a "causal" fashion,
which means that QRS complexes are detected in temporal order. This is done
for example by comparing the linearly filtered signal with two amplitude
thresholds, exponentially updated from the amplitude of previously found
complexes (Engelse and Zeelenberg, 1979). If a certain pattern of threshold
crossings occurs within an interval of 160 msec, a QRS complex is detected.
In order to reject large T-waves, some workers have introduced a time-
dependent amplitude threshold. The most common form of such a dependency is
found in detectors which incorporate a so-called "eye-closing" interval.
This means that subsequent to each detected beat the threshold is set equal
to infinity, typically in an interval of length 200-300 ms, and is then decreased to the current update of the threshold. The length of the interval
chosen must not be too large due to the obvious risk of missing early PVCs.
A very short interval, and of course the exclusion of eye-closing, however,
will not only increase the number of false alarms due to T-waves, but will
also allow the detector to produce false alarms due to wide PVCs. There is
thus a trade-off in the choice of eye-closing interval. Compromises between
these conflicting demands are found in a report from Shah et al. (1976),
who suggest a finite, but larger, amplitude threshold in this interval.
Dillman et al. (1978) apply an eye-closing interval of 200 ms, followed by
a linearly decreasing threshold. The slope of the threshold is determined
from the average R-wave amplitude and the average R-R interval. Additional
threshold tests are included to ensure that the detected beat is not a P-
wave.

A detector which, to a certain degree, incorporates future as well as
past signal properties is described by Börjesson et al. (1982). An observation interval is delimited within which QRS complexes are detected in the
order of magnitude in the pre-processed signal, not in temporal order. Due
to this "non-causal" property, eye-closing is equally applied before, as
well as after, each detected beat. Adaptivity is introduced by letting the

properties of the complexes which delimit the interval control the
thresholds. This approach allows the detector to find the QRS complexes
even when a sudden decrease in amplitude occurs.

We will finally mention some additional techniques which may be employed in QRS detectors.

a. Since the spectral content of the muscle noise has considerable overlap
   with that of a QRS, such noise will cause the performance to deterio-
   rate. In that case, a noise detector or noise measurements may be of
   great value. Various strategies for using the noise measurements can be
   adopted. One way is to exclude disturbed parts of the recording from
   analysis, another is to indicate for the end-user that detections are
   more unreliable than usual (Engelse and Zeelenberg, 1979; Fancott et al.,
   1981). A third approach is to use the noise measurements in the updating
   of thresholds. A combination of the last mentioned approaches can of
   course be employed.

b. The QRS detection process results in a table of R-R intervals. The properties of this table can be used to control a "second pass" or "look-
   back" in the algorithm (Pahlm et al., 1978; Mead et al., 1979). In cases
   of a stable basic rhythm, the occurrence of an R-R interval of approximately twice the length of the typical interval may be due to e.g. a
   missed low-amplitude ectopic beat. The processing of that interval with
   a lower threshold, or even with another linear filter in the pre-processor, may result in detection in the second pass.

c. In many applications, it is important to define a stable fiducial point
   of the detected QRS complex. Unfortunately, commonly used definitions
   such as the peak of R-wave or the maximum negative slope are not suitable (Ripley and Murray, 1980). These definitions will suffer from dis-
   continuities for certain QRS shapes, and they are vulnerable to noise.
   Recent techniques which offer a more stable definition are found in
   Gradman et al. (1980) and Nygårds and Sörnmo (1983).

EVALUATION OF DETECTOR PERFORMANCE

In the preceding sections we have outlined various approaches to QRS
detection. Within each detector structure there is usually a large number

of parameter values that must be fixed before use in a clinical setting.
For the most part, the choice of parameter values has been an integral part
of the algorithmic development, rather than the result of a separate optimization. In doing so, the designer runs the risk of choosing values which
are too attuned to the training material. If one aims at an optimization of
all parameters with respect to some performance measure, one is faced with
an impracticable amount of computations. A natural way to cope with this
problem is to optimize those parameters which have the most profound effect
on performance; this may result in feasible computations (Thakor and Webster, 1981; Sörnmo et al., 1982).

Due to the lack of a unified ECG data base suitable for evaluation of
QRS detectors, different workers have collected their own material (Mead
et al., 1979; Okada, 1979; Thakor and Webster, 1981; Bolton and Coleman,
1981; Sörnmo et al., 1982). Since e.g. the signal quality or the number of
PVCs varies from material to material, a comparison of published results is
not meaningful. It is hoped that the now available MIT/BIH data base as
well as the one from AHA will fill the needs for detector evaluation, at
least in certain respects (Schluter et al., 1980; Hermes et al., 1980). In
most studies, the performance is measured in terms of false alarm rate and
detection rate for a given set of parameter values. Although these statistical numbers yield a measure of the over-all performance, no knowledge is
achieved about the sensitivity of the detector for different parameter values. In order to accomplish this, one can display the detection rate towards the false alarm rate in a so-called receiver operating characteristic
(ROC), calculated for different values of a certain parameter, see Fig. 3.
Such diagrams have been calculated by Sörnmo (1982) by varying parameters
which determine amplitude and width criteria and for three different filter
parameters (K,L) in (1). Furthermore by adding different levels of band-
limited noise to a noise-free ECG, the ROC for an analog detector was calculated for different amplitude thresholds (Thakor and Webster, 1981). The
generation of such signals allows the designer to easily investigate the
robustness of the detector to various kinds of noise and artefacts. This
is of particular interest in ambulatory monitoring in which noisy signals
are often found.

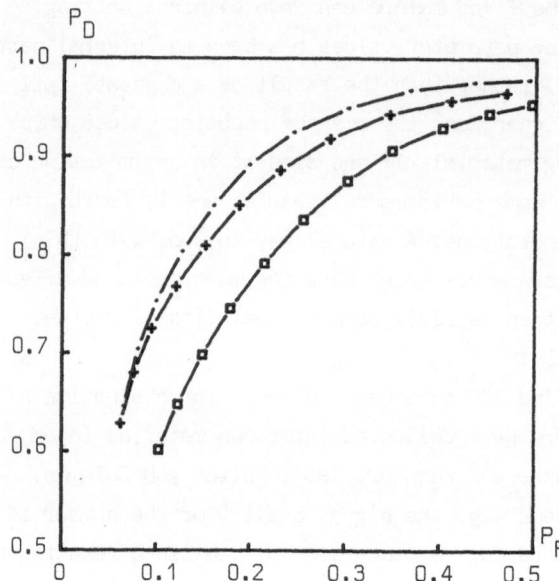

Fig. 3 ROC curves obtained for three different QRS detectors. Each point is calculated for a certain value of an amplitude threshold.

MULTI-CHANNEL ECG RECORDINGS

The present paper has provided an overview of approaches to QRS detection in one-channel recordings. The use of multi-channel recordings is currently becoming more widespread in long-term ECG analysis. By taking advantage of the fact that several channels are available, the performance of the QRS detector will be substantially improved. Since noise often occurs independently in different channels, an improved noise immunity can be obtained (Zywietz et al., 1981). Moreover, detection of PVCs will be more reliable, since a low-amplitude PVC in one channel is usually much larger in another channel. So far, few articles have been published, which present detectors designed for multi-channel recordings. A detector which employs simple majority decision logic has been implemented by Bragg-Remschel and Harrison (1980) in a two-channel system. The logic uses decisions obtained separately from each channel and from a third channel deduced by summing the rectified signals.

REFERENCES

Bolton, M.P. and Coleman, J.D. 1981. "Detection of QRS complexes in ECG signals and the evaluation of instantaneous heart rate" in Pinciroli, F. and Anderson, J. (eds.) Proc. of Changes in health care instr. due to micropr. techn., North-Holland Publ. Comp., IFIP, pp. 249-256.

Bragg-Remschel, D.A. and Harrison, D.C. 1980. "A computerized two channel
    ambulatory arrhythmia analysis system". Proc. IEEE Comput. Cardiol.,
    1980, pp. 197-200.
Brydon, J. 1976. "Automatic monitoring of cardiac arrhythmias". IEE Med.
    Elec. Monographs 18-22, pp. 27-41.
Börjesson, P.O., Pahlm, O., Sörnmo, L. and Nygårds, M.E. 1982. "Adaptive
    QRS detection based on maximum-a-posteriori estimation". IEEE Trans.
    Biomed. Eng., BME-29, pp. 341-351.
Caceres, C.A. 1963. "Electrocardiographic analysis by a computer system".
    Arch. Intern. Med., Vol. 111, pp. 196-202.
Dillman, R., Judell, N. and Kuo, S. 1978. "Replacement of AZTEC by correla-
    tion for more accurate VPB detection". Proc. IEEE Comput. Cardiol.
    1978, pp. 29-32.
Engelse, W.A.H. and Zeelenberg C. 1979. "A single scan algorithm for QRS-
    detection and feature extraction". Proc. IEEE Comput. Cardiol. 1979,
    pp. 37-42.
Fancott, T. and Wong, D.H. 1980. "A minicomputer system for direct high-
    speed analysis of cardiac arrhythmia in 24h ambulatory ECG tape re-
    cordings". IEEE Trans. Biomed. Eng., BME-27, pp. 685-693.
Fancott, T., Wong, D., Guimond, C. and Lemire, J. 1981. "Design considera-
    tions for noise immunity in the Concordia high-speed ambulatory ECG
    tape analysis system". Proc. IEEE Comput. Cardiol. 1981, pp. 343-346.
Gradman, A.H., Lewis, J.W. and Mayer, J.L. 1980. "An improved method for
    computer measurement of the R-R interval on the ambulatory electrocar-
    diogram". Proc. IEEE Comput. Cardiol. 1980, pp. 213-216.
Hermes, R.E., Geselowitz, D.B. and Oliver, G.C. 1980. "Development, distri-
    bution, and the use of the American heart association database for
    ventricular arrhythmia detector evaluation". Proc. IEEE Comput. Car-
    diol. 1980, pp. 263-266.
Holsinger, W.P., Kempner, K.M. and Miller M.H. 1971. "A QRS pre-processor
    based on digital differentiation". IEEE Trans. Biomed. Eng., BME-18,
    pp. 212-217.
McClelland, K.M. and Arnold, J.M. 1976. "A QRS detection algorithm for com-
    puterized ECG monitoring". Proc. IEEE Comput. Cardiol. 1976, pp. 447-
    450.
Mead, C.N., Clark, K.W., Potter, S.J., Moore, S.M. and Thomas Jr. L.J. 1979.
    "Development and evaluation of a new QRS detector/delineator". Proc.
    IEEE Comput. Cardiol. 1979, pp. 251-254.
Murthy, I.S.N. and Rangaraj, M.R. 1979. "New concepts for PVC detection".
    IEEE Trans. Biomed. Eng., BME-26, pp. 409-416.
Nygårds, M-E. and Hulting, J. 1979. "An automated system for ECG monitoring"
    Comput. Biomed. Res., Vol. 12, pp. 181-202.
Nygårds, M-E. and Sörnmo, L. 1983. "Delineation of the QRS complex using
    the envelope of the ECG". Accepted for publication in Med. Biol. Eng.
    & Comput.
Okada, M. 1979. "A digital filter for the QRS complex detection". IEEE
    Trans. Biomed. Eng., BME-26, pp. 700-703.
Pahlm, O., Börjesson, P.O., Johansson, K., Jonsson, B., Petersson, K.,
    Sörnmo, L. and Werner, O. 1978. "Efficient data compression and ar-
    rhythmia detection for long-term ECGs". Proc. IEEE Comput. Cardiol.
    1978, pp. 395-396.
Pryor, T.A., Russell, R., Budkin, A. and Price W.G. 1969. "Electrocardio-
    graphic interpretation by computer". Comput. Biomed. Res., Vol. 2, pp.
    538-548.
Ripley, K.L. and Murray, A. 1980. "Introduction to arrhythmia monitoring".
    IEEE Computer Society, pp. 71-87.

Schluter, P., Mark, R., Moody, G., Olson, W. and Peterson, S. 1980. "Performance measures for arrhythmia detection". Proc. IEEE Comput. Cardiol. 1980, pp. 267-270.

Shah, P.M., Arnold, J.M., Haberern, N.A., Bliss, D.T., McClelland, K.M. and Clarke, W.B. 1977. "Automatic real time arrhythmia monitoring in the intensive care unit". Am. J. Cardiol., Vol. 39, pp. 701-708.

Sörnmo, L. 1982. "Performance evaluation of an adaptive QRS detector". Technical Report TR-169, September 1982. Telecommunication Theory, University of Lund, Sweden.

Sörnmo, L., Pahlm, O. and Nygårds, M-E. 1982. "Adaptive QRS detection in ambulatory ECG monitoring: a study of performances". Proc. IEEE Comput. Cardiol. 1982.

Thakor, N.V., Webster, J.G. and Tompkins, W.J. 1980. "Optimal QRS filter". IEEE Front. Eng. Health Care, pp. 190-195.

Thakor, N.V. and Webster, J.G. 1981. "Optimal QRS detector". IEEE Front. Eng. Health Care, 1981.

Zywietz, C., Grabbe, W. and Hampel, G. 1981. "HES LKG, a new program for computer assisted analysis of Holter electrocardiograms". Proc. IEEE Comput. Cardiol. 1981, pp. 169-172.

PERFORMANCE COMPARISON OF FAST QRS DETECTION ALGORITHMS. +

A. Taddei*, C. Marchesi*, L. Landucci**

* Istituto di Fisiologia Clinica del CNR
** Universita' degli Studi di Pisa
56100 Pisa, Italia

ABSTRACT

A beat by beat evaluation of the QRS detector performance by means of an annotated ECG database is described. Fast software detectors have been compared in terms of sensitivity and specificity. Moreover the execution time is considered for accelerated time software analyses.

INTRODUCTION

The detection of the QRS complex is a basic problem in the analysis of the ECG signal; though many algorithms and devices are described in the literature, the problem hasn't yet been definitely solved because the ECG signal is affected by a large inter and intra patient variability in the morphology, rhythm and amplitude. A great versatility is particularly required in the analysis of long term ECG tracings (in CCU and in Ambulatory Monitoring). A QRS detector can work very well in several cases, but it can fail in other very significant cases in the presence of some abnormal beats. Therefore it is important to evaluate the algorithm performance in relation to the different abnormalities. This is a general problem in the development and in the application of any analysis system; in fact more and more systems are available for the analysis of the ECG signal, but often there is a lack of significant data about the assessment of their performances. The various systems are often tested in different ways and by means of different ECG databases, probably too small and sometimes "biased" in favor to the system under test (Ripley and Oliver, 1977). The topic of the performance   evaluation has been largely considered in the last years and some attempts have also been made for the solution of this problem in the field of the arrhythmia detection (Schluter et al., 1980). It is generally admitted that the best way of evaluating the performance of an analysis algorithm is the comparison with an annotated ECG database, representing the different clinical conditions

---

+ Partly supported by CNR Special Project on Biomedical and Clinical Engineering.

(Ripley and Arthur, 1975). The algorithm is tested beat by beat over the reference ECG data in order to identify the conditions in which it produces false negatives and false positives; from these results generally a performance figure is obtained in terms of sensitivity and specificity. Moreover different algorithms, tested on the same database, can be compared for the selection of the best one in a particular application.

This paper deals with the performance evaluation of QRS detection algorithms particularly suited to Ambulatory ECG analyzers. The detectors under test are evaluated in sensitivity and specificity over an annotated database, under development at our institute, which includes the most typical arrhythmias and also the ST-T change episodes. The high speed analysis of Ambulatory ECG recordings requires very efficient detection algorithms in order to minimize the computer time consumption. So fast detectors have been considered in this evaluation and a sampling rate of 100 Hz has been selected.

MATERIAL AND METHODS.

Every QRS detection algorithm has been evaluated using as a test set an annotated ECG database, under development at the Clinical Physiology Institute of Pisa (Taddei et al., 1983). The database consists of three hour ECG segments, selected from 24 hour recordings on ambulant patients, affected by the most important arrhythmias and ST-T change episodes, compatible with ischemia. The ECG signal is sampled and stored by means of a minicomputer (HP 1000). Every QRS complex of the database is identified and annotated in order to allow the beat by beat evaluation of the analysis algorithms. Two groups of cardiologists perform the selection and the annotation of the interesting cases.

As the database is still under development, the results of the detector evaluation have a significant value only as far as the comparison of different algorithms.

The detectors under test are implemented on the computer; analog devices are simulated by means of the digital filtering techniques (Antoniou, 1979).

The detection algorithm is tested beat by beat over the ECG database performing the comparison between the QRS complex annotation and the detector output. Therefore it is possible to identify the conditions in which the algorithm misses the QRS complex or produces false detections in order to derive its sensitivity and specificity.

According to the decision theory concepts (Egan, 1975), the detection process has four possible outcomes; the two detector outputs (event present and absent) are conditioned by the presence or absence of the QRS event at the input. For every ECG cycle the QRS event is judged to be present during the QRS complex interval and absent in the complementary interval. A match window extending from −50 ms before to +240 ms after the QRS onset has been established for distinguishing true from false detections (Cox et al., 1980).

EVENT

	ABSENT	PRESENT
ABSENT DETECTION	CORRECT REJECTION	FALSE NEGATIVE
PRESENT	FALSE POSITIVE	CORRECT DETECTION

Fig.1 Outcomes of the detection process.

The four possible outcomes are: correct detection and false negative in the presence of the event, correct rejection and false positive in the absence of the event (fig. 1). The sensitivity is equal to the ratio of correct detections to the total of events present and the specificity is equal to the complement to the unity of the ratio of false positives to the total of event absent. In this case the number of events present and of the events absent are equal, because every ECG cycle includes one event present and one event absent. If we call TQRS, FP and FN respectively the total of QRS complexes of the database, of false positives and of false negatives, the quantities "correct detections rate" (CDR) and "false positives rate" (FPR) are derived from the equations:

$CDR = (TQRS-FN)/TQRS$; $FPR = FP/TQRS$.

192

The sensitivity is equal to CDR and the specificity is equal to the complement to the unity of FPR.

Usually QRS detectors depend on a number of parameters, the values of which must be selected for the optimal working. So the evaluation is repeated more times for different values of the detector parameters, obtaining the corresponding values of sensitivity and specificity. The evaluation results are represented as performance graphs in terms of the coordinates "correct detections rate" and "false positives rate" (fig. 2). Every point in the representation shows the performance of the detector under test over the reference database for a particular selection of the parameter values.

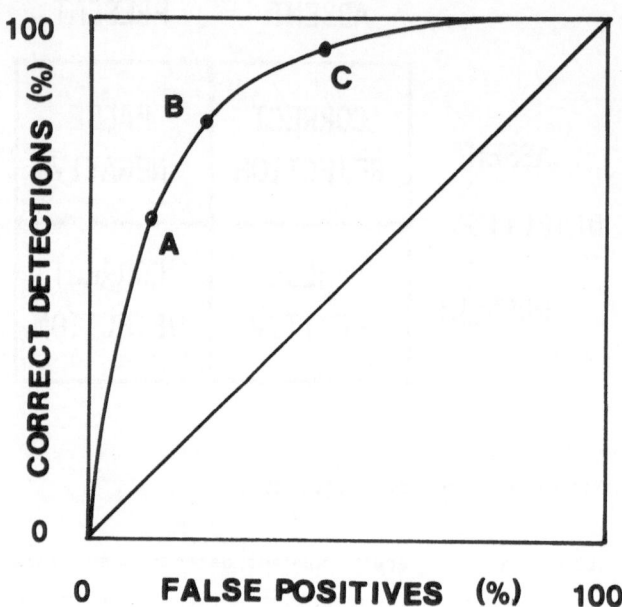

Fig.2   Performance characteristic curve.

The diagonal represents the performance of a detector operating at chance level. A typical situation is depicted from the curve, with the points A,B,C. The better the detector, the closer to the upper left its operating point will be. Following this criterion, the point B is the best one among the three operating points (A,B,C). The point A describes a detector with a moderate detection rate and few false positives while the point C corresponds to the detection of more events but also of more false positives.

However generally the performance curve of a QRS detector has a pattern deviating from the stylized situation of fig.2, because it depends on the distribution of the events detected and on the number of parameters driving the algorithm structure.

Anyway following the criterion of the best compromise between the sensitivity and the specificity, it is possible to select the optimal parameter values of every detector with reference to the used test database. The evaluation results obtained in the best conditions over the same test set are used for the comparison of different detectors; so the best detector can be individuated for a particular application.

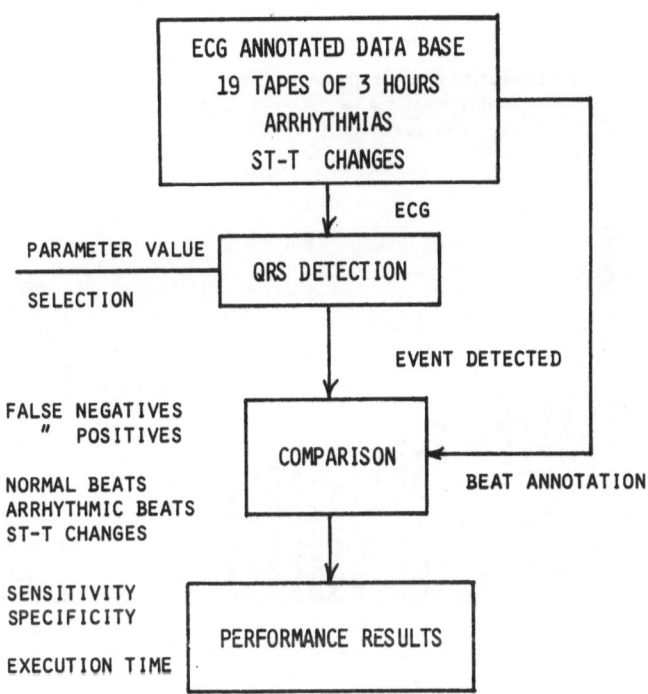

Fig.3   Evaluation of the QRS detector performance.

The detector evaluation performed on the whole QRS complex set doesn't point out in an expressive way the performance of the algorithm in the presence of some abnormal beats, which often occurr at a low rate but are very important for the diagnosis.   In fact the number of arrhythmic beats or of the ST-T change beats in our database are less than 10 % of the total.   In order to assess the algorithm capability of detecting also the abnormal events, a detailed evaluation is performed by the discrimination

194

of the normal beats and the arrhythmic and the ST-T change beats (fig. 3).

Another problem is represented by the variability of the detector performance with different ECG tracings; the detector can fail in the presence of some particular waveforms, but this isn't expressed by the average results. So the performance distribution on the various cases of the database is useful information.

The observation of these detailed results allows the identification of "difficult tapes" and so the critical waveforms can be easily individuated and the detection algorithm can be improved (Zeelenberg and Meij, 1982).

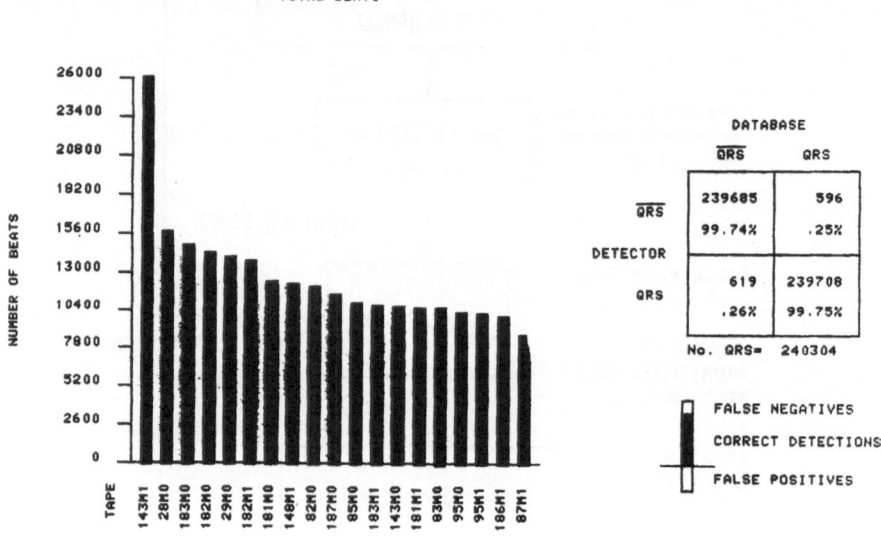

Fig.4   Tape by tape representation of the detector performance.

The fig. 4,5,6 show the performance of a QRS detector with reference to all the beats and to the classes of arrhythmic and ST-T change beats and its distribution tape by tape. We see that the tapes 182MO (fig.5) and 83MO (fig.6) are the most critical respectively in the class of arrhythmic and ST-T beats; the first tape contains episodes of atrial fibrillation and the second episodes of ST-T elevation associated to an abnormal P wave.

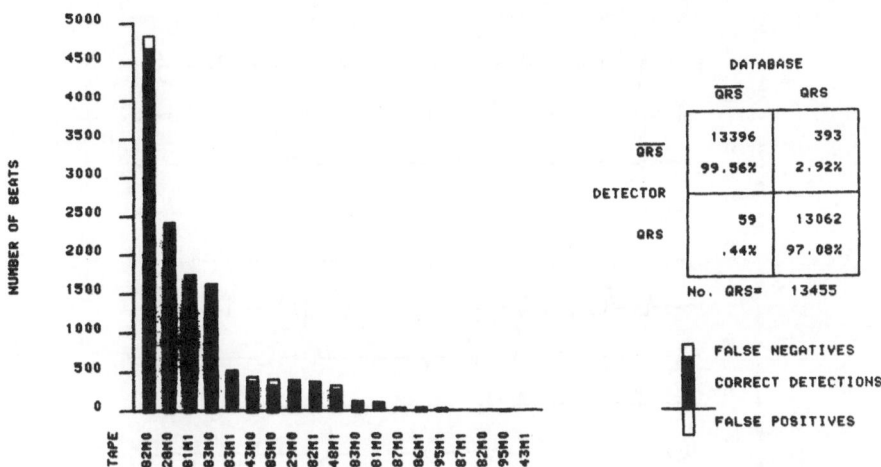

Fig.5   Representation of detector performance for the arrhythmias.

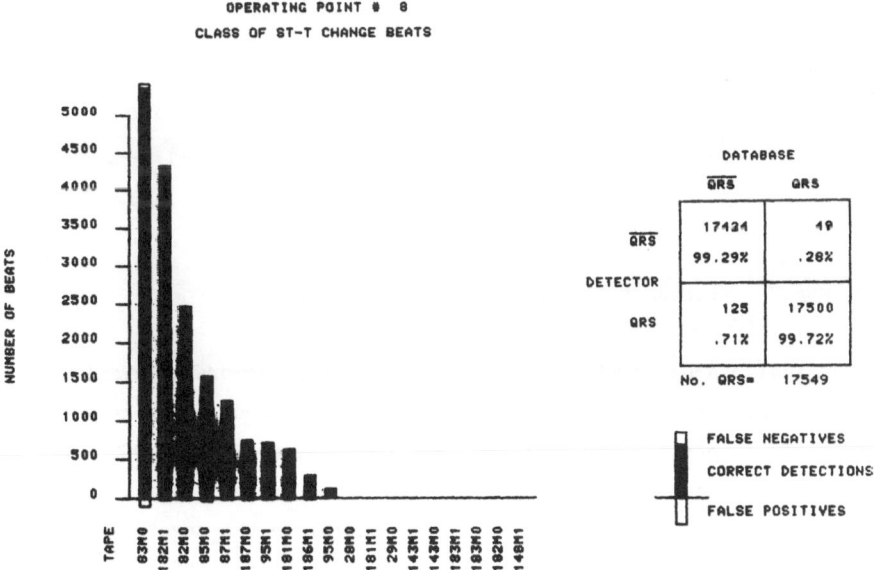

Fig.6   Representation of detector performance for the ST-T changes.

196

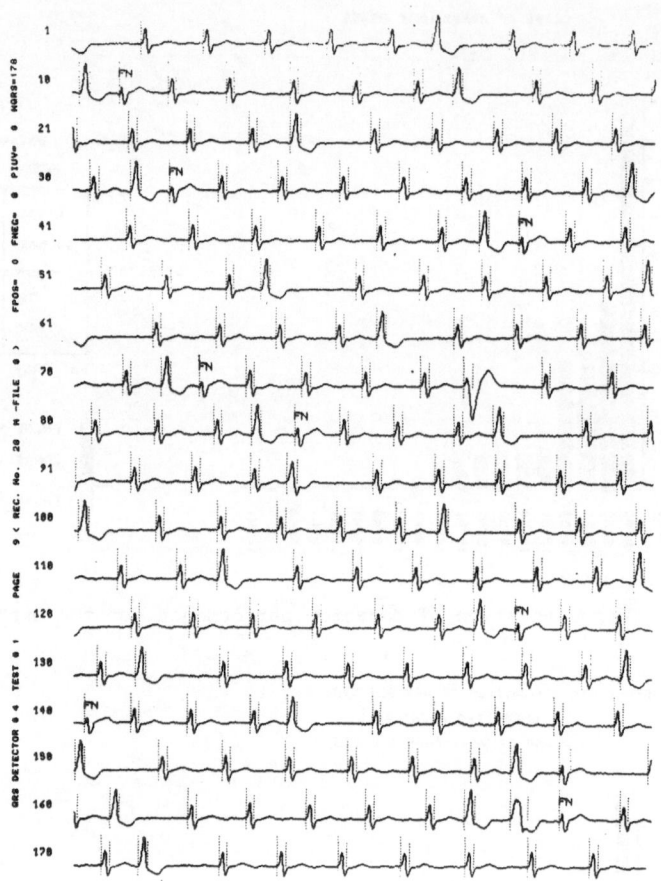

Fig.7   Representation of QRS detector errors.

A graphical representation of the QRS detector errors is available: the ECG tracing, in the format of one page for two minutes, is hardcopied by means of a graphic printer and the comments about the QRS detection outcome are associated to each beat (FN= false negative, FP= false positive) (fig. 7). This facility is useful in the development of an algorithm; however it is important to use distinct ECG sets for the development and for the test, otherwise a severe bias can be introduced (Ripley and Oliver, 1977).

APPLICATIONS AND RESULTS

The evaluation method is applicable to every QRS detector, analog or digital. Analog detectors are simulated on the computer; the characteristics of the analog filters are implemented by software using the IIR and FIR techniques (Antoniou, 1979).

At this time the method has been applied to software detectors to be used in a system for the high speed analysis of Ambulatory ECG recordings. This system requires a very efficient detection algorithm; the detector structure must be complete but also minimal in order to optimize processing efficiency.

Generally the software realization allows a more complex algorithm structure, a great flexibility, a controlled accuracy; therefore the actual trend is towards the software also because of the large diffusion of powerful and low cost microprocessor units. However, the limiting factor is represented by the algorithm execution time, to be kept low in the accelerated time analysis. Sometimes hardware is associated to software for saving the computer time.

At first eight detectors have been considered and tested on some ECG data, but only five of these have been completely evaluated over the database. In fact three detectors have been tested only on a subset of nine cases: one (Murthy and Rangaraj, 1979) is too much time consuming (70% the real time at a sampling rate of 200 Hz), the second (Okada, 1979) has a too low value of specificity (about 95%) and the other, the software version of an analog device (Remco, 1982), has low values of sensitivity and specificity (about 98%).

The general structure of a QRS detector, implemented in a computer system, is shown in fig.8. At first the analog ECG signal, obtained in line from a patient (in a real time analyzer) or off line from a reply unit (in a playback analyzer), is conditioned by means of a bandpass filter, which limits the bandwidth in order to reduce noise and to avoid aliasing. Then the signal is sampled, is A/D converted and stored on the computer. In our applications we have selected a sampling rate of 100 s.p.s. with a precision of 12 bits. Therefore the QRS detectors, working at a different sample rate, have been frequency adjusted. The numerical sequence is filtered for noise reduction, mains notching, low and high frequency attenuation (Mc Clelland and Arnold, 1976).

198

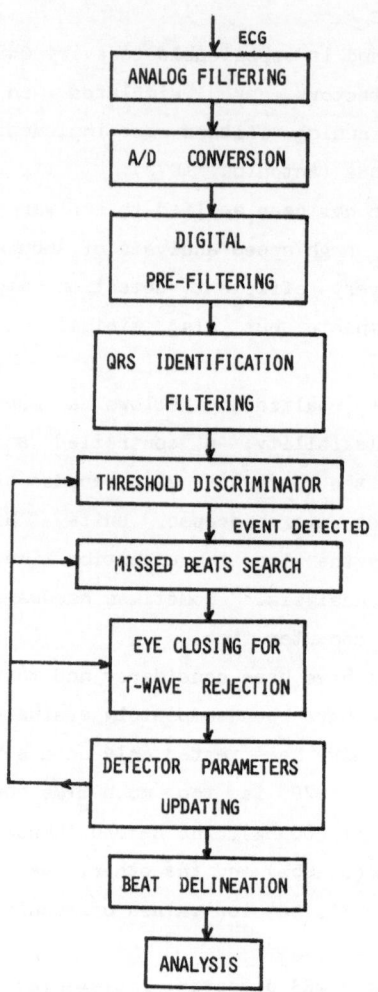

Fig.8   General structure of a software QRS detector.

The identification filter has the purpose of producing a signal that enhances the features of the QRS complex event against to other ECG events, such as the P wave, the T wave or artifacts. The signal slope is the most common feature considered in the discrimination of the QRS complex (Ripley and Murray, 1980). This is estimated by means of a differentiator with a low frequency response; often a non recursive equation is used for the realization, as in four of the detectors under test (Marchesi et al., 1982; Zeltron, 1982; Engelse and Zeelenberg, 1979) (see also appendix : detector no. 1,2,3,5). Sometimes a bandpass filter adjusted to the spectrum of the typical QRS waveform is used (Fraden and Neumann, 1980) or a "matched" filter, the impulse response of which has a QRS like pattern, is used, as in the fourth algorithm under test (Hanna, 1980). In other cases an high order transformation is applied in order to produce a single positive peak for each QRS complex (Murthy and Rangaraj, 1979; Okada, 1979).

The signal obtained from the identification filter is analysed for the event detection by the direct comparison with a voltage threshold or detecting the threshold crossings during an observation interval equal to the typical QRS duration, as in the second algorithm under test.

Some algorithms include a section for the search of the missed beats, as low amplitude beats or some ectopic beats; this section is ruled by less restrictive conditions and is activated from the overcoming of a RR time threshold. After a QRS complex has been detected, often the detector is disabled for the T wave rejection during a time interval fixed or variable with the mean heart period. If the detection algorithm is autoadaptive some parameters are modified in the course of the ECG tracing in order to follow the slow signal variations, as the mean R-R interval or the mean value of the signal derivative.

The five detection algoritms, described in appendix, have been evaluated beat by beat over the database of 19 patients; the test has been repeated more times for each detector with different values of its parameters. The results of the evaluation are graphically represented in terms of the correct detections rate and the false positives rate (fig. 9). The points, corresponding to different parameter values, in each graph describe one curve as in the first detector case or more curves, as in the second and third case, according to the number of parameters which are varied.

On these graphs we can identify the operating point corresponding to the optimal parameter values, which produce the best overall performance in terms of sensitivity and specificity.

The results obtained in the best conditions are represented in fig. 10. The sensitivity and specificity are indicated for the whole QRS population and for the classes of arrhythmic and ST-T change beats. Also the execution time is indicated because it is an important factor in an accelerated time application.

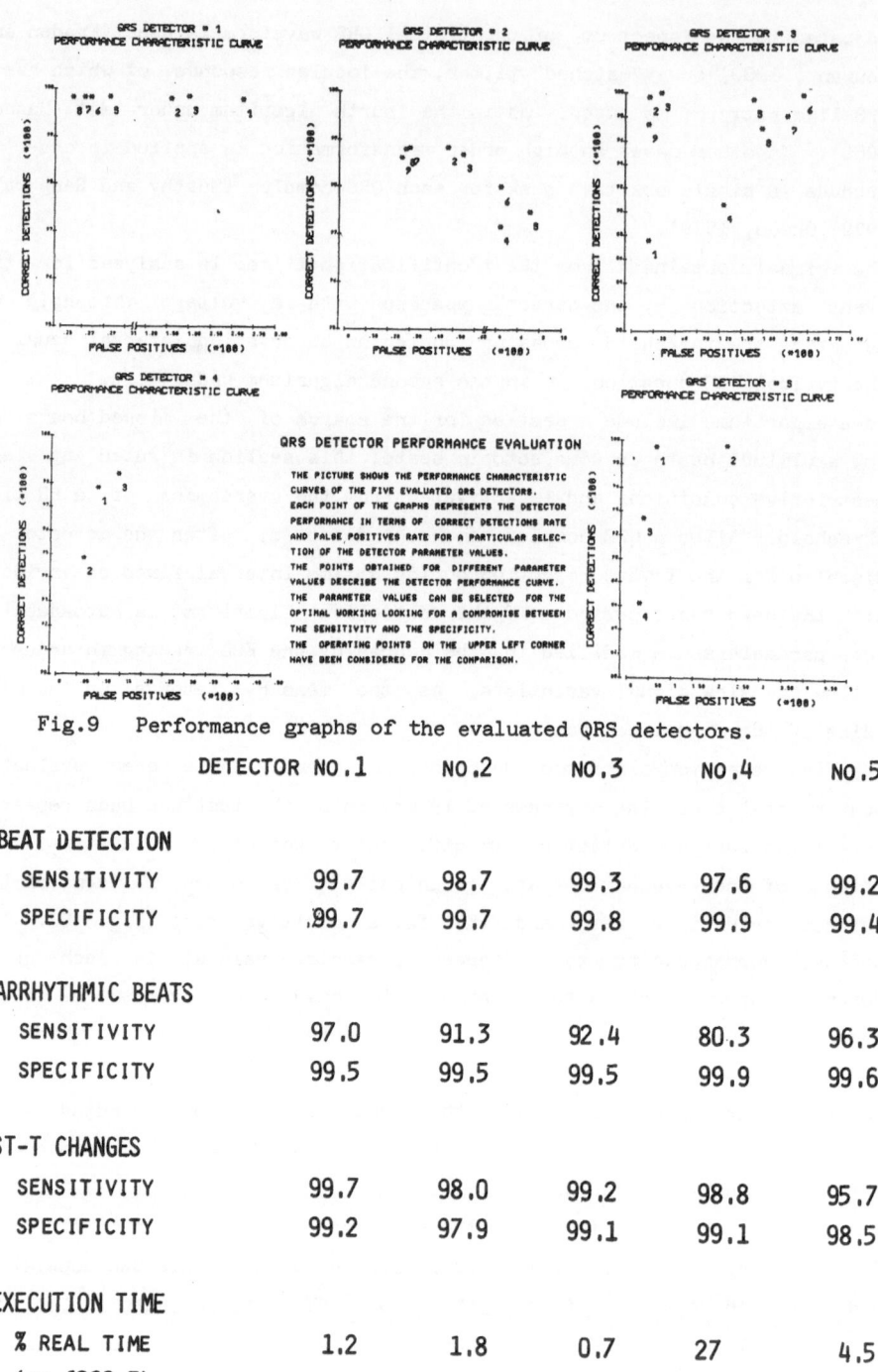

Fig.9   Performance graphs of the evaluated QRS detectors.

	DETECTOR NO.1	NO.2	NO.3	NO.4	NO.5
BEAT DETECTION					
SENSITIVITY	99.7	98.7	99.3	97.6	99.2
SPECIFICITY	99.7	99.7	99.8	99.9	99.4
ARRHYTHMIC BEATS					
SENSITIVITY	97.0	91.3	92.4	80.3	96.3
SPECIFICITY	99.5	99.5	99.5	99.9	99.6
ST-T CHANGES					
SENSITIVITY	99.7	98.0	99.2	98.8	95.7
SPECIFICITY	99.2	97.9	99.1	99.1	98.5
EXECUTION TIME					
% REAL TIME	1.2	1.8	0.7	27	4.5
(HP 1000 F)					

Fig.10   Table of performance evaluation results.. Detector no.1: developed from the authors, no.2: Marchesi et al., no.3: Zeltron, no.4: Hanna, no.5: Engelse et al.

We see that the first detector is the best in terms of sensitivity and specificity in all the classes of beats. Its execution speed is more than sixty the real time (HP 1000 F). We observe that the fourth algorithm has a very high specificity, but is less sensitive in the presence of the arrhythmic beats, which often have an abnormal morphology, probably because it is based on the matched filter technique.

CONCLUSIONS

The performance evaluation of the QRS detection algorithms is an important task in the development and application of the ECG analysis systems. This method, based on a beat by beat comparison with an annotated database, allows an easy and objective estimation of the algorithm performance. The sensitivity and the specificity obtained in the best operating conditions of the algorithm and for the various classes of ECG events give a syntetic figure and allow the comparison of different detectors. However, a detailed description of the algorithm performance in relation to the different abnormalities is useful in order to account for variability of the ECG waveforms. Probably further investigation should be done to establish more significant quantities, well suited to identify the algorithm performance.

APPENDIX

Description of the evaluated QRS detectors.

All the tested detectors are software implemented on a minicomputer in FORTRAN IV (HP 1000 F). A sampling rate of 100 Hz and a precision of 12 bits are used. The detector characteristics are described with reference to the general block diagram of fig.9.

1) Detector no. 1.
The detector is based on the analysis of the signal absolute derivative. The QRS identification filter has a bandpass characteristic and is described in the frequency domain, using Z transform notation (Rabiner and Gold, 1975), by the transfer function:

$$(1-Z^{**}-2) * (1+Z^{**}-1).$$

In the time domain, the first part $(1-Z^{**}-2)$ forms the difference between the actual input and the input delayed two samples and the second part $(1+Z^{**}-1)$ is a low pass filter.

A QRS event is detected when the estimated absolute derivative overcomes a threshold (TH), which is updated by means of a recursive averaging formula in order to follow the beat to beat variations of the QRS complex waveform. After a new beat has been detected, a time window is opened for searching the point of maximum signal slope, which is assumed the fiducial point. The window duration has been selected of 150 ms., allowing moreover the rejection of an abnormal P wave.

An eye closing period follows the QRS identification: its duration (Tm) is variable and equates the expected value of the QT time interval, which is in non linear relation with the mean heart rate.

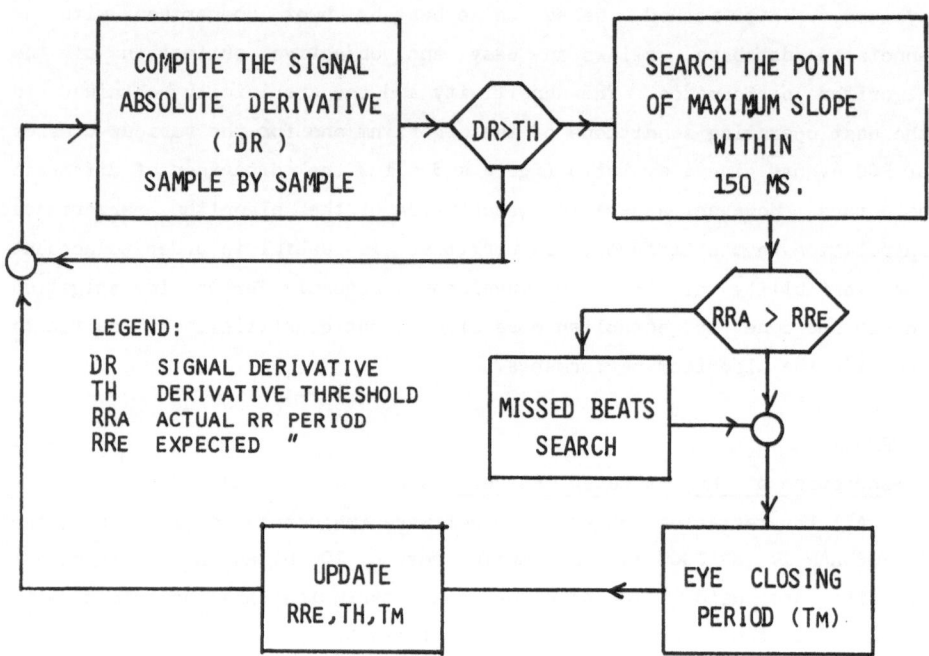

Fig.11   Block diagram of the QRS detector no.1.

The algorithm provides a look back feature for searching missed beats: this process is activated when the RR time interval of the actual cardiac cycle (RRa) has a duration longer than the expected value (RRe). In this phase the detection is ruled by less restrictive conditions.

The mean heart period (RRe) and the derivative threshold (TH), related to the mean QRS slope, are updated after each detection, with the exception of the occurrence of premature or delayed beats.

2) Detector no. 2.

This detector, described previously (Marchesi et al., 1982), is based on a first derivative/ time transform, controlled by two thresholds, on the derivative and on the observation window. The derivative is estimated by the non recursive equation:

$$DR(f(kT)) = \qquad h(nT) * f((k-n)T)$$

where DR is the digital derivative operator, $f(kT)$ is the digital signal, T is the sampling interval and $h(nT)$ $(n=0,1,...,N-1)$ is the finite impulse response. In this application: N=5, T=10 ms., $h(nT)= 2,1,0,-1,-2$.

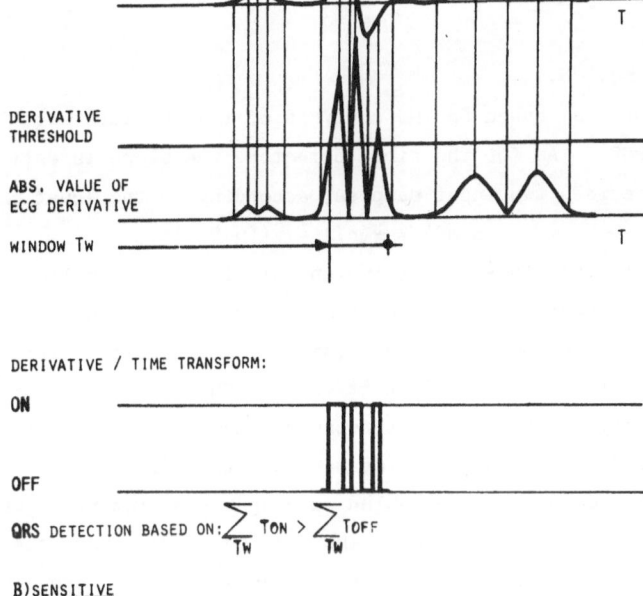

Fig.12   Decision logic of the detector no.2.

The derivative DR is rectified in order to make the algorithm independent from the polarity. The algorithm includes two steps. In the first pass, highly specific, the absolute value of the signal derivative is continuously compared to a threshold (TH). Each crossing instant initiates the measurement of the time (Ton), in which the derivative remains higher than the threshold and of the time in which it remains lower (Toff), within a time window Tw. The detection is based on the comparison between Ton and Toff (fig. 12).

The second pass, intended to increase the sensitivity, is activated when a RR interval is found higher than a continuously updated expectation limit. In this case Ton, measured in the RR intervals, is compared to an updated less restrictive time threshold, to detect possible missed beats.

The algorithm updates beat by beat the values of the parameters used for the detection (TH, Tw) and for the activation of the "missed beats" section.

3) Detector no. 3.

The detector is based on the analysis of the absolute signal derivative (Zeltron, 1982). As for the first detector, the slope is estimated by the difference between two input samples, according to the equation:

$$S(nT) = x(nT) - x((n-2)T);$$

where $S(nT)$ is the slope at the instant nT, T is the sampling interval and $x(nT)$ is the signal sample (Fancott and Wong, 1980). This filter provides a low pass attenuation following a $(\sin x)/x$ curve with a zero crossing at 50 Hz (a sampling rate of 100 Hz is used). The signal absolute derivative is continuously compared to a threshold; each crossing provides a new QRS detection and initiates the search of the first peak of the slope. Afterwards the detector is disabled during a time interval, which is in a fixed proportion to the mean heart period. Moreover the derivative threshold (TH), the mean heart period (RRm) and the eye closing period (Tm) are updated beat by beat (fig.13).

4) Detector no. 4.

The detector is based on a QRS- matched filter (Hanna, 1980). This filter is a fifteen- sample FIR filter, whose impulse response shape approximates the slope of a normal heart beat waveform. Therefore the filter has maximum absolute output when similarly- shaped waveforms are entered. The signal is conditioned by a low pass four-pole, 30 Hz, IIR filter and by a high pass 1.25 Hz filter; the corresponding transfer functions are:

$$HLP(z)= 0.57 \quad \frac{4.59+9.19*Z**-1+4.59*Z**-2}{1+0.32*Z**-1+0.06*Z**-2} \quad \frac{6.33+12.66*Z**-1+6.33*Z**-2}{1+0.45*Z**-1+0.46*Z**-2} \; ;$$

$$HHP(z)= \frac{0.94-1.89*Z**-1+0.94*Z**-2}{1-1.88*Z**-1+0.89*Z**-2} \; .$$

Then the signal is input to the QRS- matched filter; a threshold discriminator identifies QRS complexes. The threshold value decreases from the average QRS wave amplitude to half that value at a rate determined by the average QRS amplitude and average R-R interval.   An eye closing interval follows each beat. When a beat is detected, the average R-R interval and the average QRS amplitude are updated.

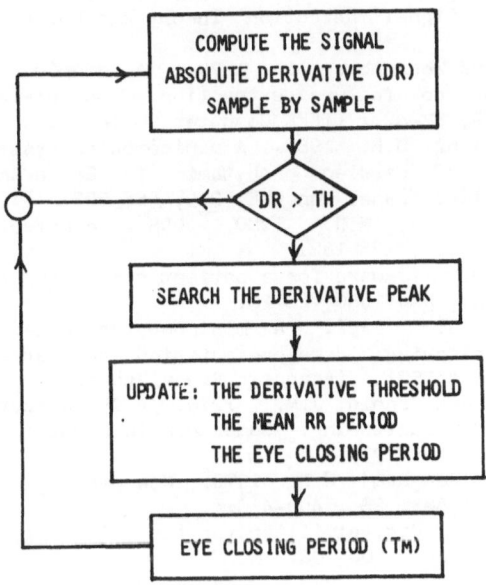

Fig.13   Block diagram of the detector no.3.

5) Detector no. 5.

The detector is based on the analysis of the signal   derivative (Engelse and Zeelenberg, 1979).   A digital filtering section provides baseline calculation, phase correction and first derivative estimation. The original version of the algorithm is designed for a 250-Hz sampling rate; so the filters have been frequency adjusted in order to perform the test at 100 Hz.

The QRS detector logic is based on the continuous comparison of the derivative with a threshold value; if this threshold is exceeded, a potential QRS onset is defined and a search is started to check the derivative pattern until a timeout occurs. Finally depending on the number of threshold crossings a baseline shift, a QRS complex or noise is recorded. After a QRS is detected the threshold value is adjusted.

REFERENCES

Antoniou, A. 1979. Digital Filters: analysis and design. (Mc Graw-Hill Book Co.)

Cox, J.R. et al. 1980. Evaluation of performance. In "Ambulatory Electrocardiographic Recording" (Ed. N.K.Wenger, M.B. Mock and R. Ringqvist) (Year Book Medical Publishers). pp. 183-197.

Egan, J.P. 1975. Signal Detection Theory and ROC Analysis. (Academic Press).

Engelse, W.A.H. and Zeelenberg, C. 1979. A single scan algorithm for QRS detection and feature extraction. Computers in Cardiology, September 1979, 37-42. (IEEE Computer Society).

Fancott, T. and Wong, D.H. 1980. A minicomputer system for direct high speed analysis of cardiac arrhythmia in 24 h Ambulatory ECG tape recordings. IEEE Trans. on BME, 27 , 685-693.

Fraden, J. and Neumann, M.R. 1980. QRS wave detection. Med. Biol. Eng. Comput., 18 , 125-132.

Hanna, K.L. 1980. Firmware for a patient monitoring station. Hewlett Packard Journal, Nov.1980, 23-28.

Marchesi, C. et al. 1982. A minicomputer based system for ECG ambulatory monitoring: data presentation and statistical evaluation. Proc. ISAM Gent 1981. (Academic Press, London). pp. 135-141.

Mc Clelland, K.M. and Arnold, J.M. 1976. A QRS detection algorithm for computerized ECG monitoring. Computers in Cardiology, 1976, 447-450. (IEEE Computer Society).

Murthy, I.S.N. and Rangaraj, M.R. 1979. New concepts for PVC detection. IEEE Trans. on BME, 26 , 409-416.

Okada, M. 1979. A digital filter for the QRS complex detection. IEEE Trans. on BME, 26 , 700-703.

Rabiner, L.R. and Gold, B. 1975. Theory and application of digital signal processing. Prentice Hall, Inc.

Remco Italia S.p.A., 1982. Personal communication. S.Pedrino di Vignate (MI), Italy.

Ripley, K.L. and Arthur, R.M. 1975. Evaluation and comparison of automatic arrhythmia detectors. Computers in Cardiology, 27-32, Long Beach, CA. (IEEE Computer Society).

Ripley, K.L. and Murray, A. 1980. Ventricular arrhythmia detectors. In "Introduction to automated arrhythmia detection". (IEEE Computer Society). pp. 71-87.

Ripley, K.L. and Oliver, G.C. 1977. Development of an ECG data base for arrhythmia detector evaluation. Computers in Cardiology, 203-209, Long Beach, CA. (IEEE Computer Society).

Schluter, P. et al. 1980. Performance measures for arrhythmia detectors. Computers in Cardiology, 267-270 (IEEE Computer Society).

Taddei, A. et al. 1983. Pilot study and preliminary experiences with a data base for the evaluation of algorithms for detection of arrhythmic and ischemic episodes. Proc. First Workshop on Ambulatory Monitoring (this volume). Pisa, April 11-12, 1983.

Zeelenberg, C. and Meij, S.H. 1982. Evaluation and optimization of an existing arrhythmia detection system by using an annotated ECG database. Computers in Cardiology 1981, 103-108. (IEEE Computer Society).

Zeltron S.p.A. 1982. Personal communication. Campoformido (UD), Italy.

DISCUSSION

Chairman: B.McA Sayers

3.1 - Algorithms for cardiac cycle detection.

MARCHESI: How do you manage, Dr. Pahlm, the problem of the duration of the observation interval? PAHLM: Concretely we take a primary selection of intervals of 300 samples and within that period we find no significant events, and that then delimits the secondary observation interval and within that we do the detection. Now 300 was just chosen because most of the RR intervals are shorter than 300 samples so we're almost sure that within that there is at least an QRS complex. Of course, you may run into the case where is no QRS complex because of the asystole. And of course you cannot lower your threshold, because then you will just adapt to the noise, so one has to be careful. I don't think the use of 300 is critical.

SAYERS: Much of what I've been hearing this morning I heard about 15 years ago. That was at the time when ECG computer processing was first approached and an enormous amount of effort put on this, and much work was done for example on the optimum choice of a band-pass filter for preprocessing and a variety of algoirthms were produced and, as far as I know, got into the system. Clearly, circumstances differ in the presence of micro-processors in the ambulatory monitoring situation. But I'm not sure there's been any new advance, that wasn't really know 10 years ago. Are you unable to explain to me where I am mis-reading the situation?

ZEELENBERG: I think you're right to a large extent, if one looks at the efforts that have been proven in arrhythmias detection in the last decade to 15 years or so. I think the last few years have concentrated on beat characterisation, rather than QRS detection. I think QRS detection systems, about 10-15 years ago, have proven to be not that easy to improve: while it's the beat classification algorithms that have improved enormously in the last 10-15 years. Probably by putting in more processing time one can improve performances, but I think this has been much more difficult for the QRS detection.

ZYWIETZ: Another reason may be that only during the last years have we collected systematically the necessary data for evaluation of those detectors, so this is maybe a reason why only during the last three years, or so, systematic analysis of performance was done.

SAYERS: I think this a very fair point. I recall many discussions leading to the establishment of data bases in the first instance, many years ago, so that probably has a lot to do with it.

ZEELENBERG: It's much easier to evaluate a beat-classification algorithm once you've done the QRS detection, because it reduces the analysis to the consideration of a few files which only contain the features for each beat. From them you get much quicker results, than trying to optimize QRS detection algorithms.

VAN BEMMEL: I think what I've heard until now in the area of ambulatory monitoring, has not reached the level of what we have reached in ECG interpretation systems, and this is mainly caused, I think, by the fact that in the early days of ambulatory monitoring, you just coped with R-R intervals. Only now you're going to improve and optimize it, and learning and testing data bases are becoming available. That's one thing: and a second thing is in order to improve that last 0.1% you need five or ten more years, and that is what we have experienced in ECG interpretation as well. Of course the ideas were there 10, 15 years ago, but the improvment of the last percentages requires a lot of effort. The other point is whether it's worth the effort. That's another question.

TADDEI: I would observe that in the QRS detection evaluation it is important to evaluate the algorithms, also under the presence of ST changes episodes, because I think so far we have evaluated the detectors only during arrhythmias episodes.

PINCIROLI: I have a question for Taddei: you have considered 4 different algorithms and you found different results for each of these. To your knowledge, inside the definition of the algorithm, is there any characteristic, able to justify the results you've obtained. Some theoretical reason of the results.

TADDEI: I think that an important feature in QRS detection is the look-back analysis feature. In this way we can work with high specificity in the first phase of detection. and in second phase we can work with larger sensitivity, because of the look-back feature. Among the algorithms we've considered thre are based on a differentiation and another on the match filter. We observed that in the fourth case with the match filter, the specificity was very high, because the correlation with the typical QRS is made. In the other cases, the introduction of the look back feature gives a larger sensitivity.

COUMEL: I go back to Van Bemmel's intervention. As a clinician, my opinion is that either you are dealing with very nice tracing and you may have 99.9 confidence in the results of the computer, or you are dealing with bad tracing. You have only to reject them and take others. I think that we have to deal not with one, or two, but with three channels. I know the names of these channels, X,Y and Z.

TOPIC: 3.2

Feature extraction for ECG waveforms characterization

FEATURE EXTRACTION FROM ECG WAVEFORMS;
TECHNIQUES USED BY AUTOMATIC ANALYSIS SYSTEMS AND CLINICAL OBSERVERS
COMPARED AND CONTRASTED

A. Murray

Regional Medical Physics Department
Freeman Hospital
Newcastle upon Tyne, UK

ABSTRACT

Techniques in current use for automatic feature extraction are examined and comparisons are made with visual techniques in an attempt to discover new approaches to automatic analysis of 24 h ECG recordings.

INTRODUCTION

The reliable automatic detection of cardiac arrhythmias from continuous ECG recordings is vital for the satisfactory analysis of these recordings. Such recordings are usually 24 h in duration and hence contain on average approximately 100 000 complexes. The process of isolating the relevant arrhythmias is often seen as 3 separate, even if interrelated, problems. They are as follows,

QRS detection

QRS feature extraction

QRS classification.

Sometimes the 3 are lumped together as in the operator identification of arrhythmias (Gymoese et al., 1975) from computer generated screen pages; and in this case the operator carries out all 3 functions simultaneously.

More often than not there is feedback from later functions to improve the overall reliability. For example, if T waves are identified as "QRSs", the QRS detection process can be modified automatically.

This paper deals with feature extraction as a independent process, with details of its association with the other processes given when necessary. Emphasis is placed on the role of the cardiologist interpreting ECG write-outs and of the operator interacting with semi-automatic analysis systems, in a search for possible ways of improving feature extraction, and hence overall system performance, in future systems.

THE EARLY ANALYSERS

The earliest analyser (described by Holter, 1961) superimposed QRSs on

an oscilloscope screen, allowing the operator to note feature differences
visually. This visual display allowed differences in QRS shape and
coupling interval to be observed, even if in a somewhat crude approach when
compared with that of today's technology.

Initially all analysers were based on this visual approach, but there
soon followed an introduction of some automatic feature extraction. Timing
was the first feature to be dealt with. Although this is not a feature of
the QRS itself it does describe how the QRS is coupled to the previous
complex. Cashman and Stott (1974) described the use of hardware to detect
early QRSs, late QRSs, bradycardia and tachycardia. Neilson (1974) was one
of the first to store the "normal" shape and then compare all subsequent
QRS shapes with it. Both examples used standard electronic techniques
without the aid of a computer. Later, more complex analysis followed with
the ever increasing use of computers.

CLINICAL FEATURE EXTRACTION

There are a number of aspects of ECG analysis which a cardiologist
reporting on an ECG write-out or an operator using a semi-automatic
analysis system will consider, often perhaps unconsciously. These include
the following,

> knowledge of ECG waveforms
> experience in interpreting ECG waveforms
> context of waveform in continuous recording
> patient information
> clinical relevance of arrhythmias.

RELATION BETWEEN CLINICAL FEATURE EXTRACTION AND AUTOMATIC MACHINE ANALYSIS

The automatic machine obviously undertakes the repetative and tiring
parts of analysis better than a human observer would, and successful
efforts have been made in producing machines to undertake analysis of 24 h
recordings. In an attempt to improve automatic analysis further, there is
much that can be learnt from the more complex aspect of human analysis.

FEATURE EXTRACTION - THE QRS

There are two main features which describe the QRS; they are its
timing from the previous QRS, and its shape. Both require the QRS to have
been reliably identified and a consistent timing marker point to have been
found. This point should preferably, but not necessarily, be the start of

the QRS.

Timing is the simplest since it requires no complex feature extraction. Although timing allows tachycardia, bradycardia and asystole to be identified, its most important role has been in the detection of early ventricular ectopic complexes. By far the majority of ventricular complexes are early, even although a few are late escape complexes or fusion complexes.

Shape is a much more complex feature to handle. This can be done by either of two approaches, and sometimes by both. The first requires identification of specific features, while the second looks at the whole waveform as a single shape feature. In the first, the following have been examined: QRS width, amplitude, area, offset, perimeter, first voltage moment and initial T slope. Table 1 lists a number of centres using these techniques.

In the second approach, difference from a single "normal" complex or from families of different complexes have been used. Two techniques are in use: shape difference and correlation. Table 2 identifies the technique in use in some centres. It should be noted that some centres appear in both Tables 1 and 2, as they use a combination of both approaches. Further details and a comparison between the different approaches have been given by Ripley and Murray (1980).

One further technique which has been used is to extract features associated with frequency components. Mead et al. (1979) have carried out some work in this area, although it has been primarily associated with QRS detection. Anderson et al. (1980) has used frequency analysis of cross-correlated waveforms for QRS classification. The time domain approaches, nevertheless, are by far the most common techniques used.

There are some basic problems associated with feature extraction techniques - artifact, natural changes in features and the large variety of ectopic complex shapes. Artifact can distort the QRS and can cause misrecognition of the start of the QRS. This latter can be particularly troublesome for subtraction and correlation techniques which are sensitive to any inconsistency in the alignment of waveforms.

Of the feature extraction systems, that of Washington University in St. Louis is the most well known (Clark et al., 1977). Its ARGUS system has been used in a number of other centres including Rotterdam (Ripley et al., 1980) and Vienna (Joskowicz et al., 1979). Of the template analysis systems, that of Edinburgh (Neilson, 1974) has been used in a number of

215

TABLE 1 QRS feature extraction techniques in use.

Centre	amplitude	width	area	offset	polarity	other	
Boston, USA	X	X					Armington et al., 1978
Chicago, USA	X	X					Kinias et al., 1978
Hannover, Germany	X	X		X		T amplitude	Zywietz et al., 1981
Indianapolis, USA	X	X	X			T slope	Knoebel and Lovelace, 1978
Los Angeles, USA	X		X			perimeter, moment	Hansmann and Sheppard, 1975
Montreal, Canada		X					Fancott et al., 1980
New York, USA	X	X	X		X		Birman et al., 1978
Paris, France		X				mean deflection	Attuel et al., 1981
Pisa, Italy		X					Biella et al., 1979
Rotterdam, Netherlands	X	X	X	X			Ripley et al., 1980
St Louis, USA	X	X	X	X			Clark et al., 1977
Vienna, Austria	X	X	X	X			Joskowicz et al., 1979
West Haven, USA	X	X	X	X	X		Gradman and Lewis, 1978

TABLE 2 QRS shape comparison techniques in use.

Centre	technique used	
Copenhagen, Denmark	correlation	Gymoese et al., 1978
Edinburgh, UK	difference	Neilson, 1974
Harrow, UK	difference	Cashman, 1978
Nashville, USA	difference	Higgins et al., 1978
Philadelphia, USA	difference squared	Monster et al., 1978
Pisa, Italy	difference	Biella et al., 1979
Stanford, USA	correlation	Spitz et al., 1977
Sudbury, USA	correlation	Feldman et al., 1980
Tel-Aviv, Israel	correlation	Rosenberg and Tartakovsky, 1979
West Haven, USA	correlation	Gradman and Lewis, 1978

other systems, such as that of Newcastle upon Tyne (Murray et al., 1979) and Glasgow (Macfarlane et al., 1979).

FEATURE EXTRACTION - THE IMMEDIATE QRS CONTEXT

Features of the ECG waveform close to the QRS have to be taken into account. This may be to ensure that the detected "QRS" is a genuine QRS and not a large T wave or P wave. The artifactual noise level can also be assessed so that decision criteria can be altered if it is considered that there is noise which would influence feature extraction. Noise could include muscle artifact whose peaks might be mistaken for QRSs and baseline instability which might distort QRSs forcing them to be allocated to a different family.

Other non-QRS features which are worth examining are P waves, evidence of an artifical pacemaker, and ST changes. P waves are notoriously difficult to detect and little progress has been made in their detection, even although this is obviously the way of distinguishing ventricular from supraventricular complexes, such as bundle branch block. A cardiologist will always examine an ECG write-out for P waves in front of complexes with normal RR intervals. Some work on automatic P wave detection needs to be undertaken, perhaps from a second ECG channel with a lead deliberately chosen to have large P waves. Evidence of an artifical pacemaker is not easy to extract because the very high frequency pacing pulse is filtered out during the recording process. ST changes can also be difficult to detect if they are small (0.1 mV) because of ST segment distortion introduced by the relatively poor low frequency response of the recorder (Bragg-Remschel et al., 1982). However changes of more than 0.2 mV can often be accepted as genuine.

Techniques are, however, available for simplifying to some extent these problems. P waves can be detected if a small oesophageal electrode is swallowed and the wires secured so that the electrode lies close to the atria (Jenkins et al., 1979). This technique is not always reliable or acceptable to patients. If a special recorder is used with patients who have artificial pacemakers a relatively long marker pulse can be recorded synchronously with the pacing pulse on a second channel of the recorder (Murray et al., 1981; Kelen et al., 1980). If faithful ST recordings are required a recording process with good low frequency response (down to 0.05 Hz) is required. Although some of the newer recorders are beginning to approach this frequency, only recorders which use a frequency modulation process actually reach it. These recorders however do not tend to be as reliable as those using the more common direct recording process.

FEATURE EXTRACTION - THE OVERALL CONTEXT

Occasionally it is not easy to decide if an "arrhythmia" captured by an analyser is genuine. This might be when a broken lead results in an asystolic pause or when fast "VT like" baseline movement is produced by the patient scratching on top of the ECG electrode. Sometimes with a single ECG write-out it is impossible to decide if it is genuine. If artifactual events have happened it is likely that they will have occurred at other times in the recording, and other examples might look less genuine, confirming the artifact. The examples found must be put into the context of the whole recording.

As an extention of context, if more than one ECG lead is recorded the other lead must obviously be examined for confirmation of the findings on the first. In only the last few years have attempts been made to analyse more than one lead simultaneously (Bragg-Remschel et al., 1980; Rosenberg and Tartakovsky, 1979).

Another problem which can be overcome if context is taken into account is that in which a number of shape families are created for one type of complex. For example, this might be because of a change in QRS shape resulting from different patient postures, or might arise from fusion complexes. Both might have a continuous change in shape between the families stored, which would be lost if the continuum is represented by say only 2 families.

FEATURE EXTRACTION - KNOWLEDGE OF PATIENT

Knowledge of the patient's clinical condition would always be taken into account by a cardiologist reviewing the results of an ECG analysis. For example it would be helpful to know if the patient has an artificial pacemaker, or syncope had been experienced, indicating the possibility of asystolic pauses.

It is also helpful if information relating to patient symptoms is available.

FEATURE EXTRACTION - WIDER CLINICAL EXPERIENCE

The wider clinical experience of a reporting cardiologist should also be considered. While reporting he will have two general background pieces of information which will colour his assessment. These are the frequency with which an arrhythmia would be expected, and the diagnostic significance of any arrhythmia. An uncommon or diagnostically important arrhythmia would be examined more carefully. An analysis system could imitate this.

A cardiologist reporting on a clinical recording, does not make use of information about every ectopic complex. In research work, even if the research workers would like 100% accuracy, this would be of little relevance because of the now well established large variation from hour to hour and from day to day (Morganroth et al., 1978). Perhaps those who are providing the technical and computer facilities are trying too hard to achieve unrealistic accuracies for the detection of single venticular complexes.

WHAT CAN WE LEARN?

The cardiologist and the human operator of a semi-automatic analysis system inevitably approach analysis differently from the automatic feature extraction of a computer system. This is borne out by the fact that it is considered important to introduce an element of quality control into automatic analysis - we still need the human check. Although we have learnt much there might be a number of areas which could bear continued or further research -

> use special recording techniques to simplify analysis
> develop techniques for P wave identification
> be aware of QRS shape changes
> use 2 channel analysis if 2 channels recorded
> keep examples of artifact to compare with "pseudo arrhythmias"
> notify the system of "expected" arrhythmias
> use different sensitivity for more important arrhythmias
> reduce efforts into achieving highly accurate detection rates
> > for single ventricular complexes.

There is much that automatic analysis might achieve in improving and simplifying the analysis of ambulatory ECG recording.

REFERENCES

Anderson, C.M., Sanders, W.J. and Harrison, D.C. 1980. Comparing the morphologies of ECG waveforms in frequency space. In "Computers in Cardiology" (Ed. K.L. Ripley and H.G. Ostrow). (IEEE Computer Society, Los Angeles). pp. 15-19.
Armington, R.M., Graboys, T.B., Lown, B. and Lenson, R. 1978. Semiautomated data reduction of ventricular ectopic activity:

methodology and clinical application. Med. Instrum., 12, 340-342.

Attuel, P., Rosengarten, M., Leclercq, J.F., Milosevic, D., Mugica, J. and Coumel, Ph. 1981. Computer quantitated evaluation of cardiac arrhythmias. PACE, 4, 23-35.

Biella, M., Contini, C., Kraft, G., Marchesi, C., Mazzocca, G.F. and Taddei, A. 1979. A minicomputer based system for automatic analysis of 24 hour ECG and its evaluation. In "Computers in Cardiology" (Ed. K.L. Ripley and H.G. Ostrow). (IEEE Computer Society, Long Beach, California). pp. 201-204.

Birman, K.P., Rolnitzky, L.M. and Bigger, J.T. 1978. A shape oriented system for automated Holter ECG analysis. In "Computers in Cardiology" (Ed. K.L. Ripley and H.G. Ostrow). (IEEE Computer Society, Long Beach, California). pp. 217-220.

Bragg-Remschel, D.A., Anderson, C.M. and Winkle, R.A. 1982. Frequency response characteristics of ambulatory ECG monitoring systems and their implications for ST segment analysis. Am. Heart J., 103, 20-31.

Bragg-Remschel, D.A. and Harrison, D.C. 1980. A computerized two channel ambulatory arrhythmia analysis system. In "Computers in Cardiology" (Ed. K.L. Ripley and H.G. Ostrow). (IEEE Computer Society, Long Beach, California). pp. 197-200.

Cashman, P.M.M. 1978. A pattern-recognition program for continuous ECG processing in accelerated time. Comp. Biomed. Res. 11, 311-323.

Cashman, P.M.M. and Stott, F.D. 1974. A semi-automatic system for the analysis of 24 hour ECG recordings from ambulant subjects. Biomed. Eng., 9, 54-57.

Clark, K.W., Hitchens, R.E., Ritter, J.A., Rankin, S.L., Oliver, G.C. and Thomas, L.J. 1977. Argus/2H: a dual channel Holter-tape analysis system. In "Computers in Cardiology" (Ed. H.G. Ostrow and K.L. Ripley). (IEEE Computer Society, Long Beach, California). pp. 191-198.

Fancott, T., Wong, D. and Lemire, J. 1980. A software implementation of a high speed Holter ECG tape analysis system for a single small processor. In "Computers in Cardiology" (Ed. K.L. Ripley and H.G. Ostrow). (IEEE Computer Society, Los Angeles). pp. 131-134.

Feldman, C.L., Hubelbank, M., Lane, B. and Valvo, V. 1980. Performance enhancement of a Holter processing system with microprocessor controlled over-reading stations and remote terminals. In "Computers in Cardiology" (Ed. K.L. Ripley and H.G. Ostrow). (IEEE Computer Society, Los Angeles). pp. 127-130.

Gradman, A.H. and Lewis, J.W. 1978. YALECG: a new system for computer analysis of ambulatory electrocardiograms. In "Computers in Cardiology" (Ed. K.L. Ripley and H.G. Ostrow). (IEEE Computer Society, Long Beach, California). pp. 211-214.

Gymoese, E., Andersen, J.D. and Sandoe, E. 1978. Random access mass storage ECG-analysis system (RAMSES): a new system for quantitative analysis of long-term ECGs. In "Computers in Cardiology" (Ed. K.L. Ripley and H.G. Ostrow). (IEEE Computer Society, Long Beach, California). pp. 221-224.

Gymoese, E., Larsen, I.A., Andersen, J.D. and Sandoe E. 1975. A system for high-speed scanning of electrocardiographic tapes based on sequences of computer generated static TV pictures. In "Computers in Cardiology" (Ed. K.L. Ripley and H.G. Ostrow). (IEEE Computer Society, Long Beach, California). pp. 3-6.

Hansmann, D.R. and Sheppard, J.J. 1975. The new Dyna-Gram system for high speed analysis of ambulatory ECG. In "Computers in Cardiology" (Ed. K.L. Ripley and H.G. Ostrow). (IEEE Computer Society, Long

220

Beach, California). pp. 155-159.
Higgins, S.B., Woosley, R.L., Herrin, C.B., Compton, J.L. and Harris, T.R. 1978. A minicomputer based system for the quantification of ventricular arrhythmias. In "Computers in Cardiology" (Ed. K.L. Ripley and H.G. Ostrow). (IEEE Computer Society, Long Beach, California). pp. 355-358.
Holter, N.J. 1961. New method for heart studies. Science, 134, 1214-1220.
Jenkins, J.M., Wu, D. and Arzbaecher, R.C. 1979. Computer diagnosis of supraventricular and ventricular arrhythmias. Circulation, 60, 977-987.
Joskowicz, G., Balatka, H., Glogar, D., Weber, H. and Steinbach, K. 1979. A high speed digital Holter tape analysis with full editing capability. In "Computers in Cardiology" (Ed. K.L. Ripley and H.G. Ostrow). (IEEE Computer Society, Long Beach, California). pp. 277-280.
Kelen, G.J., Bloomfield, D.A., Hardage, M., Gomes, J.A., Khan, R., Gopalaswamy, C. and El Sherif, N. 1980. A clinical evaluation of an improved Holter monitoring technique for artificial pacemaker function. PACE, 3, 192-197.
Kinias, P., Norusis, M. and Fozzard, H.A. 1978. A dual-processor computer for arrhythmia analysis. Med. Instrum., 12, 330-331.
Knoebel, S.B. and Lovelace, D.E. 1978. A two-dimensional clustering technique for identification of multiform ventricular complexes. Med. Instrum., 12, 332-333.
Macfarlane, P.W., McClung, J., Irving, A., Watts, M.P., Taylor, T.P. and Lawrie, T.D.V. 1979. Computer assisted analysis of dynamic (24-hour) electrocardiograms. In "Progress in Electrocardiography" (Ed. P.W. Macfarlane). (Tunbridge Wells, Pitman Medical). pp. 123-126.
Mead, C.N., Cheng, J-S, Hitchens, R.E., Spenger, B.F. and Thomas, L.J. 1979. Recent progress in frequency-domain analysis of the ECG. In "Computers in Cardiology" (Ed. K.L. Ripley and H.G. Ostrow). (IEEE Computer Society, Long Beach, California). pp. 43-47.
Monster, A.W., O'Connor, D. and Chan, H. 1978. Rapid scanning of ambulatory EKG recordings using several computers operating in parallel. In "Computers in Cardiology" (Ed. K.L. Ripley and H.G. Ostrow). (IEEE Computer Society, Long Beach, California). pp. 33-38.
Morganroth, J. Michelson, E.L., Horowitz, L.N., Josephson, M.E., Pearlman, A.S. and Dunkman, W.B. 1978. Limitations of routine long-term electrocardiographic monitoring to assess ventricular ectopic frequency. Circulation, 58, 408-414.
Murray, A., Campbell, R.W.F. and Julian, D.G. 1979. Operator-controlled computer system for analysis of 24 hour electrocardiographic recordings. In "Computers in Cardiology" (Ed. K.L. Ripley and H.G. Ostrow). (IEEE Computer Society, Long Beach, California). pp. 197-199.
Murray, A., Jordan, R.S. and Gold, R.G. 1981. Pacemaker assessment in the ambulant patient. Br. Heart J., 46, 531-538.
Neilson, J.M. 1974. High speed analysis of ventricular arrhythmias from 24 hour recordings. In "Computers in Cardiology". (IEEE Computer Society, Long Beach, California). pp. 55-59.
Ripley, K.L. and Murray, A. 1980. Introduction to automated arrhythmia detection. (IEEE Computer Society, Long Beach, California).
Ripley, K.L., Okkerse, R.J., Engelse, W.A.H., Vinke, R.V.H. and Zeelenberg, C. 1980. Implementation of Argus/2H at the Thoraxcentrum. In "Computers in Cardiology" (Ed. K.L. Ripley and

H.G. Ostrow).   (IEEE Computer Society, Long Beach, California). pp. 135-138.

Rosenberg, N.W.   and Tartakovsky, M.B.   1979.   The TELAVIV system   - Three-channel Evaluation of Long-term ECG records for Atrial and Ventricular Identification and Verification of arrhythmia.   In "Computers in cardiology" (Ed. K.L. Ripley and H.G. Ostrow). (IEEE Computer Society, Long Beach, California). pp. 29-32.

Spitz, A.L., Fitzgerald, J.W.   and Harrison D.C.   1977.   Ambulatory arrhythmia quantification by a correlation technique. In "Computers in Cardiology" (Ed. H.G. Ostrow and K.L. Ripley).   (IEEE Computer Society, Long Beach, California).   pp. 225-231.

Zywietz, C., Grabbe, W. and Hemple, G. HES LKG, a new program for computer assisted analysis of Holter electrocardiograms. 1981. In "Computers in Cardiology" (Ed. K.L. Ripley). (IEEE Computer Society, Los Angeles). pp.169-172.

PARAMETER EXTRACTION FOR AUTOMATIC ANALYSIS OF ECG TRACES

R. Balzarotti, F. Bartoli, G. Baselli, S. Cerutti, D. Liberati

CNR Centro di Teoria dei Sistemi, Dipartimento di Elettronica
Politecnico di Milano, Piazza Leonardo da Vinci, 32, 20133 Milano, Italy

ABSTRACT

The present paper aims at introducing original techniques of linear digital filtering (traditional and optimal ones) for the automatic processing of ECG traces. Innovative feature extraction methods are also described in the area of parametric identification (feasible both using stochastic and deterministic signals) and of spectral estimate (Maximum Entropy Spectrum, Pisarenko Harmonic Deconvolution and Prony method). Results are shown in the field of automatic measurements of P, QRS, T waves and of heart rate variability on the basis of the time series constituted by the R-R intervals. The obtained parametrizations are discussed together with interesting applications foreseen in the future by the further development of methodological and technological means towards the implementation of new equipment for diagnosis and patient monitoring.

INTRODUCTION

The fundamental problem in biological signal processing is to determine a relation between the biological system under examination and the signal (or signals) produced by it (Sayers, 1977). Such a relation is achieved both by exploiting the anatomo-physiological knowledge of the system and by making an analysis of the produced signals. The signal processing procedure aims, therefore, at capturing the information which travel, in a dynamic way, inside the signal itself. The present paper wants to introduce a few methodologies of parameter extraction for ECG traces, with particular emphasis on digital filtering, identification and spectral estimation. The applications are in the area of P, QRS, T waves recognition and in the measurement and display of heart rate variability (HRV).

ECG SIGNAL PROCESSING AND PARAMETERS EXTRACTION

The whole procedure of ECG signal processing is described in the general block diagram of Fig. 1. The step of pre-processing is fundamental to obtain the transformed signals on which to carry out the phase of parameter extraction. These parameters are used to classify the signals and give objective elements to take a decision on the patient.

It is not the aim of the paper to deal with the general acquisition and A/D convertion aspects (reference may be made to (AHA, 1975; Ruttiman, 1977) at this regard). Basically, digital filtering applications will be

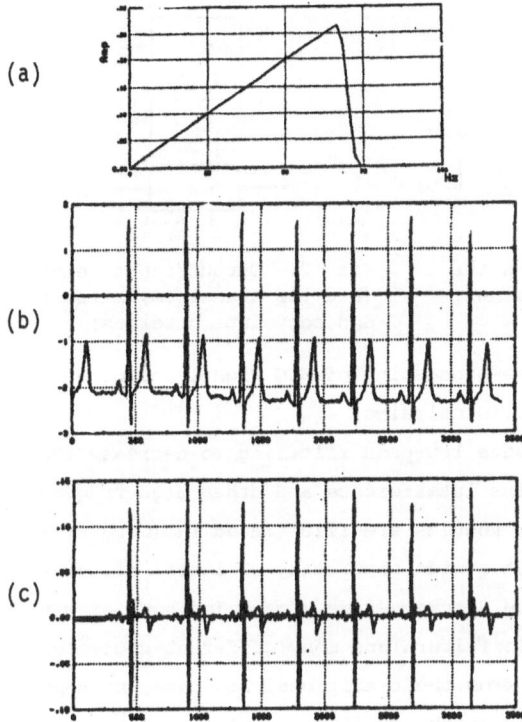

(a)

(b)

(c)

Fig. 3 - (a): Characteristic of derivative filter (low-pass 70 Hz); (b): original X lead signal; (c): filtered signal using (a).

A further step is the correction of the baselines drift: for details see (Bartoli, 1983a). Fig. 4 illustrates a fitting of the baseline using a sum of a polynomial and a sinusoid via non linear regression algorithm. Simpler algorithms of linear regression may be applied cycle-by-cycle using elementary fitting curves like straight-line, parabolic and cubic ones on a set of points estimated to be isoelectric (i.e. between T and P waves): the residual variance along the correction curve is an indicator of the baseline removal. Other approaches such as cubic splines (Meyer, 1977), Fourier expansion (Wellner, 1976), etc. are also possible.

In order to test the sensitivity of the wave recognition algorithms to different values of low-pass filtering, the results shown in Fig. 5 have been obtained The basic hypothesis is that the beat-to-beat variations in the wave durations for short time length are due to the noise superimposed on the tracings (the considered patients have no rhythm disturbancies). Fig. 5 shows the mean values with standard deviation of the durations

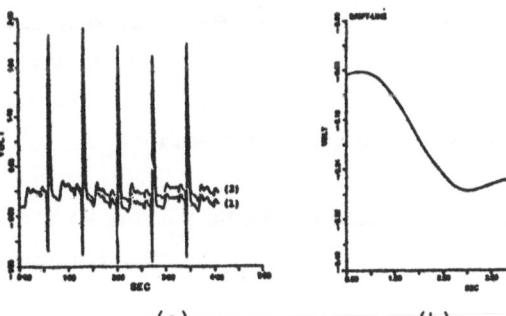

(a)

(b)

Fig. 4 -(a): Original signal (1) and corrected signal (2) using a non-linear regression algorithm ("pattern-search" method). The fitting curve (straight-line + sinusoid) is shown in (b).

of P, QRS and T waves for an X trace (7 sec. sampled at 500 Hz): the ori-

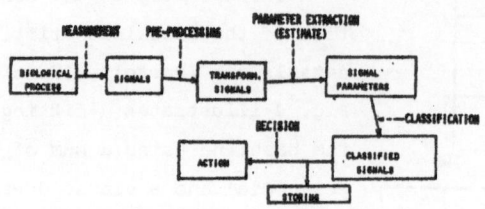

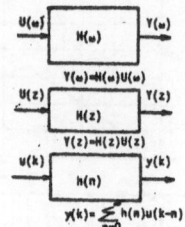

Fig. 1 - General block diagram with the steps of biological signal processing.

Fig. 2 - Output/input relation (Fourier transform, z-transform and convolution series)

described both for the phase of pre-processing of ECG signal and of enhancement of information useful for clinical aims.

The pre-processing step includes low-pass filtering to decrease the presence of myoelectric noise, mains interference and other high frequency noises on the tracings themselves. Results are illustrated in (Cerutti,1982); here it is important to remark that a wide generality of linear filter with linear phase may be designed in the discrete-time domain (methods of windowing, frequency sampling, equiripple filters) and many different characteristics may be implemented starting from the traditional low-pass, high-pass, band-pass, stop-band filters as far as the derivative filter and the ones realized via Hilbert trasnforms (Bartoli 1982a; Bartoli 1982c). The concept of digital filtering is in this way more extended, including a wide set of general algorithms and mathematical operations which, given an input time series, do correspond an output time series with enhanced or processed characteristics in the discrete-time domain (see Fig. 2). The output/input relation is expressed via $H(\omega)$ (frequency response of the filter expressed in terms of its Fourier transform), or via $H(z)$ (relation in z-transform domain), or via $h(k)$ (coefficients of the impulse response) by means of the convolution with the input time series.

APPLICATION OF DIGITAL FILTERING FOR THE WAVEFORMS RECOGNITION

It is well known that the fiducial points of most of the automatic processing procedures on the ECGs are constituted by the QRS occurrence. Classical derivative + threshold techniques are used as well as different ones like templates, pattern recognition etc. (Ripley, 1980). In Fig. 3 the frequency response of a derivative filter is shown with the original and filtered signals together with a threshold value which may be tuned according to the various needs of recognition, (QRS or P-T waves).

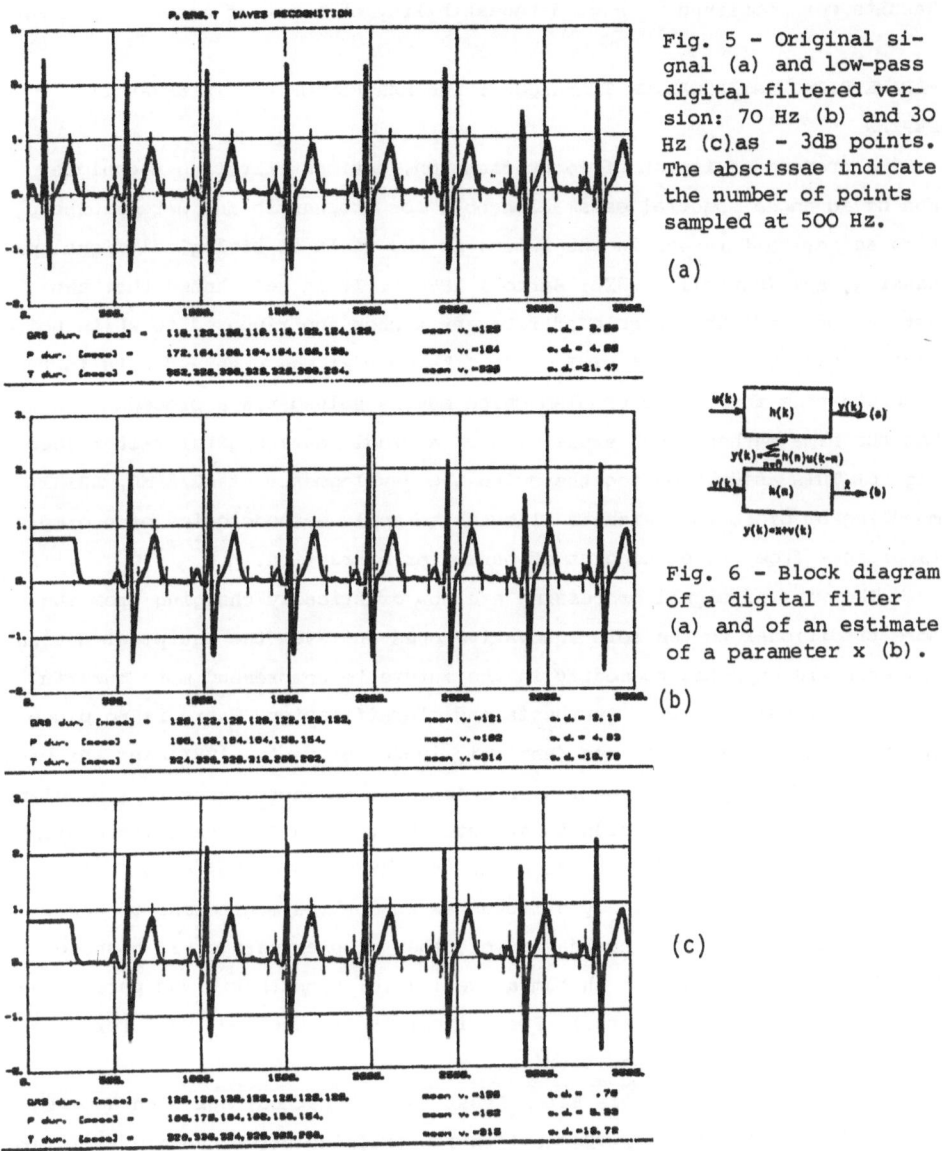

Fig. 5 - Original signal (a) and low-pass digital filtered version: 70 Hz (b) and 30 Hz (c) as - 3dB points. The abscissae indicate the number of points sampled at 500 Hz.

(a)

(b)

(c)

Fig. 6 - Block diagram of a digital filter (a) and of an estimate of a parameter x (b).

ginal signal is indicated together with the low-pass filtered versions of it for various values of cutoff frequencies. It is possible to think of a selective digital filter to improve the measurements of the various ECG com plexes as demonstrated in (Cerutti, 1982): 70 Hz low-pass filter does not corrupt P and T waves and improves the QRS duration measurement in most of the cases, while, for example, 30 Hz low-pass filter introduces strong distortions especially at onset, offset and maximum of QRS while improves considerably the measurements of T wave and, with less evidence, of P wave.

Results were obtained with good repeatability on a set of about 20 patients.

PARAMETRIC IDENTIFICATION TECHNIQUES: THE EXAMPLE OF R-R INTERVAL TIME SERIES

A tremendous impact of identification, optimal filtering techniques and of advanced spectral estimation both for stochastic and deterministic time series is foreseen in the future in the field of biological signal pro cessing, see (Bartoli, 1982b; Bartoli 1982c). It is well known that the estimation $\hat{x}$ of the variable of interest x when superimposed to white noise $v(k) = |0, \lambda^2|$ (where $x + v(k) = y(k)$, being $y(k)$ the observed data in the discrete-time form) is a problem which may be solved via a procedure which has the same mathematical expression of a traditional digital filter (see Fig. 6).This assumption together with the developments of AR/ARMA, ARMAX modeling of biological signals allow us to apply methodologies of enormous importance from the standpoint of parameter extraction.

The ways of signal processing are now drastically changing from the more traditional to the more innovative ones and even the equipment design criteria are expected to modify in the future to comprehend more powerful tools of signal analysis, synthesis and classification. There is no place to mention such methods, see (Bartoli, 1982c; Bittanti, 1981) for the basic concepts. In the present section an example of AR (autoregressive) modeling is applied to the time series constituted by the R-R intervals (tachogram) as a method of parameter extraction for the HRV. Such method of ECG signal processing is becoming widely diffused as an on-line monitoring of heart rate and a non-invasive evaluation of other complex parameters bounded to the fluctuation of cardiac rhythm as well (i.e. sympathetic and parasympa- thetic influences on ECG etc.). See (Kitney 1980; Akselrod 1981) for detai- led information of such applications.

The identification (via Batch Least Squares Method) has been applied to about 30 patients under rehabilitation training after myocardial infarc tion or acute ischaemic disease at the Don Gnocchi Foundation Medical Center. The detected epochs were: A - standing and resting condition; B - uncon- strained exercise test; C - cyclette exercise test. The results of the i- dentification on a period of about 350 complexes are shown in Fig. 7, under the form of pole diagrams of the estimated model, while Fig. 8 depicts the more traditional tachogram (a), amplitude histogram (b) and scattergram (c). Five order model (and therefore five coefficients) are sufficient to fit the data of the tachogram: the position of the poles on the z-complex plane

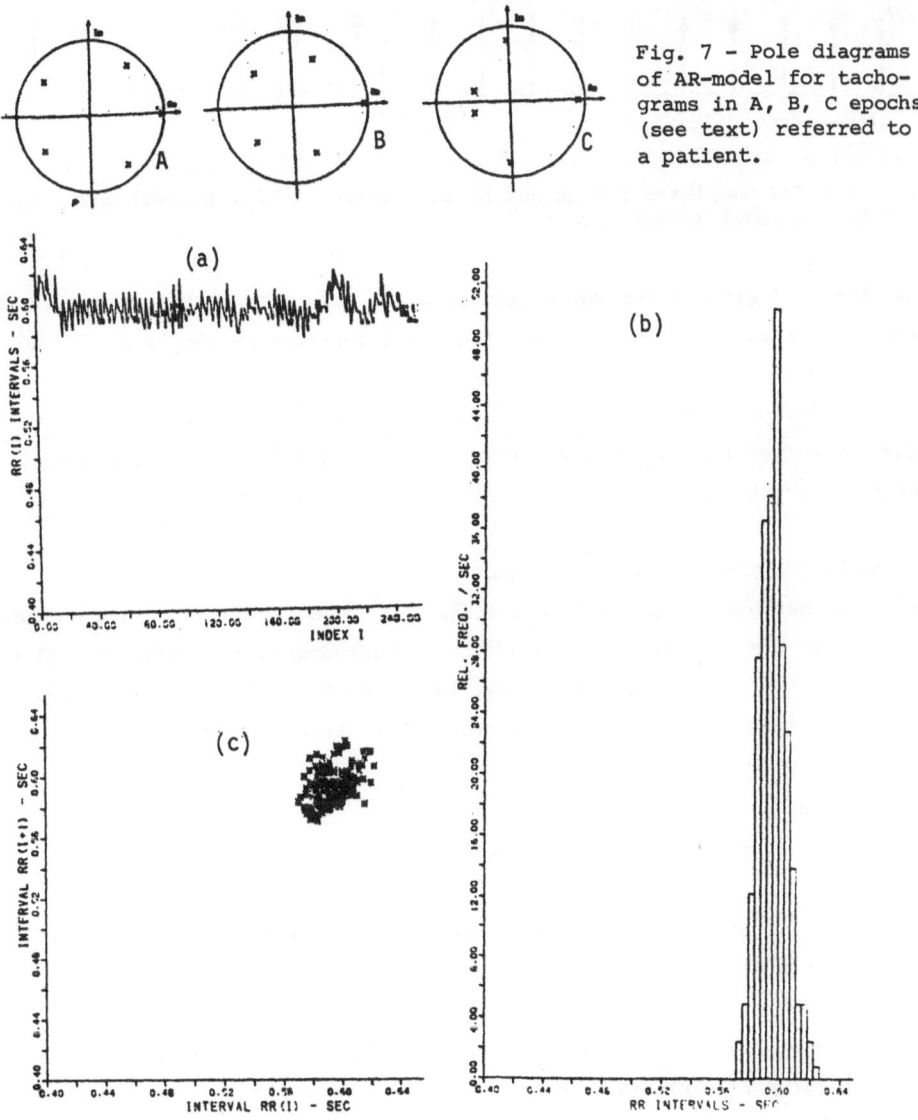

Fig. 7 - Pole diagrams
of AR-model for tacho-
grams in A, B, C epochs
(see text) referred to
a patient.

Fig. 8 - Plotting of tachogram (a), amplitude histogram (b) and
scattergram (c) for a R-R interval time series constituted by 350
complexes.

(Fig. 7), together with the information shown in Fig. 8, are extremely sensitive to the variations of cardiac rhythm and such a technique of parametri
zation appears interesting both for research and clinical purposes.

The identification approach allows another interesting parametrization for the HRV. Fig. 9 shows a time record of an ECG lead with superimposed

228

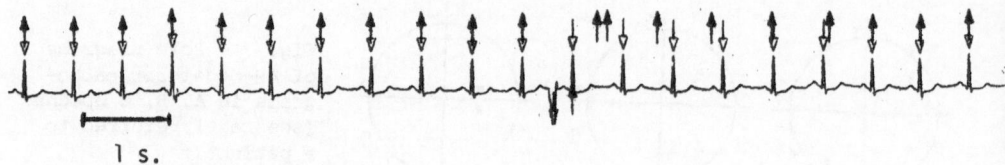

1 s.

Fig. 9 - QRS complexes recognized by the program (white arrows) and predicted by the model (black arrows).

two kinds of arrows: the white ones show the recognized QRS complexes while the black ones indicate the predicted QRS occurrence on the basis of the fifth order model introduced above. It is worth noting that the plotting of the prediction error (difference between the actual and the predicted values) may function as a quantitative mean for classification of abnormal beats or rhythms.

ADVANCED SPECTRAL ESTIMATION METHODS

Advanced methods of spectral estimation have recently been introduced which are indeed competitive to the traditional periodogram approach, generally carried out via FFT algorithms (Kay, 1981; Cadzow 1982). As an example, the so called maximum entropy spectrum (MES) may be obtained by AR identification coefficients:

$$P(f) = \frac{\lambda^2 \, \Delta t}{\left| 1 + \sum_{i=1}^{N} a_i \exp \left(-2\pi f j i \Delta t \right) \right|^2}$$

where P(f) is the power density spectrum as a function of frequency, λ^2 is the variance of the identification input white noise, a_i are the N coefficients and Δt is the sampling interval. Fig. 10 shows the MES relative to the cases of Fig. 7 by using 18 points of the autocorrelation function (the spectrum is expressed in cycle/beat and the amplitude is in arbitrary units). A more correct estimation is thus available with respect to the FFT approach with an enhancement of information about the underlying physiological mechanisms reported in literature (effects of respiratory arrhythmia, blood pressure and termoregulatory control mechanisms). The same spectrum is also estimated by using two other parametric methods: Pisarenko Harmonic Deconvolution (PHD) and Prony method (Kay, 1981). The former estimates the main n sinusoids of the spectrum with a good accordance to the MES (the points in Fig. 10 shows the relative positions of the estimated four principal sinusoids), while the latter confirms the trend of the data, in another

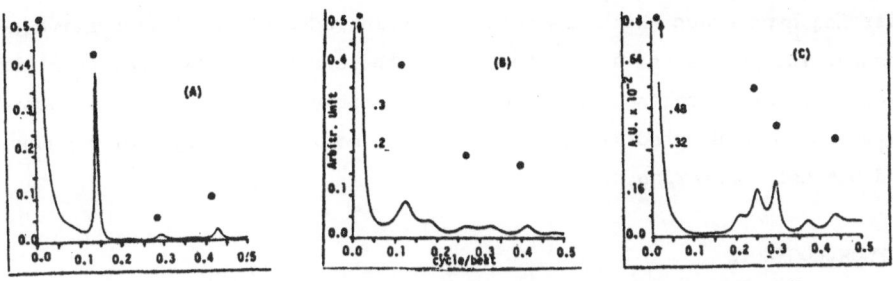

Fig. 10 - ME-spectrum referred to A, B, C epochs of Fig. 7.

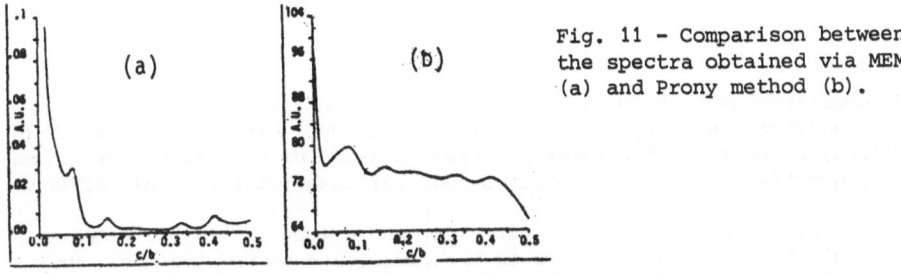

Fig. 11 - Comparison between the spectra obtained via MEM (a) and Prony method (b).

case, with a less resolutive power (see Fig. 11). Refinements of such spectral estimation methods and a more extensive use of them on a larger set of ECG signals are in course of execution.

Finally, it is important to remark that while such advanced techniques require rather sophisticated methodologies of signal analysis, they may have execution times in a dedicated machine (with reasonable coefficients order),which are comparable with the FFT techniques in the same situations. On the other hand, given the same number of parameters, the former techniques present a higher resolution,with respect to the latter, no need to window the data and more correct starting hypotheses.

CONCLUSION

Only a few examples of digital linear filtering, identification and spectral estimate have been described in the present paper as means of parameter extraction from ECG tracings. Such advanced and powerful techniques are believed to change considerably the methodologies and applications in biological signal processing with respect to the already available ones. Important aspects to further investigate at this regard are the validation of clinical significance of such parameters on a larger amount of cases, the connection with other indicators which cardiologists and physicians in general are more familiar to and, finally, the accurate testing of the

starting hypotheses which are required in introducing these innovative a-
spects. The problem of execution time of the algorithms does not seem particularly heavy, taking into account a possibly larger and more widespread
diffusion of dedicated microprocessor-based equipment design for diagnosis
and patient monitoring.

ACKNOWLEDGMENTS

The present paper was partially supported by a grant from Italian Mini-
stry of Education - Special Project on Cardiovascular Systems.

REFERENCES

AHA Committee. 1975. Recommendations for standardization of ledas and of
    specifications for instruments in ECG and VCG. Circulation, 52, 20-87.
Akselrod, S. et al. 1981. Power spectrum analysis of heartrate fluctuation:
    a quantitative probe of beat-to-beat cardiovascular control. Science,
    213, 220-222.
Bartoli, F., Cappelletti, T., Cerutti, S. and Crippa, M. 1982a. Effects of
    digital filtering procedure on the processing of ECG tracings. Proc.
    World Congr. Med. Phys. and Biom. Engin., Hamburg.
Bartoli, F. and Cerutti, S., 1982b. Identification and filtering programs
    for the biosignals processing. Proc. World Congr. Med. Phys. and
    Biom. Engin., Hamburg.
Bartoli, F. and Cerutti, S. 1982c. Methodologies and techniques of digital
    filtering for the ECG signal processing. Rass. di Bioingegn., 7: 8-34
    (in italian).
Bartoli, F., Cerutti, S; and Gatti, E. 1983d. Digital filtering and re-
    gression algorithms for an accurate detection of the baseline in ECG
    signals. Med. Inform. (in press).
Bittanti, S. 1981. Parametric identification, ed. CLUP, Milano (in italian).
Cadzow, J.A. 1982. Spectral Estimation: an overdetermined rational model
    equation approach. Proc. IEEE, 70: 907-939.
Cerutti, S., Gatti, E. and Masciadri, L. 1982. An automatic procedure of
    pre-processing ECG/VCG signals. Int. Journ. Bio-Med. Comp., 13: 329-
    342.
Kay, S.M. and Marple,S.L. 1981. Spectrum analysis: a modern perspective.
    Proc. IEEE, 69: 1380-1419.
Kitney, R.I. and Rompelman O. 1980. The study of heart rate variability.
    Clarendon Press, Oxford.
Meyer, C.R. and Keiser H.N. 1977. ECG baseline noise estimation and removal
    using cubic splines and state-space computation techniques. Comp.
    Biomed. Res., 10, 459-470.
Ripley, K.L. and Murrey, A. eds. 1980. Introduction to automated arrhythmia
    detection. IEEE Computer Soc. Press.
Ruttiman, U.E. and Pipberger, H.V. 1977. The effect of bandwidth limitation
    on measurements of the vector ECG. Proc. IEEE SCAMC, Washington D.C.
Sayers, B. McA. 1977. Processing and analysis of biological signals. In
    "Biomedical Computing" (Ed. W.J. Perkins). (Pitman Medical, London).
Wellner, U. and Brodda, K. 1976. Sensitivity of VCG parameters to baseline
    adjustment procedures. Adv. Cardiol., 16 (Karger, Basel).

DISCUSSION

Chairman: B. McA Sayers

3.2 - Feature extraction from ECG waveforms.

WOLFF: If you in a bio-chemistry laboratory use a flame-photometer, the way you get a very good signal to noise ratio is that you introduce an element like Lithium, or something of this kind, which isn't normally present to any great extent, and you look at everything in relation to the concentration of Lithium that you find in the flame. Now could one not imagine a recording analysis system where you quite deleberatly, from some other part of the body, like two electrodes stuck on the back, fed from a high impedance generator, injecting a very highly standardized, very predictive signal, like fast pulses controlled with a quartz oscillator of some kind. Then you train your analysis system to look for these, to predict these, because it knows exactly what the time accurance is going to be and it knows what the amplitude ought to be. And use that to test the reliability and sensitivity of the algorithm your detection system uses? Because if for instance the system was unable to recover this very predictable signal, we would also, I think, have no chance of recovering the signal you want.

MURRAY: I think we must keep our minds open to look for new concepts and new ideas. I've no strong feelings for that particular idea. In the first instance, I'd like to keep things as simple as possible, but if that was to be looked at, and to be found useful I see no reason why it shouldn't be adopted.

ROSENFALCK: The methods you, Dr. Cerutti, mentioned here are very commonly applied to EEG recordings. There I can see they have a great value because usually, in the EEG analysis, you want to extract the information about the frequency content. In EKG you actually have a series of single events and you really want to know something about the changes in the shape of the event. I'm really somewhat in doubt whether it's worthwhile to use the ARMA model because you actually hide your results very much with such complicated feature extraction method.

CERUTTI: On the other hand are of common use in EEG analysis, the Wiener or Kalman filters to detect some transient change, such as Epilectic seizure. I'm working now on this kind of situation, the problem is, how is the information that you really want to capture? I think that Kalman filter (it is the optimal filter on the basis of the mean square error) is the right method because it is able to classify some very fast rhythm under basal condition, whose statistics you are really aware of. So, I think, the approach I have shown on the figure regarding the plotting of the prediction error, is able to give us some quantitative information, in case of very fast variations of the rhythm. I think the autoregressive models may be not applicable in the problem you mentioned. The optimal filtering is the best method and the prediction error is a quantitative information any way.

ROSENFALCK: I'm sure that even the Kalman and Wiener filtering are getting a little more doubt now. I don't know if you know Dr. de Weerd's article, where it is shown they really have a very limited value in single events analyis. It is very applicable for continuous signals of a more stochastic character.

SAYERS: The difficulty about that argument, Dr. Rosenfalck, is that the sequence that Dr. Cerutti is talking about, is in effect treated as if it were a continuous component, It is not treated on a single event basis. This I think does change somewhat the sort of critical comment that you would make. Is that fair, Dr. Cerutti?

CERUTTI: Sure. I think the paper you mentioned of Dr. de Weerd is undoubtably putting clear some problems. My opinion is that if you want to study evoked response, obviously the first response is different from the last one, and if you carry on an averaging method you lose completely this adaptation mechanism. I think that some optimal ways of dealing with signal processing are worthwhile to apply in this kind of signals. As regards the ECG, my form of parametrization takes into account the complexity of the system over a period of time you may choose. Of course the problem is the stationarity of the signal: but you may test it on basis of the well know test for stationarity. So the parameterization you get is not on a single beat, not on a single rhythm, but you may have record of variable length.

TALMON: I'm a little bit puzzled about the clinical implication of the methods you have proposed. I don't see how we can use this kind of information in a diagnostic sense, and I have a feeling, although I have no evidence for it, that perhaps the approach suggested by Gustavsson, where he's trying to model arrhythmias and trying to fit the models and select the best model for a particular rhythm is not a useful approach in clinical practice.

CERUTTI: Yes. I think the form of the autoregressive estimation gives you a very important form of spectral estimation for biological signals in general. I do believe that in some sense we could carry on some parallel processing of different signals. My opinion is that, for example, you may get some parameterisation of the blood pressure, together with the ECG and find out some cross correlation, or some statistical description of them that may be useful to interpret the system also in clinical terms. I mentioned, the necessity of direct comparison between the black-box approach, and the approach more familiar to physicians, the transparent box. If we are working in finding out the effect of the sympathetic and parasympathetic nervous system on the heart-rate variability and if you had some information about the black box approach, that simply means it gives me, let me say only 7 parameters, well suited to the data for a particular record, and we found that in other different situations the model upgrades or degrades, and the same thing is confirmed by the traditional clinical evidence, I think that the method really shows its convenience.

TOPIC: 3.3

Feature extraction for hemodynamic signals characterization

AMBULATORY BLOOD PRESSURE SIGNAL FEATURES: IDENTIFICATION, MEASUREMENT AND IMPLICATIONS

B.McA. Sayers, Loretta R. Cicchiello*

Imperial College, London SW7 2BT, UK.
*Istituto di Fisica,
Facoltà di Ingegneria, Università di Napoli, Italy.

ABSTRACT

Long term records of blood pressure (mean, systolic or diastolic) and of heart rate are subject to fluctuations that can be regarded as naturally subdividing into five components: a circadian pattern, linear segmental baseline movements, short duration positive or negative unidirectional transients, vasomotor activity and respiratory-linked effects. These components are, in broad terms, unrelated.

The problems of quantification created by these components is discussed; it is argued that the most appropriate response may be to isolate and measure the components separately and, following up this approach, the contribution of each in short-length sample measurements is assessed.

The similarities between heart rate and beat-variable pressures in respect of certain of these components is considered as a basis for utilising HR measurements for the possible detection of potentially significant occurrences in blood pressure

INTRODUCTION

Long-term records of intra-arterial blood pressure exhibit considerable fluctuation. Disregarding the trivial case when episodes of a specific type are sought, the major problems of interpretation depend upon a proper quantitative description of the data. This is difficult to achieve for two reasons: the large, apparently erratic variability of the records, and their substantial correlational structure. We examine these two matters, their implications and the means for circumventing their effects.

THE VARIABILITY OF BLOOD PRESSURE AND HEART RATE RECORDS

An examination of systolic or diastolic pressure records, or of heart rate (SP, DP, HR) shows the problem (Figure 1): in the seemingly erratic and substantial fluctuations of each of the variables. On the short time scale, all three variables are affected by relatively fast activity attributed to respiratory, pressure vasomotor or thermal vasomotor origins (Sayers, 1973) but these components will be disregarded here. On the longer time scale, circadian variations, slow baseline movements and transient fluctuations are also evident in all three variables. They have

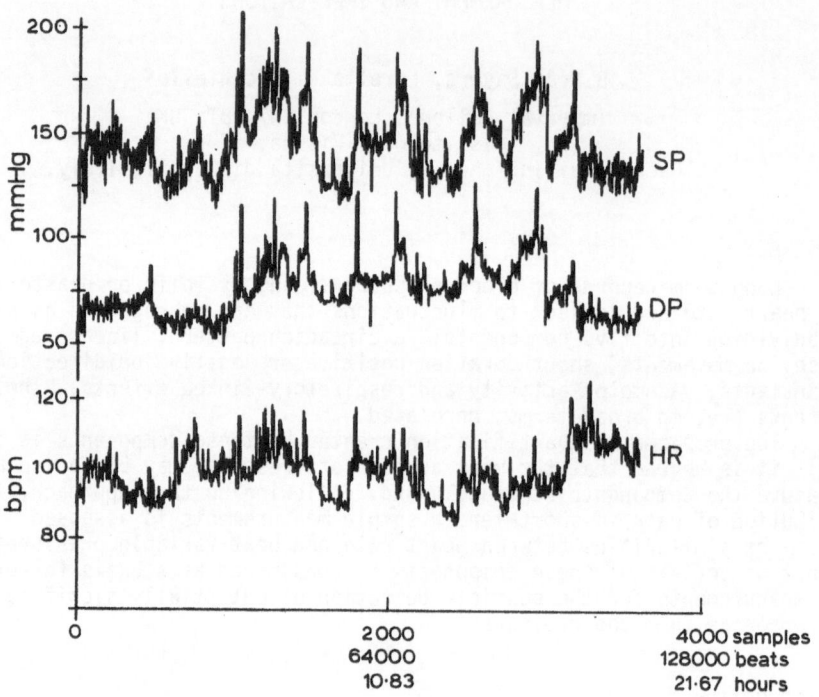

FIGURE 1. A record of systolic and diastolic blood pressure and heart rate, measured on an individual beat basis and averaged for display over 32 successive beats.

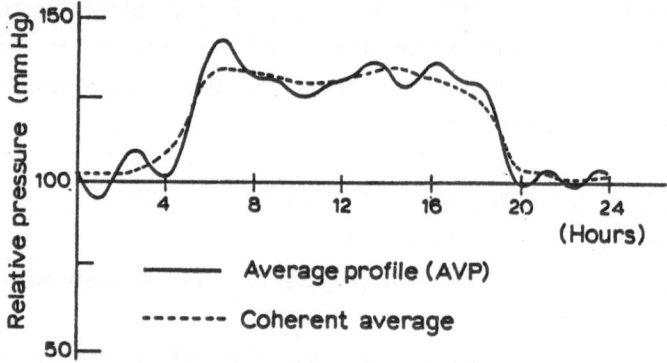

FIGURE 2. Average profile, determined by spectral averaging of 38 records and reconstituted to the 10-th harmonic, and the coherent average of the same records, using the 0.8 minute mean blood pressure.

already been described for 0.8-minute mean blood pressure measurements
(Sayers et al., 1982), and the study has now been extended to SP DP HR
and other beat variables in 55 patients.

Circadian variations

The main task in identifying the circadian pattern is to recognise the
main features of interest underlying the individual characteristics of the
specific patient and the particular 24-hr period chosen. Some kind of
inter-patient, or perhaps intra-patient, average pattern is needed. But
patient sleep periods alter from day to day, and start at different times
on different days. So standardisation is needed if general features are to
be detected.

Standardisation of a kind can be achieved by aligning one feature or
another in each of many daily records - such as the waking time. However
this requires a subjective decision in which the choice affects the alignment of other features, so this approach is regarded as unsatisfactory.
An alternative is to fix the proportion of the record occupied by the sleep-
ing cycle, and to employ an objective method for alignment. Averaging in
order to detect major features can then be readily carried out in a single
operation. We have preferred this approach.

It depends upon the fact that, in frequency domain terms, pattern
details in a signal are dictated by the phase spectrum. This has two consequences. First, if several records are misaligned, they can be brought
into alignment by a 'regression-spinning' procedure involving the phase
spectrum which has the effect of 'spinning' the signal on its time-base to
its most nearly symmetrical position. This can be a fully objective process. Second, common features in the resulting ensemble of records contribute a specific phase spectrum; if statistical variations exist, or if
the common pattern is combined with additive noise, the phases of each
relevant spectral component will have a more-or-less sharply unimodal
histogram. The modal value of phase, or in some circumstances the mean
phase, can be taken as a guide to the phase due to the common pattern.
Accordingly, an estimate of the common pattern can be formed by inverse
transforming a signal spectrum made up of the average amplitude spectrum of
the ensemble of individual records combined with the mean phase spectrum of
the 'spun' records. This results in the so-called spectral average of the
records. The spectral average of the circadian pattern of the records

examined here has been formed in the following way.

For this operation, a 32 x data reduction is routinely used, by averaging 32 successive values of the individual SP, DP or HR beat magnitudes. The resulting signals were then low-pass filtered to 10 harmonics of 1 cycle per 24 hours. The sleep period part of each record was extended to 8 hours by interpolating replicated values in the middle of the nighttime period record, and adjusting the total record length to 24 hours - if necessary by removing a small number of values in the mid-daytime region. The Fourier phase spectrum was obtained for each record and 'unwrapped' by an algorithm due to Sutton and Cheung in our Laboratory. A linear regression was carried out to estimate the best-fit linear curve describing the unwrapped phase spectrum for each record, and that best-fit line was subtracted from the unwrapped phase spectrum. The resulting values were entered into the spectral averaging procedure, which was carried out by the phase-vector method due to Cheung. The time-domain 'spectral average' was reconstituted from the average amplitude and phase spectra.

Figure 2 shows the form of the spectral average for BP, in comparison with the best choice of coherent average from the same group of records. The main differences lie in the more detailed representation of early matudinal overshoot and some later fluctuations provided in the spectral average. The validity of these features can be assessed by a statistical analysis of the ensemble mean deviation in the light of the ensemble SE, taken locally near the maximum point of the feature; in the records showing this feature (virtually all), the matudinal overshoot ensemble mean deviation is some 3.5x ensemble SE, and is accordingly judged to be significant. This feature must therefore be regarded as potentially interesting, even though it does not appear in the coherent average of the records (because of the low-pass filtering effect of the variable latency). A simple high pass filtering will remove the circadian patterns from the record, leaving other components for investigation in the so-called 'residual signal'.

Segmental baseline movements

It is a *sine qua non* that sporadic baseline movements of these variables is common - if only for mechanical reasons linked to changes of posture or effort, but presumably to other causes as well. However this does not preclude the isolation and quantification and, of course, suppression of this component in the residual signal.

The slow baseline movements can be isolated by lowpass filtering the

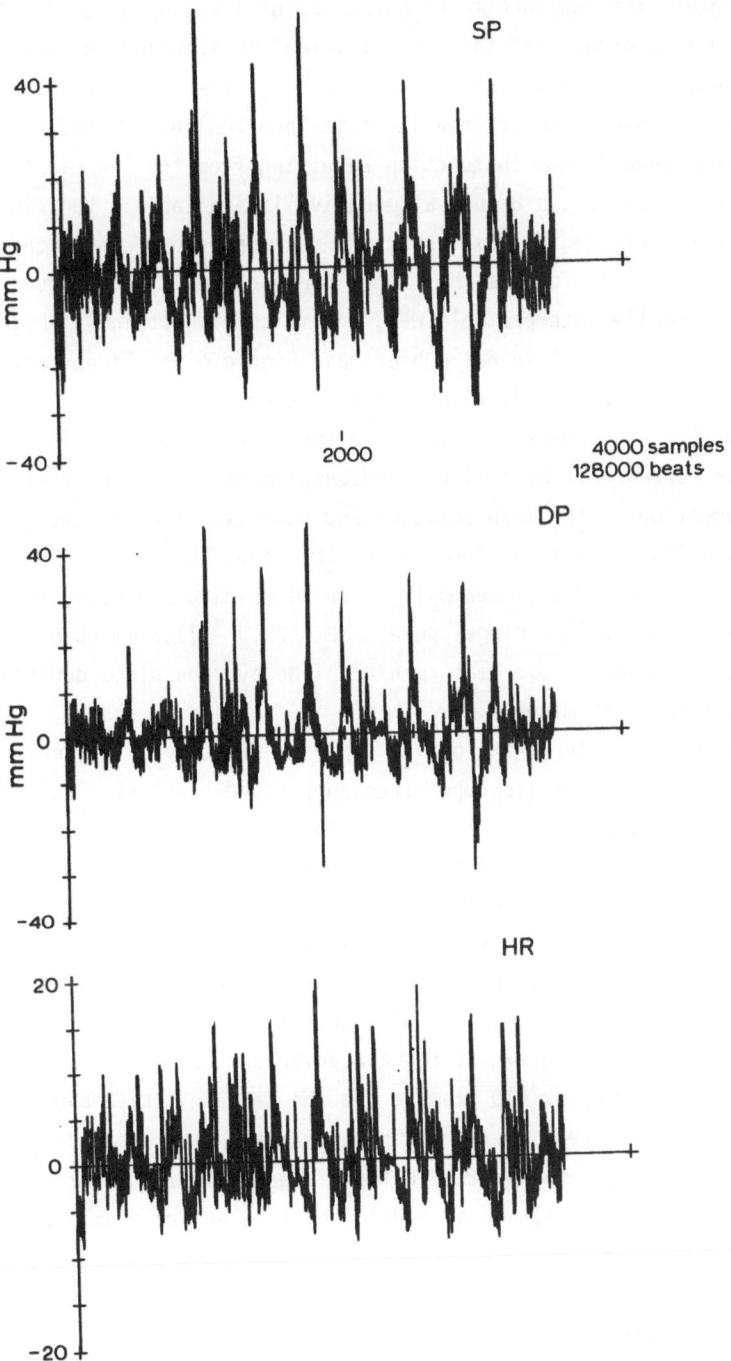

FIGURE 3. The residual signal in SP, DP (mmHg) and HR (beats per min.) after removal of the circadian feature by HP filtering. The notable feature is the irregular baseline movements.

residual signal, for instance to 60 harmonics of 1 cycle/24 hours. It is evident from inspection that this is sufficient to accommodate most of the slow fluctuations in the residual signal although there is scope for optimisation of this choice. Nevertheless, it is inconvenient to handle the irregular continuously smooth function resulting from the low pass filtering operation. However, a usable alternative is available: the linear segmental curve obtained by joining up the successive extrema of the continuous function. It follows the smooth curve closely, can be quantified readily in an easily interpretable way, and is simply obtained. Figure 3 shows the residual signal in one subject and Figure 4 the linear segmental pattern obtained, for the SP, DP and HR variables.

As a matter of pragmatic convenience therefore, slow baseline movements can be represented by a linear segmental model; the relevant quantitative information is the mean positive and negative slope values (almost always within 2%) the average duration of the slope segments, and the CV values (between 0.5 and 0.7, commonly). In 24 resting subjects, the mean values of average baseline slopes were: SP = 29.9 ± 11.3 mm Hg/hr; DP = 22.3 ± 9.3; HR = 16.7 ± 3.3 beats/min/hr. The average slope duration of a segment was about 25 minutes.

The choice of filter that, on its low pass frequency side, selects the circadian pattern, and on its upper frequency (band-pass) side selects the baseline fluctuations, is open to discussion. In our work, the choice has resulted from a close examination of the spectral average profile to identify component fluctuations that are attributable to all or most records. Increasing the cutoff frequency for the circadian pattern about about H10 of 1c/24 hrs results in a sharp decrease in the mean/SE ratio of the extra components that start to emerge, showing that these extra components are not significant in the context of the circadian pattern itself. Reducing the cutoff frequency below H10 smooths out the matudinal rise and overshoot; but the components thereby lost from the circadian pattern are nevertheless linked to it, and appearing in the residual signal, merely alter the statistical base of the linear segmental model (which is entirely able to accomodate these extra components thus transferred from the circadian pattern). As a matter of interest, Figure 5 shows a circadian pattern for one subject, one of the least significant examples which, nevertheless, still exhibits the main circadian-linked fluctuations.

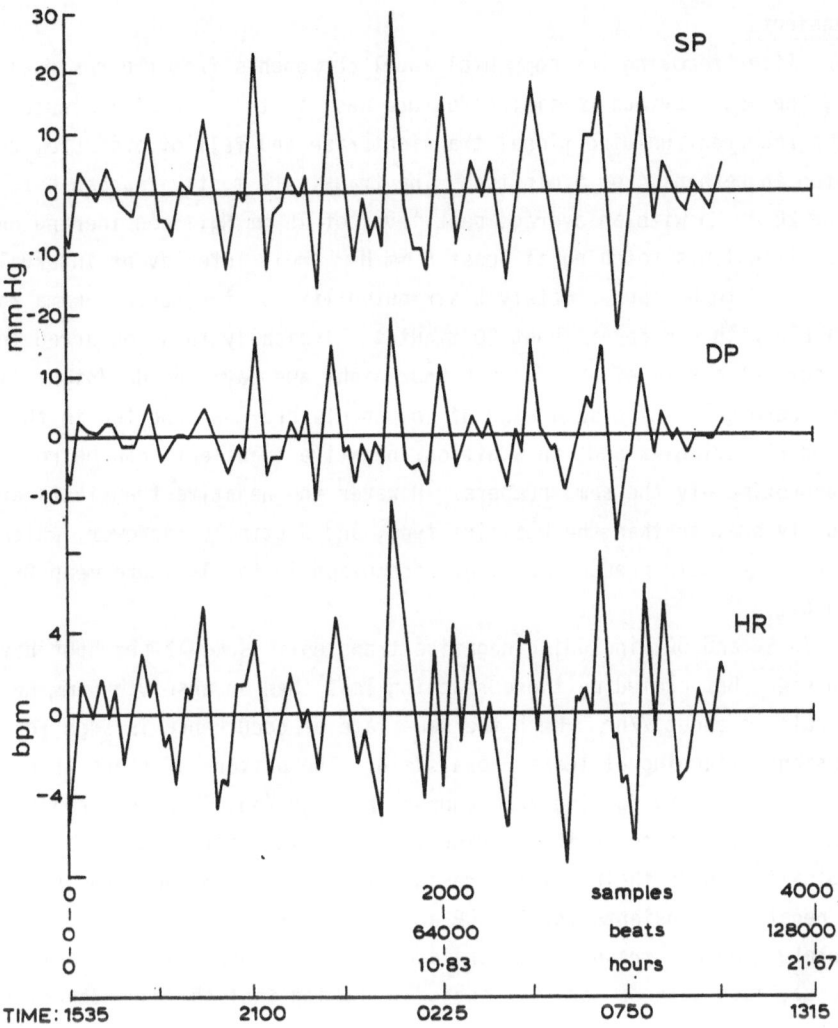

FIGURE 4. The baseline movements in SP, DP and HR modelled as a sequence of linear segments, obtained from the low-pass filtered version of the residual signals shown in Figure 3.

Transients

After removing the segmental model components from the residual signal, the most obvious remaining feature was, in the case of 1-minute mean
BP, a recurrent unidirectional transient rise and fall of pressure, completed in perhaps 4 or 5 minutes. The transients mostly reached between
5 and 20 mm Hg with an average peak level of 15 mm Hg; considering only
those transients reaching at least 5 mm Hg, their inter-event intervals
were found to be approximately distributed like a first-order gamma random
variable with a mode of about 20 minutes. Typically these occurred in all
subjects at a rate of about 3 per hour night and day; no day/night differences were seen. The same kind of components are now reported in the SP,
DP and HR variables and, in addition, negative transients can be recognised
in approximately the same numbers. However the negative transients are
slightly smaller than the positive type, and distincly narrower, which may
explain why their presence was not recognised in the 1-minute mean BP
records.

In SP and DP, including negative transients, some 12 per hour have
been seen, but excluding those reaching less than an absolute 5 mm Hg.,
the rate is about 7/hr. Much the same rate of occurrence is seen for HR
transients reaching at least 5 beats/min. The pattern of these transients
can be compared by forming the coherent average (ensemble average) of many
examples, aligned to their individual maxima, in exactly the same way as
originally led to their initial recognition. Figure 6 shows the positive
and negative transients for SP, DP and HR- as with the other curves, each
discrete sample corresponds to the average of 32 successive beats (on
average, 19.5 seconds for this subject, showing that the duration of the
positive-going transient is perhaps about 4 minutes or so and that of the
negative-going transient somewhat less at about 2 minutes. The peak transient reaches approximately 8xSEav or more in each of these variables, where
SEav is the average figure across the set of pre- and post-reference samples
shown in the Figure. A preliminary estimate of the serial correlation coefficients of the (positive transient interevent interval sequence suggests
that any correlation is insignificant. The histogram of intervals is, as
for the 1-minute mean BP transients, unimodal and of approximately first-
order gamma shape with a mode of about 17 minutes, for both the positive
and the negative transients taken separately.

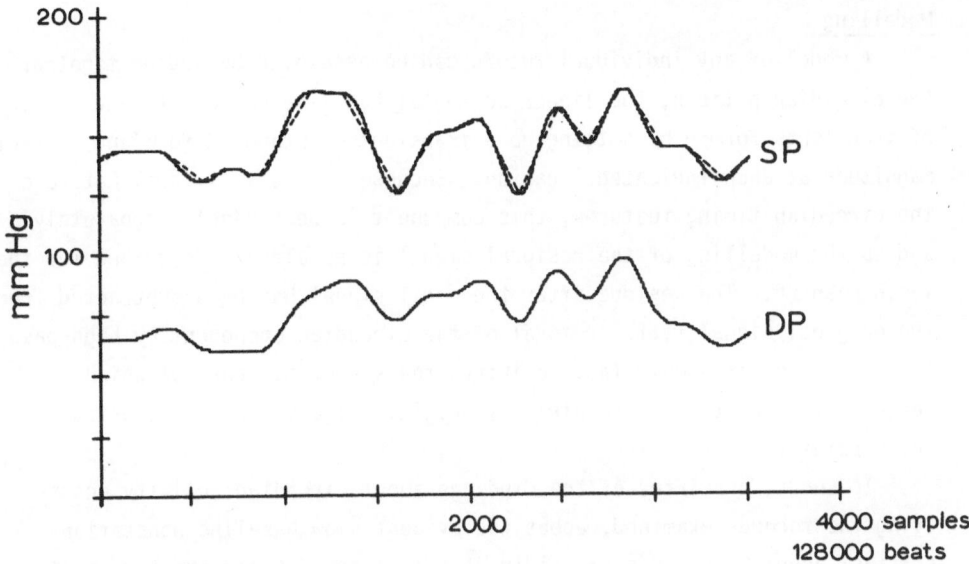

FIGURE 5. The circadian features of the SP and DP records, band limited to H/10: note that the linear segmental approach could also be used for describing individual components of these records.

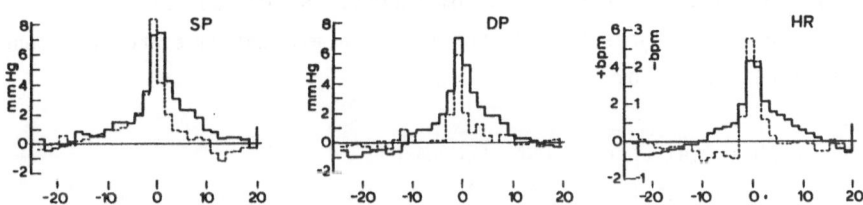

FIGURE 6. Average transients in SP, DP and HR in 55 subjects; both positive-going and (absolute) negative-going transients (apparently occurring independently) are shown. Note that the negative transients (shown dashed) are generally of shorter duration.

Modelling

A model of any individual record can be assembled by adding together
the circadian pattern, the linear segmental baseline component, and the set
of transients formed by setting up a transient of standard form and correct
magnitude at each indicated location. Because of the individual nature of
the circadian timing features, this component is best handled separately,
and so the modelling of the residual signal is as already described for the
1-min mean BP. The residue after the model signal has been subtracted from
the original signal (after removal of the circadian component by high-pass
filtering) contains only fast activity, the systematic part of which is
largely of vasomotor and respiratory origin. Figure 7 a,b,c illustrates
these points.

In short, by virtue of the findings about circadian activity underlying the records examined, about the evident slow baseline nonstationarities, about both types of unidirectional transient and about vasomotor
and respiratory contributions, it appears that a very detailed resolution
of the beat variable signals is feasible. The various components thus constitute the main features of these signals. It is argued that the presence
of these spontaneous components offers a natural basis for separating the
blood pressure or heart rate signals into different contributions. Broadly
speaking, it is easy technically to accomplish such a separation and to
quantify individually the separate components. So two questions arise:
what are the consequences of adopting this scheme, and what are the consequences of not doing so?

SEPARATE QUANTIFICATION OF SIGNAL COMPONENTS

Restricting attention to the slow baseline segmental and transient
components, quantification in the individual record can be summarised as
follows: the segmental component can be described by its average slope and
duration values and the corresponding coefficients of variation (CV); the
transients can be described by their statistics (ensemble mean peak height
and CV; average rate; interval distribution - which can probably be taken
from population estimates). With these two sets of data, it is possible to
estimate the influence of these components by direct measurement. The
important point is that, in the presence of the large variability which is
exhibited by each of the variables, satisfactory quantification depends on
longitudinal averaging to suppress the local fluctuations. So the question
is: how do the isolated components affect the values obtained by longitu-

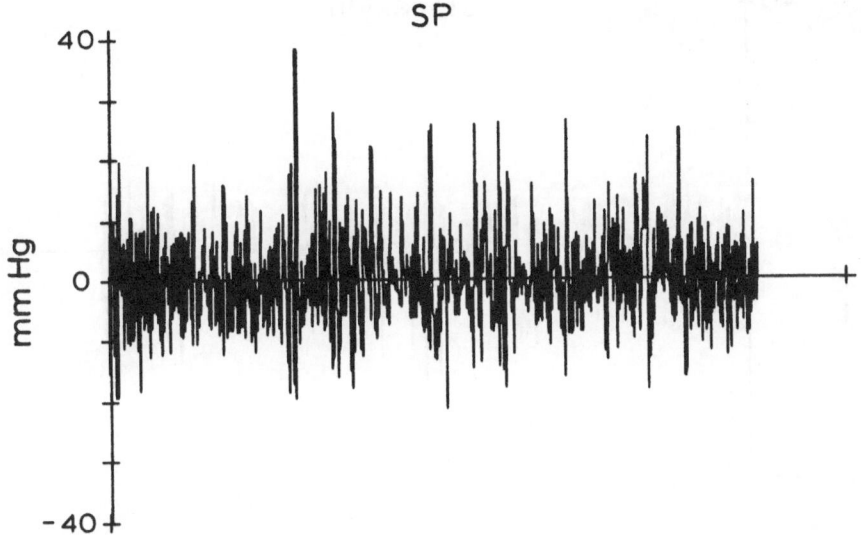

FIGURE 7a. Systolic pressure signal after removal of circadian features and of the baseline segmental components.

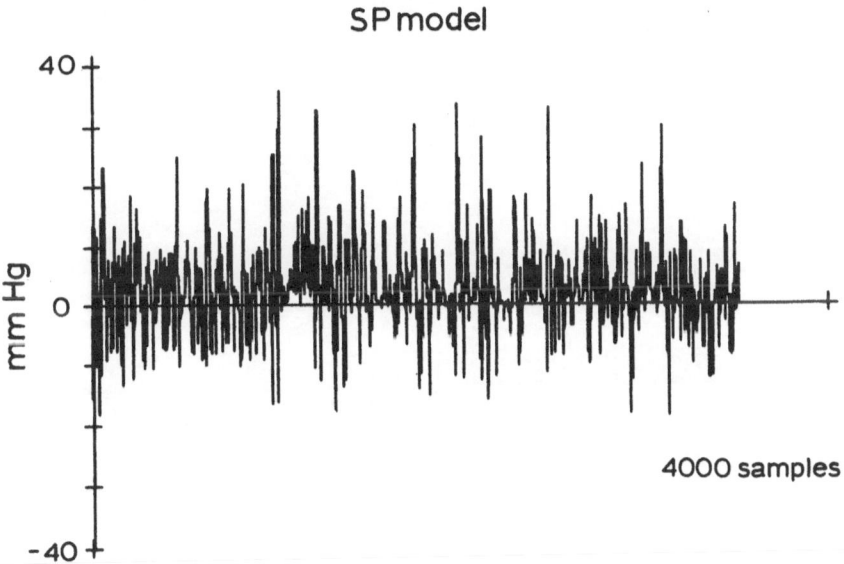

FIGURE 7b. Model of the signal in Figure 7a, constructed by summating average SP transient waveforms as shown in Figure 6, located and magnitude scaled in accordance with the result of inverse filtering the signal in Figure 7a.

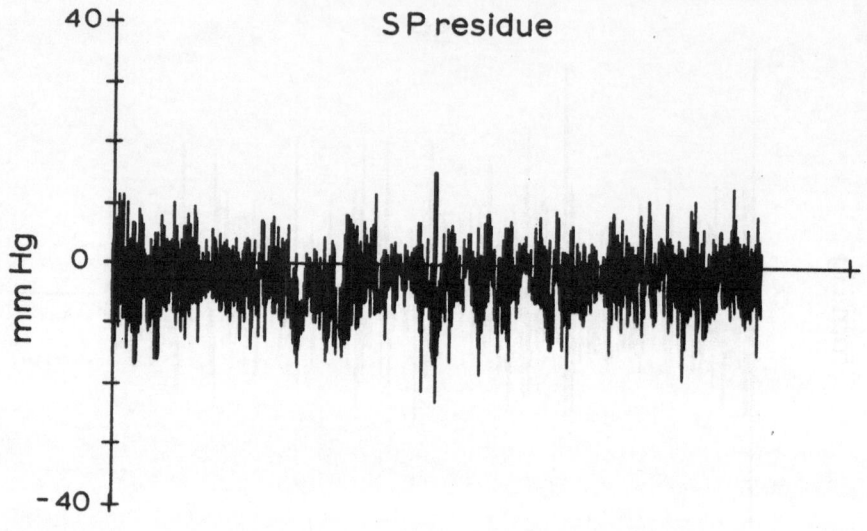

FIGURE 7c. The residue after the model signal of Figure 7b is subtracted from the SP signal of Figure 7a.

dinal averaging over various representative averaging times (i.e., signal sample sizes)?

In the segmental model, the mean of various lengths of signal can be taken directly to represent the effect of averaging over various durations, so that scanning through the complete 24-hr record leads to an estimate of the resulting mean and its variability due to this component. In the case of the transients, the method adopted has been to use the available statistical information to generate representative simulated signals formed of recurrent transients having the same statistical properties as in the real data. Again, averaging over many examples of the simulated signal at the chosen duration leads to an estimate of the contribution to averaged measurements.

The report on 1-min mean BP (Sayers et al., 1982) shows two things from this kind of investigation: that both components contribute in a sample-size dependent way to both mean BP and its variability. But the effect is certainly not merely a monotonically-decreasing function of the sample size over which averaging is conducted. If measurements are made on the whole signal, very great variability can occur because of the possible additive or subtractive conjunction of transients and segmental slopes, further complicated by the fluctuations visible in the circadian pattern. (If point measurements are used, short-period SP differences of up to 75 mm Hg are not uncommon; in HR this figure may be 30 bpm). Furthermore, there is nothing to indicate that the separate components share a common source, so for this reason also, separate quantification would seem to be appropriate.

SIMILARITIES BETWEEN SP, DP AND HR ACTIVITY

It would be overstating the similarities to argue that BP fluctuations can be fully detected in a parallel HR record. However, many of the transients occur in both SP or DP and HR (we will report the details elsewhere) and the transient patterns are similar. The slow nonstationarities of baseline are quite well parallelled in the two types of record, and it is generally true in our records that all substantial excursions of SP or DP are represented in HR, although not in a fully proportional way. Turning to the circadian pattern, the main features are common except, usually, at the start of the resting period at night; it is noticeable that the HR records do, however, more closely parallel the pulse pressure circadian components than those of SP or DP. This raises the possibility of recognising extrema of SP or DP from the occurrence of HR extrema, and given sufficient data to generate statistical confidence levels, this may be feasible. But if so, the procedure would certainly require that observations be interpreted in the light of ongoing activity.

THE CORRELATIONAL STRUCTURE OF LONG-TERM BP AND HR DATA

In view of the substantial variability of SP, DP and HR records, stabilisation of individual measurements is vital; longitudinal averaging is the first choice procedure and in view of the issued raised above, it is interesting to relate the difficulty of achieving satisfactory performance in this way to the underlying structure of the data and its influence on statistical estimators like averaging. Two aspects are involved. The first concerns mean-value estimates; the second concerns signal power estimates (likely to be of interest in describing unpatterned or highly-variable records).

The relevant issues are discussed in Sayers et al., 1981a, 1981b, 1981c. The key concept is that of the degrees of freedom in a sample of sequential data points (say, k-points long). The degrees of freedom content of a k-point record can be specified in terms of the reduction in dispersion of the individual data points in the k-point mean value (SE). By definition

$$DF_k = (SD/SE)^2, \qquad \text{and}$$

if all the data points can be regarded as independent, in the sense of uncorrelated, the value DF_k coincides with the number of observations k. However, if successive data points are correlated, the variability of the sample mean is not improved to the extent of the precise factor k over that of the original data. Nevertheless, it is still possible to use the relation above to describe the degrees of freedom content of the data sample, but now the relation involves the serial correlational structure of the data: R_j for $j=1,2,...(k-1)$. It is convenient to take the ratio of DF_k to the number of data points and define the degrees of freedom per point DF_k/k for the k-point sample. For uncorrelated data, DF/pt = 1; in much biomedical data it is much less and, typically, for SP, DP or HR DF/pt lies between 0.05 and 0.15. The specific relation is (Sayers et al, 1981a):

$$DF_k/k = (1+S_{kR})^{-1} \text{ where } S_{kR} = 2 \sum_{j=1}^{k-1} (k-j)R_j/k$$

The serial correlation structure thus influences the DF/pt figure and so the improvement in measurement stability due to longitudinal averaging.

All the components identified in the SP, DP and HR variables contribute strongly to the R_j sequence so, not surprisingly, there is substantial interference with the performance of simple longitudinal averaging as an estimator of signal mean values. Various strategies are available to reduce this problem; Sayers et al (1981c) discuss the possibility of subsampling to alter the correlational structure of the data, for instance.

When signal power measures are in use, the serial correlation structure of the data again influences the form and magnitude of the dispersion of sample values, and these matters turn out to be relevant to the problem of quantitative surveillance of variables like BP or HR. Again it is possible to specify the degrees of freedom content of a k-point sample in respect of power measurements, DF_p. Several problems arise. First, sample power values are biased, by a factor F, which depends upon R_j. The expected value of power is $<s^2>$

$$<s^2> = \sigma^2 (1 - S_{kR}/(k-1)) = \sigma^2 F$$ where σ^2 is the true average power. Second, DF_p is given by:

$$DF_p = 2 \Sigma P_i^2/(\Sigma P_i)^2$$ where P_i specifies the i-th Fourier harmonic power spectral value and i=1, 2...k/2. The power spectrum is, of course, related to the serial correlation sequence for the discrete data in the sample, and DF_p can be (approximately) estimated also through the R_j sequence. The particular relevance of these matters is to the comparative testing of signal samples drawn from BP or HR sources.

Because of the serial correlation structure, typical samples will unavoidably be, in effect, small-size samples in the statistical sense. If the data values are Gaussianly distributed, statistical comparison of the mean of two samples will require a t-test type of approach. In summary, in these circumstances, it is possible to specify a so-called 'compensated t-' variable (ct), which behaves for correlated data very much as a true t-variable does in uncorrelated data. The formula for 'ct' takes account of bias and DF_k effects, through a compensating factor CF, given by:

$$CF = F^{\frac{1}{2}}/(1 + S_{kR})^{\frac{1}{2}}$$

and the t- tables are entered with the value ct at DF_p degrees of freedom. (It has been shown that power in a correlated sample is distributed approximately Chi-^{2} with DF_p degrees of freedom, and this is the key factor in determining DF for the t-distribution.)

So, statistically based testing for signal differences can be made using the above information, even in strongly correlated data, as in the present variables. Naturally, the same applies to the separate component signals - with different parameters, of course.

CONCLUSION

These findings, which are qualitatively comparable for all the records examined, confirm that isolated point observations of BP - however measured - are liable to large variability; worse, in unfavourable (but not uncommon) circumstances, they may be uninterpretable. This results from the behaviour of the different contributing components that have been identified in both BP and HR.

Since there is no evidence at present that these components are generally linked to any significant extent, it is argued that the most illuminating measurements are likely to be those that depend on the separate quantification of the different components. And even where this is not possible it is clear that the appropriate protocol of measurement would require a sufficient number of repeated observations to identify the current dynamic state of the variable: what is happening to the baseline? is a transient present? In some circumstances it may also be desirable to ask about the circadian pattern and perhaps also: what is the power of the fast components?

At least some of these questions could easily be answered with the aid of simultaneous (and continuing) HR measurements, because of the extent to which the presence and dynamic state of the important components in BP is signalled in HR.

ACKNOWLEDGEMENTS

This work was supported by the U.K. Medical Research Council. Figure 2 is reproduced by permission from Medical Informatics (Sayers et al., 1982).

REFERENCES

Sayers BMcA. (1973). The analysis of heart rate variability.
Ergonomics, 16, 17 - 32.

Sayers, B.McA., Cicchiello L.R., Raftery E.C., Mann S.R. and Green H. (1982)
The assessment of continuous ambulatory blood pressure records.
Medical Informatics, 7, 93 - 108.

Sayers B.McA., Ruggiero C. and Feuerlicht J. (1981a).
Statistical variability of biomedical data: Part 1. The influence of
serial correlation on mean value measurements.
Medical Informatics, 6, 1 - 11.

Sayers B.McA., Ruggiero C. and Feuerlicht J. (1981b).
Statistical variability of biomedical data: Part 2. The influence of
serial correlation on power estimates.
Medical Informatics, 6, 207 - 220.

Sayers B.McA., Sandoval L.S. and Ruggiero C. (1981c).
Statistical sampling strategies for averaging purposes in serially-
correlated biomedical data.
Medical Informatics, 6, 271 - 278.

HOW SHALL WE ANALYSE THE
AMBULATORY BLOOD PRESSURE SIGNAL?

P.M.M.Cashman
Clinical Research Centre, Harrow ,England

ABSTRACT
    Can an internationally coordinated approach be formulated for the analysis of ambulatory invasive blood pressure recordings? This question is considered in regard to data storage,data presentation,analyser implementation and analyser performance specification. The methods used in several major centres are reviewed; there is already a good degree of standardisation of raw data recording methods, but as yet no consensus on data presentation. Analyser implementation is very unlikely to become unified. It would, however, be worthwhile to attempt to agree on ways of specifying the performance requirements for the central feature extraction algorithms, however implemented. At present very little quantitative data is available on the accuracy, repeatability or artefact rejection of the various analysers already being used.

1.INTRODUCTION

Since the theme of the present Workshop is to plan a concerted action on ambulatory monitoring, it is appropriate here to consider whether a totally unified approach to the analysis of the ambulatory intra-arterial blood pressure signal is possible, or indeed desirable. This question can best be answered if the current state of ambulatory intra-arterial BP monitoring is examined in four main areas:

> Data storage
> Data presentation
> Implementation of analysis systems
> Specification of performance requirements for
> > analysis systems

2. DATA STORAGE

For the purposes of this paper the most important element of data storage is the recording of the raw arterial blood pressure signal. One of the strengths of the current worldwide effort in ambulatory BP recording is that the raw data are nearly all being stored in the same format. Table 1 shows the recording methods used by the major organisations

active in the field; it is evident that the CRC Mark 2
transducer and the Oxford Medilog 4-24 recorder are widely
employed. Some aspects of the basic recording systems will
now be briefly reviewed.

TABLE 1   Recording Methods used in Ambulatory Invasive BP
           (Note: only representative references are cited)
----
a) Brachial/radial artery cannula : CRC Mk2 transducer :
   Medilog 4-24 recorder.

Location	Reference
Oxford	Floras et al,1982
Harrow	Millar Craig et al,1978
Belfast	Murnaghan et al,1980
New York	Wertheimer et al, 1978
Cleveland	Mehta et al,1980
Birmingham	Watson et al,1980
Padova	Pessina et al,1978
Sydney	Hunyor et al,1980
Newcastle	Murray and Sanders, 1980
Pisa	Palombo et al (verbal only)
Ghent	Clement et al(verbal only)
Amsterdam	van Montfrans et al,1982
Milan	Mancia et al,1982

b) CRC Mk2 transducer with modified Oxford MR-20 recorder

Harrow	Davies et al,1982
Tampere	Saranummi et al,1982

c) Radiotelemetry Recording

Berlin	Schultze et al,1978
Erlangen	Zerzawy and Bachmann,1981
Yokohama	Kaneko et al,1982(verbal only)

d) Pulmonary artery cannula : solid state recorder

London	Perry et al, 1982

2.1. The 4-24 Recording System and Modifications

The blood pressure signal is generally obtained from a
cannula inserted percutaneously into the non-dominant brachial
or radial artery. The cannula is connected by a fluid-filled
tube to a combined transducer- perfusion unit produced at the

Clinical Research Centre, Harrow (Millar-Craig, Hawes and Whittington, 1978) which develops a differential signal of some 30-40 mV which is passed to a Medilog 4-24 cassette tape recorder (Oxford Medical Systems Ltd.). The recorder contains plug-in modules allowing up to four tracks to be simultaneously recorded on a C120 cassette for at least 24 hours. The BP signal is recorded using mark-space modulation of a 40 Hz carrier; usually only the the differentiated edges of the carrier waveform are applied to the recording head (AM4 system), although in the original AM2 system the full carrier waveform was recorded. Another tape track is generally occupied by a 60Hz crystal-derived time/event signal and the remaining two tracks are often used to record the surface ECG. The recommended track allocations are : 1,2 = ECG ; 3= BP ; 4 = time/ event, to minimise the effect of tape transport disturbances on the BP signal, which is the most critical. The recorder is powered by four RM1 mercury batteries which also provide d.c. excitation for the blood pressure transducer. Recent work (Kenny et al,1980; Grimbergen et al,1982) indicates that for optimum BP drift and noise performance a voltage stabiliser should be fitted to the recorder. Other suggested modifications have involved separate battery packs for transducer and recorder (Murray and Sanders,1980) or the use of a different transducer with separate excitation (Goldberg et al,1980).

Even if none of the above changes are made, the standard 4-24 recorder MUST be modified for blood pressure recording by bringing the negative supply line out to the transducer connector, otherwise the signal-to-noise ratio will be seriously compromised.

2.2. The MR-20 Recording System.

Although the 4-24 recorder is generally reliable for BP work if carefully maintained, it suffers from limitations which make it necessary to restrict the bandwidth of both the ECG and the blood pressure signal. We have recently explored the possibility of using an FM recorder, the Oxford Medilog

MR-20, to overcome these limitations (Davies et al,1982 ; Davies, Cashman et al, in press). Though the modified MR-20 has proved to be capable of excellent BP and ECG performance, the required modifications were difficult in practice and the system is unlikely to be suitable for widespread use. Alternative options are currently under development, including a fully digital recording technique.

2.3. Radiotelemetry Recording

In the Berlin system described by Schultze et al (1978), the brachial artery cannula is continuously flushed by a Fenwal pressure infusion system and the blood pressure is measured by a Statham P37 transducer; the signal is transmitted to a tape recorder at a central station while the subjects are allowed to move about within the confines of the ward. The Erlangen system of Zerzawy and Bachmann (1981) has a range of up to 1000m and uses a similar system to obtain the signal. Telemetry must obviously restrict the subject's freedom unless the raw data can be stored on a portable recorder of some kind.

2.4. Solid State Recording and the Future

The large memory capacity required to acquire a complete raw blood pressure signal for 24 hours (some 15 megabytes) has so far not been realised in a patient-borne recorder. However, a recent paper by Perry et al (1982) described an ambulatory instrument which obtains pulmonary artery pressure from an indwelling catheter, processes the signal and stores average values in a solid state memory. It seems likely that the next few years will see advances in memory technology sufficient to allow a patient-borne recorder for the raw data to become a practical proposition. At the same time, the knowledge gained about the BP signal using existing tape recording techniques may by then allow the processing to be reliably performed before storing the results, so that the need for saving the raw BP signal will have been eliminated altogether.

2.5. Data Storage Subsequent to Recording

Although it might at first sight seem that digital computer media such as magnetic tapes and disk cartridges could provide the basis of an international standard for storage of blood pressure data and intermediate results, it is unlikely that any standardisation will be achieved other than in storage of the raw signal values. The reason for this, as will be demonstrated later, is that a wide range of different analyses is already being carried out all over the world, using generally incompatible systems and methods.

2.6. Conclusions on Data Storage

Returning to the recording media we presently have available, it is clear from Table 1 that many centres are currently using the Medilog 4-24 system as a common standard. This naturally encourages the hope that exchange of data between organisations will become a more regular feature of this type of study. Certainly if it is possible to prevent a proliferation of different BP recording standards, the technical obstacles to data sharing will be minimised. (It is nevertheless essential to take advantage of major improvements in recording technique that may become available from time to time.)

3. DATA PRESENTATION

Table 2 gives a summary of the major contributions to the development of ambulatory intra-arterial blood pressure data presentation.

TABLE 2   Developments in Ambulatory BP Data Presentation.

Date Location   Method   Reference

1969 Oxford   Visual chart writeouts   Littler et al,1972
1972 Oxford   24-hour histograms.   West et al,1976
1976 Harrow   1-hour histograms,trends   Millar Craig 1978
1976 Belfast   1-minute means,trends   Mitchell et al,1978
1977 Belfast   Circadian spectral analysis   Mitchell et al,1978
1977 Imperial   Effects of nonstationarity   Sayers et al,1978
     College
1979 Belfast   Circadian cosine fitting   Murnaghan,1980
1981 Harrow   3 variability indices   Mann et al, 1982
1982 Imperial   Identification of patterns   Sayers et al, 1982
     College

It can be seen that so far as machine-assisted analysis
is concerned, the periods of interest became steadily shorter
from 1972 to 1977, decreasing from 24-hour histograms to
1-minute averages of systolic and diastolic pressure. This
was partly due to the falling cost of mass data storage and
computers, but also reflects an increasing awareness of the
significance of short-term blood pressure variability.
Throughout this period, 24-hour trend plots and basic
statistical measures such as the mean and variance of systolic
and diastolic pressure were used as the basis for patient
characterisation and comparison, for example in evaluating
anti-hypertensive drugs.

At this point a group at Imperial College, London
published the results of a detailed examination of resting and
ambulatory blood pressure records (Sayers,1978 ; Sayers, Ellis
and Green, 1978). In essence, this statistical analysis
showed large and frequent shifts in the mean ambulatory BP and
a high degree of serial correlation in the data. This led to
the conclusion that simple statistics would not provide a
reliable measure of within-subject and between-subject
variability until the various pattern features in the
long-term records had been identified, measured and removed.

A start had already been made in this direction by the
Belfast group who had obtained descriptions of the broad

24-hour ('circadian') pattern of blood pressure in terms of Fourier spectral components (Mitchell et al, 1978).This was later focused down to a method of fitting a simple cosine function to the 24-hour pattern and observing changes in amplitude, phase and frequency associated with pre-eclampsia (Murnaghan et al,1980; Mitchell et al, 1982). An alternative way of quantifying the circadian pattern was suggested by Mann et al(1982) who developed three indices of variability which were used to characterise normotensives, hypertensives and patients with autonomic failure.

Most recently, the Imperial College group has reported the results of its continued efforts to identify robust patterns in the long-term data (Sayers et al, 1982). Besides the broad circadian pattern, there are several°clear features including medium-term trends and rapid unipolar transients as well as the more familiar vasomotor and respiratory oscillations. The features are described in more detail elsewhere in these Proceedings.

Conclusions on Data Presentation

From the foregoing it is apparent that there is as yet no generally accepted standard way of presenting ambulatory blood pressure data. Many approaches have been tried, and new ones are still being proposed as more becomes known about the properties of the signal. It is also well known that this type of study is very labour-intensive, so that development on a broad front should be encouraged while at present it would be inappropriate to try to lay down any standard form of data presentation.

4. IMPLEMENTATION OF BLOOD PRESSURE ANALYSIS

It has already been pointed out that at least 16 organisations are now active in ambulatory invasive BP monitoring. Though Table 1 showed widespread standardisation as far as recording is concerned, the situation is very different when data analysis is considered. Each of the organisations in Table 1 has more or less independently developed its own techniques for analysis, tailored to meet the clinical objectives of the studies being carried out, and also to give the most effective solution within the constraints imposed by local resources. The clinical objectives of the various organisations appear to be converging (Clement et al, 1982); but the resource constraints are likely to remain a major cause of diversity in analyser implementation. These will include such factors as the time and manpower available for developing and operating the analyser, the hardware (particularly computers) to hand and the amount of software expertise which can be readily called upon. A further and very important factor is the scale of the operation to be undertaken, i.e. the number of 24 hour tapes to be processed each day, which can range from less than one to five or more. Depending upon the manpower available to operate the analyser and check the results, this will determine whether a fully automated system with its inherent risk of unnoticed errors, or an interactive system with its lower processing speed, should be chosen. Our experience at Northwick Park has been that it is desirable for each tape to be reviewed at least once before the cannula is removed from the patient, i.e. that the first stage of analysis should be accomplished within 24 hours of recording. To achieve this with a load of five or more tapes per day, the processing must either be performed at maximum speed on one analyser or else divided into separate stages, with storage of intermediate results. Both options are currently being explored.

Extrapolating from this experience to other centres, it is not surprising that since 1972 there has appeared a wide range of different and incompatible hardware and software configurations, some of which have had many man-years of development invested in them.

Conclusions on Analyser Implementation

Now that analyser development has proceeded independently at so many centres over a considerable period, it would be unrealistic to attempt to impose any standard implementation on existing users. This implies that compatibility between organisations will be very limited. In contrast to ambulatory ECG monitoring, it is highly unlikely that any commercially produced analyser will arrive to change this situation, because of the inherent hazards and restricted application of invasive ambulatory blood pressure monitoring.

5. SPECIFICATION OF BP ANALYSER PERFORMANCE REQUIREMENTS

5.1. Aims of Standardisation: accuracy and artefact rejection
----

Although this wide range of blood pressure tape analysers has been used to produce clinical results which have been compared at many international meetings, virtually no validation data is available to indicate how much confidence can be attached to the results from the different organisations. At present there is no common specification for the performance that can be expected from a BP tape analyser; this is an area in which international coordinated action is both desirable and possible. To specify and validate a system would require answers to two main questions: first, how accurately and reproducibly does the system measure the features of interest? and second, how effectively does the system reject or take account of artefact? This latter question in particular has received almost no attention in most of the published descriptions; it is probably even more important for blood pressure analysis than for ambulatory ECG, since in BP work the emphasis is on measuring absolute values rather than classifying waveshapes. It is also important because the Medilog 4-24 tape recording system used for the majority of these studies can introduce specific distortions and artefacts which could reduce the accuracy of blood pressure measurement. To obtain best results, strict quality control is necessary at all stages of the process so that artefacts are minimised during recording, detected during analysis, and excluded during compilation of the results.

5.2. Artefacts Common on Blood Pressure Recordings

TABLE 3   Sources of Artefact on Ambulatory BP Recordings.

Artefact	Worst Effect on BP
8 Hz gearbox ripple	10mmHg peak-to-peak
Tape speed variation	6 mmHg peak-to-peak
Transducer drift	25 mmHg over 24 hours
Non-linearity	10 mmHg at 0 or 300 mmHg
10 Hz bandwidth limitation on replay	
Intermittent cannula occlusion	

Table 3 indicates the problems most commonly encountered on recordings made with the CRC Mk 2/Medilog 4-24 system. It must be emphasised that this is a 'worst-case' list and recordings are unlikely to suffer from all the defects at once. In fact many of these sources of artefact can be much reduced by correct installation and regular maintenance of the recording and replay equipment. The 8 Hz ripple and the effects of tape speed variation are often amenable to careful adjustment of the recorder; installing the manufacturer's flutter compensation system can give a further 3 dB improvement in the signal- to-noise ratio. Transducer drift and non-linearity must be minimised by correct setting of the offset and gain controls; in a few cases, bad results have also been obtained because the users did not realise that the standard 4-24 recorder needs wiring modifications (as mentioned in Section 2.1) before it can be used for blood pressure. It is also important to remember that if a modified 4-24 recorder is returned to the factory for servicing, these wiring modifications will routinely be removed unless the recorder is specifically labelled to the contrary.

A different source of distortion which is sometimes overlooked is the fact that although the recorder uses a carrier frequency of 40 Hz, the replay demodulator contains a final low pass filter which limits the overall system response to 0-10 Hz. This is done in order to remove as much of the carrier as possible, but it also implies that any measurements on BP signal components above about 8 Hz are likely to be dominated by the phase and amplitude characteristics of this replay filter. Therefore the usefulness of parameters such as dP/dt (e.g. Hassen 1976) must be regarded as severely limited.

The final major source of artefact on these recordings is intermittent obstruction of the brachial artery cannula. If the blockage is total, the result is an increasing ramp in pressure as the perfusion pump tries to clear the cannula. This positive transient may have any duration, from one second to several hours. In the case of partial obstruction, the pulsatile arterial signal becomes damped and the periodic pressure fluctuation caused by the perfusion pump becomes more apparent. This interfering signal most commonly takes the form of a sawtooth at either 3 or 6 cycles per minute, showing regular sharp drops in pressure rather similar to those produced by ectopic beats (Littler,1980; Millar Craig et al, 1981). These effects are usually easily recognised visually on a chart record of the raw signal, but they may present problems for an automatic blood pressure tape analyser.

5.3.   Feature Extraction Methods in Existing BP Analysers

Having indicated the main problems posed for the feature extraction algorithm which might be included in an automated analyser, it is now appropriate to look at those systems which have so far been published. Twelve systems are listed in approximately chronological order in Table 4; it should be pointed out that only the essential characteristics of the central feature extraction process are included in the Table.

TABLE 4   Feature Extraction Algorithms Used for
Long Term Blood Pressure Recordings

(Note: '+' = presence, '0' = absence of item.)

	A	B	C	D	E	F	G	H	I	J	K	L
REQUIRED:												
Hardware preprocessor	+	+	0	0	0	+	0	0	0	0	+	+
Mass Storage	0	0	+	+	+	0	0	0	+	+	0	0
ECG Trigger	0	0	0	+		0	0	+		+	0	0
Other timing criteria	0	0	0				+					+
PROVIDED:												
Beat by beat output	+	0	+	+	0	0	0	+			+	0
Artefact checking	+	0	+	+	+	0	+	+				0
Interactive editing	0	0	0	+	+	0	0	+				0
Tape speed correction	+	0	+	0	0						0	
PERFORMANCE:												
Effective speed x real time	25	25	12								60	60
Raw precision (bits)	8	8			11					9		
Diff. cf. hand meas. (mmHg)	5/3						3%					
ALGORITHM DETAILS	+	+	+	+			+	+				

SYSTEM REFERENCES:

A	1975 Harrow	Cashman et al 1979
B	1976 Belfast	Mitchell, Ruff and Murnaghan 1979
C	1978 Cleveland	Walsh, Thomas and Goldberg 1978
D	1978 Imperial College	Sayers, Ellis and Green 1978
E	1979 Oxford	Sleight, Floras and Jones 1979
F	1979 Sydney	Hunyor, Larkin and Kenny 1980
G	1980 Birmingham	Littler 1980
H	1980 Belfast	Ruff, Mitchell and Murnaghan 1980
I	1980 Padova	Semplicini et al 1981
J	1980 Pisa	derived from (Marchesi 1980)
K	1981 Tampere	Saranummi et al 1982
L	1982 Milan	Di Rienzo et al 1982

For the purposes of this review, "feature extraction" will be taken to mean the extraction of measurements from every cycle of the raw waveform, although this information may not be available on a beat-by-beat basis to the rest of the analysis program. Most of the algorithms listed extract systolic and diastolic pressure; others use a beat-by-beat mean arterial pressure (MAP) derived by integrating the whole waveform or by using the triangular approximation. Pulse pressure is measured in a few cases, beat-to-beat interval in nearly all. A very few systems are deriving additional variables such as left ventricular ejection time, dP/dt and a peripheral resistance index.

The Table lists first the essential requirements for the different algorithms, followed by the extra facilities provided which would be relevant to their validation. Finally the performance figures are given, together with an indication as to whether full details of the algorithm have been published.

Several points are readily apparent from the Table. Firstly, there is a wide diversity of methods in use as evidenced by the different requirements of the various algorithms. Secondly, in several cases no detailed description of the algorithm is available. Thirdly, there is very scanty information about the accuracy of each system, for example as compared to hand measurements from a chart tracing. Although hand measurements do not provide a very good "gold standard", they can at least give an indication that the automatic system correctly detects the systolic and diastolic points in the presence of recorder noise. Furthermore, the systems in which these algorithms are embodied all use different means of calibrating the blood pressure data, in an effort to overcome the residual non-linearity of the recording system. If the calibration signal itself is noisy, then it is possible that an analyser with a highly sophisticated automatic calibration program may give less accurate results than an analyser using simple two-point linear approximation: at the moment there is no way of knowing.

Artefact rejection is mentioned in most of the descriptions cited in the Table. Interactive editing, where available, obviously provides the best chance of protection against gross distortion and interference.However, there is no standardised means of quantifying the automatic rejection of submaximal interference such as recorder noise and partial cannula occlusion. The logical way for this to be done is by means of standard test tapes which could be distributed to all centres active in the field. One such tape has recently become available (Crosby and Hunyor 1982).

It is also important to know what happens to the algorithm's output when the blood pressure is disrupted by arrhythmias; clearly a system which looks at the ECG should discriminate genuine changes from artefact much more effectively than one which relies on the BP signal alone. On the other hand, an algorithm which relies on the ECG for correct blood pressure detection may fail if the ECG is intermittent or noisy. Similarly, if the algorithm puts constraints on the values of systolic, diastolic or pulse pressure which will be accepted, cycles may be missed if the blood pressure suddenly changes profoundly, for example in drug-induced postural hypotension.

It is easy to see why the accuracy and repeatability of these algorithms must be evaluated, when one looks at the literature on real-time blood pressure feature extraction algorithms intended for use in intensive care. Space does not allow an exhaustive review here, but the differences quoted between computer and hand measurement range from 5 to 17 mmHg (Shubin et al,1967; Fozzard et al,1974; Endresen et al,1975). It is reasonable to suppose that these performance figures were obtained using BP signals that were much less noisy than the ambulatory recordings currently being discussed, although perhaps physiologically more extreme.

An interesting incidental point emerges from the intensive care literature; in some algorithms the systolic point is defined as preceding the diastolic point, whilst in others the diastolic precedes the systolic. Pulse pressure may therefore be defined as the amplitude of either the upstroke or the downstroke, a distinction which becomes significant if the effects of arrhythmias on the beat-by-beat blood pressure are being measured. It would be desirable to reach a consensus on which definition should be used before detailed ambulatory studies in this area become widespread.

6. SUMMARY AND CONCLUSIONS

The viability of international coordinated action on ambulatory invasive blood pressure recording has been examined in regard to data storage, data presentation, implementation of analysers and the specification of analyser performance.The following conclusions are drawn:

1. At present we are in a good position to preserve compatibility of raw data recording formats between organisations.

2. Data presentation is still under development; no standard method is likely to emerge for some time.

3. There are already so many different and incompatible analyser implementations that international coordination on analyser design is unlikely.

4. By contrast, it would be appropriate to try to formulate target specifications for the feature extraction algorithms.

5. Before this can be done, the existing analysers should be evaluated using standard test tapes such as that offered by Crosby and Hunyor at Royal North Shore Hospital,Sydney.

6. Agreement should be sought on the definition of pulse pressure for beat-to-beat studies.

REFERENCES

Note: "ISAM 1977, ISAM 1979 and ISAM-GENT 1981"
      refer to the following publications:
ISAM 1977, Proceedings of the Second International Symposium
      on Ambulatory Monitoring (Eds.F.D.Stott, E.B.Raftery,
      P.Sleight and L.Goulding).(Academic Press,London 1978)
ISAM 1979, Proceedings of the Third International Symposium
      on Ambulatory Monitoring (Eds.F.D.Stott,E.B.Raftery and
      L.Goulding).(Academic Press,London 1980)
ISAM-GENT 1981, Proceedings of the Fourth International
      Symposium on Ambulatory Monitoring and the Second Gent
      Workshop on Blood Pressure Variability (Eds.F.D.Stott,
      E.B.Raftery,D.L.Clement and S.L.Wright).(Academic
      Press,London 1982)

Cashman,P.M.M.,Stott,F.D. and Millar Craig,M.W. 1979. Hybrid
      system for fast data reduction of long-term BP
      recordings. Med. & Biol.Eng. & Comput. 17,629-635.
Clement,D.L. 1982. Round Table Discussion: How Shall We Define
      Blood Pressure Variability? ISAM-GENT 1981,607-619.
Crosby,P.A. and Hunyor,S.N. 1982. A test tape for evaluation
      of continuous blood pressure analysis techniques.
      ISAM-GENT 1981, 426-432.
Davies,A.B.,Balasubramanian V.,Cashman,P.M.M.,Stott,F.D. and
      Raftery,E.B. 1982. Accurate and simultaneous recording
      of ST segment,heart rate and blood pressure in patients
      with ischaemic heart disease. ISAM-GENT 1981,68-76.
Davies,A.B.,Cashman,P.M.M.,Balasubramanian,V. and Raftery,E.B.
      Simultaneous recording of arterial blood pressure,heart
      rate and ST segment in the ambulant patient: a new
      system. Med. & Biol.Eng. & Comput. (in press)
Di Rienzo,M.,Cioffi,P.,Pedotti,A. and Mancia,G. 1982. Blood
      pressure and heart rate variability at normal and high
      blood pressure. ISAM-GENT 1981,626-631.
Endresen,J.,Gamble,A. and Hill,D.W. 1975. A Comparison of two
      methods for computer analysis of arterial BP waveforms.
      Europ.J.Intens.Care Medicine 1, 125-128.
Floras,J.S.,Jones,J.V.,Hassan,M.O.,Osikowska,B.A.,Sever,P.S.
      and Sleight,P. 1982. Differences between cuff and
      direct ambulatory BP in patients with essential
      hypertension. ISAM-GENT 1981, 515-521.
Fozzard,H.A.,Kinias,P.D. and Pai,A.L. 1974. Algorithms for
      analysis of on-line pressure signals.
      Computers in Cardiology, Bethesda 1974, 77-80.
Goldberg,A.D. 1980. In:Blood pressure workshop.
      ISAM 1979,448.
Grimbergen,C.A.,van Montfrans,G.A.,Pos,M.,Borst,C. and
      Dunning,A.J. 1982. Temperature dependence of the
      Oxford-Medilog BP measuring amplifier.
      ISAM-GENT 1981,433-443.
Hassen,A. 1976. Monitoring ECG and BP in the intensive care
      unit with portable instruments.
      Postgrad. Med. J.52 (Suppl 7), 142-146.

Hunyor,S.N.,Larkin,H. and Kenny,P. 1980. Comparative 24 hour
    antihypertensive efficacy of once and twice daily
    prazosin therapy. ISAM 1979, 189-196.
Kenny,P.,Hunyor,S.N. and Renwick,J.A. 1980. An appraisal of
    technical characteristics of the Oxford Medilog
    ambulatory BP recording system. ISAM 1979,445-448.
Littler,W.A.,Honour,A.J.,Sleight,P. and Stott,F.D. 1972.
    Continuous recording of direct arterial pressure and
    ECG in unrestricted man. Br. Med. J. 3, 76-78.·
Littler,W.A. 1980. In: "Clinical Ambulatory Monitoring"
    (Ed. W.A.Littler).(Chapman & Hall,London). pp. 96-109.
Mancia,G.,Pomidossi,G.,Parati,G.,Bertinieri,P. et al. 1982.
    BP response to labetalol in twice and three times daily
    administration during a 24 hour period.
    Br.J.Clin. Pharm. 13 (Suppl 1), 27S-35S.
Mann,S.,Millar Craig,M.W.,Gould,B.A.,Altman,D.G. and
    Raftery,E.B. 1982. The assessment of BP variability
    from hourly mean values. ISAM-GENT 1981, 572-581.
Marchesi,C.,Varanini,M. and Guidi,M. 1980. Reliable
    identification of acute episodes during ECG and
    haemodynamic monitoring in ICU . Computers In
    Cardiology,Williamsburg 1980,315-318.
Mehta,S.K.,Walsh,J.T.,Moni,K. and Goldberg,A.D. 1980. Single
    daily dosage of acebutolol in hypertensives.
    ISAM 1979,197-202.
Millar Craig,M.W.,Bishop,C.N. and Raftery,E.B. 1978. Circadian
    variation of blood pressure. Lancet 1, 795-797.
Millar Craig,M.W.,Hawes,D.W.C. and Whittington,J. 1978. New
    system for recording ambulatory BP in man.
    Med.& Biol. Eng.& Comput. 16, 727-731.
Millar Craig,M.W.,Mann,S.,Cashman,P.M.M. and Raftery,E.B.
    1981. Continuous tape recording of ambulatory BP :
    technical considerations.
    Biotelem. Pat. Monitg. 8, 56-66.
Mitchell,R.H.,Ruff,S.C. and Murnaghan,G.A. 1978. Computer
    processing of long-term BP and pulse rate variations.
    ISAM 1977,195-200.
Mitchell,R.H.,Ruff,S.C. and Murnaghan,G.A. 1979. A system for
    determining long term variations of BP and pulse rate.
    IEEE Trans. Biomed. Eng. BME-26 (5), 310-311.
Murnaghan,G.A.,Mitchell,R.H. and Ruff,S.C. 1980. BP rhythms in
    normotensive and pre-eclamptic pregnancy.
    ISAM 1979,157-166.
Murray,A. and Sanders, G.L. 1980. Improving the reliability
    and accuracy of ambulatory BP recordings.
    ISAM 1979,456-461.
Perry,S.G.,Nathan,A.W.,Cochrane,T.,Gosling,P.T. and Camm,A.J.
    1982. A solid state recorder for ambulatory monitoring
    of pulmonary-artery pressure.
    J.Med.Eng. & Technol.6(6),231-235.
Pessina,A.,Palatini,P.,Veronese,P.,Ardigo,A. and Dal Palu,C.
    1978. Value of ambulatory monitoring in the diagnosis
    and management of hypertension. ISAM 1977,185-191.

Ruff,S.C.,Mitchell,R.H. and Murnaghan,G.A. 1980. Heart rate
    variability and its relationship to BP in pregnancy.
    ISAM 1979,261-270.
Saranummi,N.,Kalli,S.,Suuronen,J.,Turjanmaa,V. and Uusitalo,A.
    1982. Analysis of ambulatory BP recordings with a
    microcomputer.
    Computers in Cardiology, Florence 1981,119-122.
Sayers,B.McA. 1978. In: Data Processing Workshop.
    ISAM 1977,315-319.
Sayers,B.McA.,Ellis,N.W. and Green,H.L. 1978. "Minimum and
    Maximum Requirements for Physiological Measurement :
    Intra-arterial Blood Pressure".A Pilot Study Report.
    (Imperial College,London).
Sayers,B.McA.,Cicchiello,L.R.,Raftery,E.B.,Mann,S. and
    Green,H.L. 1982. The assessment of continuous
    ambulatory BP records. Med. Informatics $\overline{7}$(2),93-108.
Schultze,G.,Hauff,A.,Hullmeine,D.,Isichei,E. and Dissman,T.
    1978. Economic digital analysis in long term arterial
    BP telemetry. ISAM 1977,173-184.
Semplicini,A.,Pessina,A.C.,Palatini,P.,Mormino,P.,Casiglia,E.,
    Ventura,E. and Dal Palu,C. 1981. Computer analysis of
    continuous BP recordings in essential hypertension.
    Biotelem.& Pat.Monitg. $\underline{8}$, 100-105.
Shubin,H.,Weil,M.H. and Rockwell,M.A. 1967. Automated
    measurement of arterial pressure in patients by use
    of a digital computer. Med.& Biol. Eng. $\underline{5}$,361-369.
Sleight,P.,Floras,J. and Jones,J.V. 1979. Automatic analysis
    of continuous intra-arterial BP recordings. In: "Blood
    Pressure Variability" (Ed. D.L.Clement).(MTP Press,
    Lancaster, England). pp 61-66.
Van Montfrans,G.A.,Grimbergen,C.A.,Pos,M.,Borst,C. and
    Dunning,A.J. 1982. How to identify cuff-responders.
    ISAM-GENT 1981,504-514.
Walsh,J.T.,Thomas,C.W. and Goldberg,A.D. 1978. Computer
    analysis of continuously recorded BP in ambulant
    hypertensives. Computers in Cardiology, 1978.
Watson,R.D.S.,Stallard,J.J. and Littler, W.A. 1980. Effects of
    once daily administration of beta adrenoceptor
    antagonists on arterial pressure and its variability.
    ISAM 1979,203-208.
Wertheimer,L.,Bandu,I. and Amerasinghe,S. 1978. Blood pressure
    in normal subjects. ISAM 1977, 143-148.
West,M.J.,Sleight,P. and Honour,A.J. 1976. Statistical
    analysis of the 24 hour BP using pressure frequency
    histograms. Postgrad. Med. J. $\underline{52}$ (Suppl.7),100-103.
Zerzawy,R. and Bachmann,K. 1981. Radiotelemetry of Direct BP.
    Biotelem. & Pat. Monitg. $\underline{8}$, 7-14.

DISCUSSION

Chairman: B. McA Sayers

3.3 Feature extraction for haemodynamic signals characterisation.

COUMEL: I enjoyed very much your presentation. Is your message that there is no further information in the blood-pressure than in the heart-rate itself? Are they always closely correlated, as you nicely showed, or is there some-exception, which is, as always, of very great importance?

SAYERS: Yes, I didn't elaborate that point. The main issue I think, as far as the comparison is concerned, lies in this particular point. If particular values of blood-pressure are reached, as a result of the rate of change of pressure rising towars some maximum, and are transients superimposed on it, there's a fairly strong probability that the heart-rate is doing the same sort of thing. If you regard high values of systolic pressure as indicators of anything that might be of interest, not necessary for cardiovascular reasons, but for several reasons, then it may well be possible to identify that sort of feature in the heart-rate much more easily than it would be if you had to make a blood pressure measurement. And the point I suppose I'm making in that particular direction is that you probably wouldn't ever suggest that you can get blood-pressure information of any detailed quantitative character out of heart-rate, but you can learn a lot about what's going on at that particular time from looking at the heart-rate.

VAN BEMMEL: Did you look at those patterns for different days and nights for the same subjects? And did you find, certain standard patterns for an individual, or families of patterns, can these families be generalized? We found, and again you see that this is a very fruitfull workshop, in EEG sleep records, and also EEG's during hemo-dyalisis over days and nights, that these patterns were very individual.

SAYERS: It depends on what you mean by a pattern in this context. The basic point is that virtually all the records one see exhibit the features I've spoken about. What differs is the quantitative description in each case what the average slope of the base-line movements is, what the average amplitude or average duration is. That is rather different between normotensive individuals and hypertensive individuals for obvious reasons. And furthermore, it differs before and after therapy if you're using beta-blocker on the individual. The occurence of some cardiovascular events, cardiac trauma, also influences the issue. I would rather not be drawn on the question of the extent to which you have got characteristic feature which are characteristic of individuals, here, because I haven't got enough data to answer that question. I think we probably have got enough data, and I indeed sent off a paper recently, to distinguish what really does look normotensive from what probably does'nt. It is an operational distinction that matches the rather more extreme clinical distinctions as well. So I think the short answer is that we're on the way to try and achieve definitive measurements, but they really do boil down to statements about the average height of the transient, the average frequency, the average slope and duration of the base line and the characteristics of the circadian features. Incidently, there's a morning overshoot very often, which is quite interesting, in the circadian pattern. That also is fairly definitive of the state. To what extent the individual is individually characteristic, I can't say at the moment.

WOLFF: You have made a very good case for ambulatory monitoring. But for me the much more important philosophical questions is: let us say that this had been an acoustic conference not one about cardiology, and we had been discussing the kind of signal you would have got from a microphone mounted on the roof of this building. It would have looked rather similar, and using your technique you could have separate out of the bell ringing every hour, the fact that siesta occurs, very periodic events. You would have ended up with some kind of minimum signal which was really rather like the more or less random pertubations which you got at the end. Now it seems to me there ought to be a difference between that kind of signal and one for which one believes there is an underlying purpose. Now, I would have thought there was a mechanism which tended to control the blood-pressure for the benefit of something. There would be no such mechanism for controlling the noise level of Pisa, for the benefit of something. Now I see a qualitative difference between a series of the kind which you've been describing, behind which there may be somebody who turns knob, influenced by a whole range of situations, and the signal, which is nearly the sum of a lot of components, which have a purpose, but which are not in any sense related. Now is that a factor which one ought to feed into one's philosophy of signal analysis, that a thing will be tending to optimize something, and which might be a further feature which you could add into this question of dissecting the signal into its components.

SAYERS: Well, I would be the last to object to that philosophical point. I don't think I agree with the basic issue that you brought forward, suggesting a difference between the two situations, the acoustic and the physiological one. Both represent systematic activity at work, in one case it's done for different purposes, in the other case it represents systematic activity characterizing physiological activity. But basically I think when you're talking about regulational control in the classic sense you have to distinguish between the two extreme mechanisms that are at work: the long-term regulation, which is really relevant over periods of months, and the other one which is really relevant over periods of seconds, when you are talking about responses to postural disturbances and so an. So I don't think either of those two, are going to enter as classical control entities into the characterization of a 24 hour record. Nevertheless, the basic point that I'm bringing forward is really that it doesn't make sense to look at a complete signal without regard to the obvious features which you can demonstrate are common to all of these records. Because if you can establish that they are operating indipendently then it doesn't make sense, except, perhaps, for statistical reasons, to pull them together. Can I remark the reason why you cannot really get such a thing as an average blood-pressure, is quite obviously linked to the presence of the different features and their occurences, when you just smooth one of them out, there's another one coming up to make trouble for you. And there is no way, I think, to make any sensible measure of an average blood- pressure, for that reason. Well why should you try? I think you can do so on the individual components. That's a different matter, and that does make sense.

ZYWIETZ: In the methods you are applying, you are removing some systematic effects. This helps in classification and in comparison of measurements between individuals, and so you see what is the variance between individuals and in this way you are able, by this kind of synchronised measurements, to compare better, for example, the blood-pressure of normotensive or hypertensive subjects. If you are able to remove those effects by these methods, you are doing the same thing as regression analysis: to reduce variance and to understand better what is going on in different individuals.

SAYERS: Yes, in individual components, that's absolutely right.

MANCIA: I think I am belonging to the club of continuous blood-pressure recording however, we should criticise ourselves for not doing, limited as they are, casual blood-pressure measurements. That is, just a single measurement, has a fair correlation with prognosis of hypertension and predicts some of the accidents, such as strokes, to a fairly accurate extent. So before we really throw this in the basket and claim the superiority of our system we have to prove there is a better index for prognosis of cardiovascular disease. I fully agree, however, that studying transients could be a nice way of understanding some feautures of cardiovascular regulation, and I really liked your data in this regard; I am very often confused at the meaning of circadian rhythm. In my mind, it refers to the influence which can produce at the same time of the day, regardless the different conditions of the subjects, certain variations, which then can be reproduced. Now are we allowed to talk of circadian rhythm for blood-pressure when, if you change the behaviour of the subject, if the subject sleeps during the day for example, his variability changes, his mean blood-pressure may change, his blood-pressure profile may change. Shouldn't we simply limit ourselves to talk about the effect of behaviour on blood-pressure?

SAYERS: No, I think not. I can't see the force of the argument you're bringing forward. Circadian just means circa a day, not exactly, but roughly a day's recycling or repetition in general terms. This is the reason why circadian is such an attractive term. But what I wanted to make clear is when you're looking at an average profile of what an individual does, or individuals at large do, over the day, you really are talking about that circadian pattern because you have to standardize. Now I said I didn't want to get into the details of how it was done because I've already published that: the consequence of this is that you are standardising over a fixed time and you can identify the occurences, of particular features in the circadian pattern throughout the day. That's the sense in which it is a circadian pattern, even if you regard the particular example of it, the particular member of the ensemble as a diurnal variation. In order to interpret it you have to standardize it, and that's the important issue here.

WALSH: I'd like to thank you, Dr. Cashman for your very illuminating presentation of many of the problems, which have occured with the Oxford Medilog System, for recording blood-pressure. I think it is an area which, although it has received some attention at variuos ISAM conferences and at a less extent in the literature, has really been overlooked to a great degree in interpreting much of the data that's been reported. I would like to share what experiences have been in Cleveland with this system. I think the first point that must be made is that the system must be considered front to back, that is, from the point at which the catheter begins to measure blood-pressure to the last averaged out-put that comes out of the computer. And in our experience the main problems were not with the computer algorithms but were in fact with the recording system. I think many of the variuos computer algorithms, as least for the clinical purposes of half-hourly means or hourly means, and even in fact for beat to beat data as far as the computer algorithm itself is concerned, are probably reasonable. Where the real problems, in my mind, have occured is in the recording system itself, which has problems with virtually each of its components. Our first major discovery was that the transducer was extremely non-linear and thermally unstable. And what we did in Cleveland was to replace the transducer with a different unit which is temperature compensated. The next stage was to change the recording amplifier in the AM4 to one which had much better performance stability and to regulate the battery supply in that unit. Once we did this and hand-selected our recorder for noise, we found the units we had could range anywhere from 6 to 15 mmHg of noise, peak to peak, which is obviously going to bias us the systolic, diastolic pressure by that amount. We found that we could maintain the system for a hand-selected, hand-designed unit, to a maximum drift area of 5 mm. of Mercury, at all levels of calibration. The other point that needs to be considered, is that the replay system is higly non-linear. So, the problem is not so much with the computer algorithms, many of which will be satisfactory for the clinical purposes that exist today, nor perhaps for the kinds of purposes which Prof. Sayers was discussing.

CASHMAN: Well, I wouldn't argue with a great deal on that, although I woldn't in effect paint too black a picture. I think you can be unlucky in the selection of a particular transducer. As you know there is a wide spread of manufacturer's specifications. I would like also to see the computer algorithms evaluated, simply because there's little written about the way they work, and because for istance the bed-side computerized monitors seem to be so unpredictable.

BALASUBRAMANIAN: As one who has been very interested in evaluation, and feels that every system should be adequately validated, it does appear to me that the intra-arterial blood-pressure monitoring technique has still not adequately been validated, and what is disturbing is the large number of publications, particularly from my institution, which has used this system to validate home blood-pressure measurement How valid are those publications when you are comparing an unvalidated system, with so much of errors, against something which is again unvalidated?

CASHMAN: I think it's probably true to say that the error band for both systems is equally larger, it's probably larger for the home blood-pressure. That's certainly something to bear in mind. That's really why I brought this up, because I think there is a sort of assumption getting into the folklore, that the Oxford system is O.K. You can plug it in and let it go.

BALASUBRAMANIAN: I'm very glad this point has been brought up because one of the concerted actions we must take if we are going to define this as a gold standard. Is this a gold standard, or is it a brass standard, a copper standard? At least let's know what standard it is.

TOPIC: 3.4

Algorithms for the classification of biological signal waveforms

PATTERN RECOGNITION IN BIOLOGICAL SIGNALS [*)]

Jan H. van Bemmel and Jan L. Talmon
Dept. Medical Informatics
Free University
AMSTERDAM

1. INTRODUCTION

1.1. Objectives

Biological signals cover a wide range of frequencies, from almost zero, e.g. the signals representing the changes in the menstrual cycle, up to several kHz, e.g. from the electromyogram (see Table 1). In this contribution we will discuss some statistical and other operations on biological signals, especially on the ECG, not only because the latter signal is representative for a time-varying biological phenomenon, but also since the efforts made and the results obtained in electrocardiography are very illustrative for the methods applied to biological signals in general.

SIGNAL	BANDWIDTH (Hz)	AMPL.RANGE (above zero)	QUANTIS. (bits)
EEG	.2 -50	300 µV	4-6
EOG	.2 -15	4 mV	4-6
ECG	.15-150	5 mV	10-12
EMG	20-8000	5 mV	4-8
Bl.Press	0-60	400 mmHg	8-10
Spirogr.	0-40	10 l	8-10
Phonoc.	5-2000	80 dB	8-10

Table 1.

Frequency- and amplitude ranges for some biological signals.

Many strategies and techniques - preprocessing, estimation of features, boundary recognition and pattern classification - can also be applied to the electroencephalogram, the spirogram, hemodynamic and many other signals (Cox, 1972). The ultimate goal of such processing is the medical diagnosis or - in research - to obtain insight in the underlying biological processes and systems. As far as the methods applied to the ECG are concerned, not only the relationship to the analysis of other biological signals is clear, but, far wider, also to many other, non-biological signals and to image processing and pattern recognition in a wide sense.

---

*) Parts of this article are taken from ch. 23 of the
Handbook of Statistics, vol. II (see Van Bemmel, 1982)

Our main objective, therefore, will be to show the
state-of-the-art in biological signal processing and to
discuss specifically the processing of the electrocardiogram
for the interpretation of ECGs during rest or exercise as well
as for ambulatory care or monitoring.

1.2. Properties of biological signals

Biological processes - especially if we study or observe them
in patients - are highly complex, dynamic and adaptive. Only
seldom they can be described in mathematical terms or by well
established theories and models. Very often an empirical and
phenomenological approach, based on observations in the time
domain, may help to characterize the condition of the process
- the organ or the patient - in particular if it is in a
pathological state. A further hindrace on our way to a proper
understanding is the well-known fact of variability, i.e., the
fact that similar biological systems in similar circumstances
hardly ever have identical behaviour. In the feature space
this results in nebulous distributions of features instead of
obtaining clustered clouds.

If we observe and examine these non-stationary and non-linear
processes in medicine, we have to restrict ourselves most of
the time to non-invasive data acquisition methods. This
results in a disturbed and often incomplete data set - the
disturbance stemming from other, also active, processes within
or outside the body. On the other hand, the process may be
studied consecutively or simutaneously by a variety of
different techniques - physical, chemical - which yield a
certain redundancy in the information stream. For instance,
the condition of the heart may be examined by the ECG, the
phono- and apexcardiogram, by catheterization, by nuclear
imaging, by ultrasound or even real-time CT scanning.

On such incomplete, but still redundant information the
medical diagnosis is based. The physician iterates gradually
and stepwise to the final decision. In such decisions, signal
analysis and pattern recognition is a main issue.

Understanding the process is sometimes much facilitated when
we are able to stimulate the process by offering it
standardized loads; to bring it in a certain condition; or to
provoke reactions to inputs. In such cases the signals can
often be understood much easier; it diminishes disturbances,
decreases the variability and offers the possibility to
explain system responses in physiological, clinical or other
scientific terms.

1.3. Acquisition

With modern technology and its micro-sensors a host of
different transducers, instruments and data acquisition
techniques became available to study the human body and to
examine the individual patient. Electrodes for the recording
of the ECG have been much improved by new materials and
buffered amplifiers; multi-function catheters can be shifted
through veins and arteries, e.g., for the intra-cardiac
recording of the HIS-electrogram, flows and pressures;

micro-transducers can even be implanted for long-term monitoring of biological signals. Many other, non-invasive, methods have been devised to study the organism under varying circumstances, e.g., during physical exercise.

In the entire process of signal analysis, the data acquisition is of course a very important stage to obtain low-entropy information and signals with a high SNR. For this reason it must be stressed that signal processing starts at the transducer; it has no sense to put much effort in very intricate statistical techniques if the transducers are not properly located and if the disturbances are unacceptable, hampering detection, recognition and classification. During the last decade, in many instances the signals are digitized as soon as they have been acquired and amplified and are recorded in digital form or real-time processed. Data acquisition equipment is presently often brought very near to the patient, even to the bedside, for reasons of accuracy, speed, communication and possible system failure. Dependent on the specific goal, the processing is done real-time (e.g. for patient monitoring on a coronary care unit, CCU) or off-line (e.g. for the interpretation of the (ambulatory) ECG for diagnostic purposes).

After this rather general introduction we will concentrate on signal analysis, primarily by computerized methods such as digital filters, pattern recognition methods and related statistical techniques. In this respect we will follow the main steps by which computer interpretation is usually done.

2. STAGES IN INTERPRETATION

The over-all purpose of the interpretation of biological signals and images is the reduction and transformation of an often redundant but disturbed transducer output to only a few parameters, which must be of significance for subsequent human decisions. This interpretation can be subdivided along the well-known stages in Pattern Recognition (e.g. Kanal, 1974), i.e.:
(1) measurement;
(2) preprocessing or transformation;
(3) feature selection;
(4) classification (see Figure 1).
In this sense signal processing runs parallel to pattern recognition and image processing (Van Bemmel, 1979). Nevertheless, the interpretation of the ECG can also be viewed as consisting of other steps, i.e.: detection; typification; boundary recognition; feature selection and classification; data reduction. At every step it is possible to discern each of the four different stages, earlier mentioned. A practical realization of signal interpretation along such steps and stages has been realized in a few operational systems. One of these, for ECG interpretation (Talmon, 1974), is illustrated in Figure 2, of which the caption further explains the structural set-up.

280

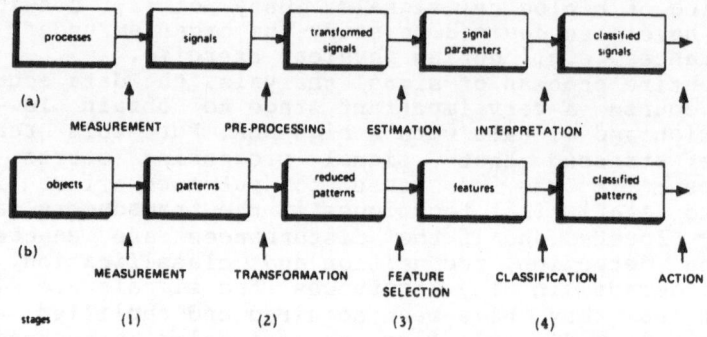

Figure 1.

Stages in pattern recognition and signal processing which run
fully parallel. In many instances, however, the processing is
not as straightforward as indicated here, but includes several
feed-back loops. In this article, several such feedback
examples are mentioned.

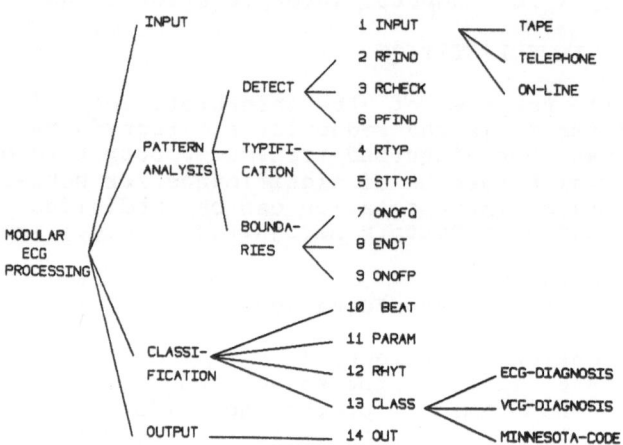

Figure 2.

Example of the set-up of a modular processing systems for the
computer interpretation of ECGs/VCGs. The different tasks can
be clearly discerned, whereas these can themselves be
subdivided in groups and modules. The advantage of a
structured set-up is its easy evaluation, maintenance and
implementation.

3. DETECTION

The detection of signals is the first step in all digital signal processing. Many examples can be mentioned, but in the following paragraphs we shall mainly treat the ECG.
ECGs are a big challenge to develop generally applicable processing methods. The first problem to be solved is to detect all QRS-complexes without too many false positive (FP) or missed beats (FN). If this problem has been solved, the question remains of how to detect the tiny P-waves amidst the always present disturbances, especially if the rhythm and QRS-waves are chaotic.

3.1. A priori knowledge

Before treating the specific problems of QRS- and P-wave detection, we want to mention the fact that any detector can only operate optimally if as much as possible a priori knowledge about the signals (shape, occurrence) has been built into it. Figure 3 illustrates this situation, often referred to as strong or weak coupling between detection and estimation. We will wherever possible make use of this in the following.

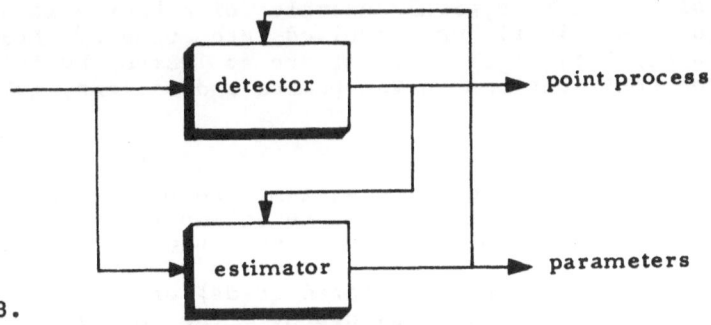

Figure 3.

Illustration of the principles of strong and weak coupling for simultaneous detection and estimation of signals. In case of weak coupling, only one feed-back loop is present. In ECG pattern recognition, these principles are frequently used.

Biological processes, such as the functioning of the heart, can frequently be considered in the time domain as a series of coupled events, as for instance the relation between the P-wave and the QRS-complex. In analyzing such signals we are interested in the occurrence of each of these events, which can be expressed as a point process. In many instances, however, it is a complicated task to derive the point process from the signal if we do not exactly know what event (waveshape) to look for. On the other hand, the determination of the waveshape itself is very much facilitated if we are informed about the occurrence of the events (the point process). Accordingly, a priori knowledge about one aspect of the signal considerably simplifies the estimation of the other.

In practice, this process of simultaneous detection and estimation as in ECGs, is done iteratively: a small part of the signal serves for a first, rough event detection and estimation of the waveshape, and based upon this, an improved point process can be computed and so on.

However, if we have to deal with only rarely occurring waveshapes as in intra-ventricular depolarization with wandering pacemakers, such a priori knowledge is not available. We can only improve the estimation if at least a few ECG-beats of identical shape are present for analysis.

It is unnecessary to state, that the optimum performance of a detector is only obtained if we also have at our disposal the prior probabilities of the occurrences of the different waves. Although the latter is seldom known for the individual ECG, a good compromise is the optimization of the detector's performance e.g. for a library of ECGs and to test it on another, independent population. We shall give a few examples of detection by means of the analysis of the ECG.

3.2. Detection of ventricular activity

The purpose of QRS-detection is to detect all depolarization waves, including premature beats, resulting from a dipolar wavefront travelling through the ventricles. The detection of QRS-complexes is a typical example of a heuristic approach, although the algorithms involved are usually trained on learning populations or at least are evaluated by independent ECGs (see contributions in Van Bemmel and Willems, 1977).

● preprocessing

Since most ECG interpretative systems are processing at least 3 simultaneous leads, also the detection functions are based on combined leads. The commonly used detection functions $d(i)$ (i the sample number) are based on derivatives (i.e., comparable to band-pass filtered leads) or - in terms of three-dimensional vectorcardiography - the spatial velocity. If the ECG(i) is expressed as

$$ECG(i) = (X_1(i), X_2(i), X_3(i)) \qquad (1)$$

then the detection function $d(i)$ can be written as

$$d(i) = \sum_k T(X_k(i)) \qquad (2)$$

with T a transformation of $X_k(i)$. The most simple formula for computing the derivative is, by taking the two-sided first difference, so that

$$T = [X_k(i+1) - X_k(i-1)]^2. \qquad (3)$$

The spatial velocity is in this case just the square root of $d(i)$. Other, simpler forms, saving processing time for $d(i)$ are, with absolute values:

$$T = |X_k(i+1) - X_k(i-1)|. \qquad (4)$$

A third detection function which is also seen, is computed
from the original amplitudes, with

$$T = [X_k(i)]^2. \tag{5}$$

The disadvantage of d(i) with the last transformation is, that
it is very sensitive to changes in baselines. Other functions
for T are, though sometimes more elaborate, essentially
identical to the ones mentioned here or combinations of it.
Figure 4 shows an example of a detection function computed
from absolute first differences according to (4).

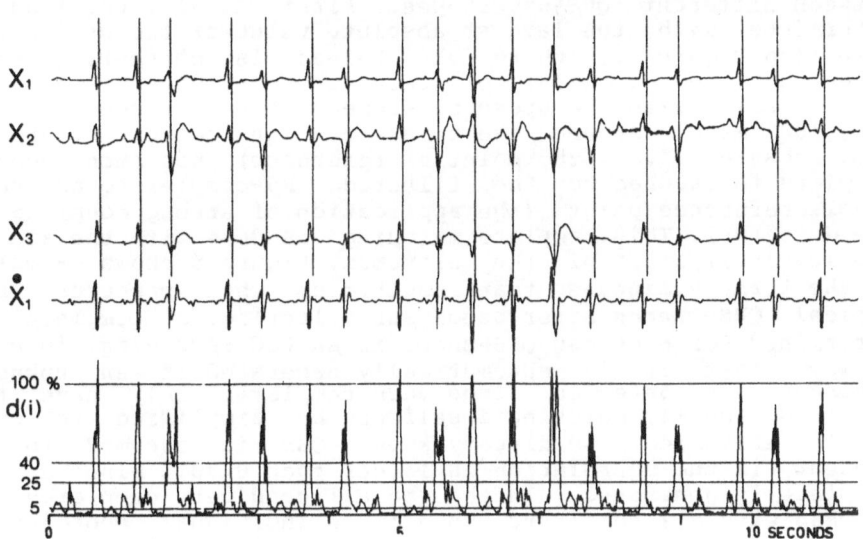

Figure 4.

Detection of the QRS-complexes in an ECG recording. From the
scalar leads X (i), the detection function d(i) is computed.
Three thresholds are applied after estimating the 100% level.
A candidate QRS is detected with these thresholds. Further
refinement, i.e. the determination of a point of reference, is
done from the derivative of one of the leads, in this case X .
Vertical lines indicate the points of reference of the
detected QRS-complexes.

● features and classification

As an example of the detection of the QRS in the latter signal
we will discuss a method reported by Hengeveld (1976) and
Plokker (1978). Detection is done by first computing the
averaged peak of all QRS-complexes in d(i). Next, thresholds
are applied at 5, 25 and 40% of this averaged peak.
A QRS-complex is labelled as a candidate wave if the detection
function fulfills the following conditions:

"d(i) > 25% during > 10 msec." AND "some d(i) > 40% (6)
during 100 msec. thereafter" AND "the distance
to a preceding candidate > 250 msec."

Other systems apply different thresholds and rules for QRS
finding, but all approaches follow one or another logical
reasoning or syntactic rule, based on intrinsic ECG
properties, expressed as statistics of intervals, amplitudes
or other signal parameters. We shall proceed with the method
described in Plokker (1978). If the candidates, mentioned
above, are found, an algorithm is applied to discriminate
between different QRS-waveshapes. First of all, the lead is
determined with the largest absolute value of the derivative
(see also Figure 4, where the X-lead is chosen). In this
selected lead, a point of reference is determined: the
zero-crossing with the steepest slope within a search interval
of ± 100 msec. around the first rough indication. After the
zero-crossing (i.e., the point of reference) has been found a
template is matched to the filtered QRS-complex to assure a
stable reference point (the application of strong coupling in
the detector). This template matching is done with the aid of
two levels at ± 25% of the extremum. Figure 5 shows examples
of the ternary signals, that result from this procedure, for
typical QRS-shapes after band-pass filtering. A template is
determined for each new QRS-shape in an ECG recording, in such
a way, that it is automatically generated if an unknown
waveshape is detected. Since such templates only have the
value 0 and +1, matching itself can be simplified to only
simple arithmics. An already known QRS is assumed to be
present if the correlation is larger than 0.70, else a new
template is generated. In the end all candidate complexes are
matched with all templates found in an individual recording to
determine the highest correlation factors. A method as
described here, yields much less than 0.1% FP (false alarms)
or FN (missed beats), see Table 2 for the results of the
evaluation derived from Talmon (1983).

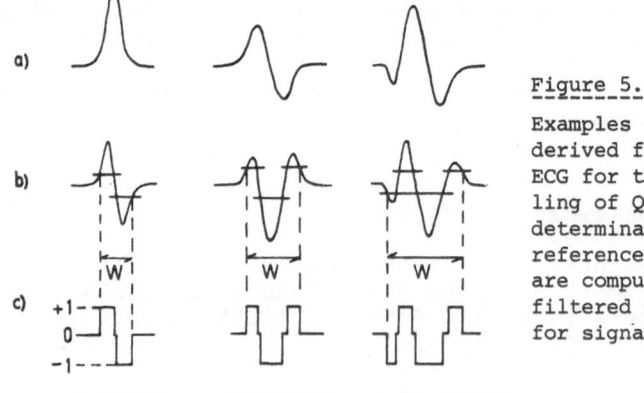

Figure 5.

Examples of ternary templates,
derived from an individual
ECG for the preliminary labelling of QRS waveshapes and the
determination of a point of
reference. The ternary signals
are computed from the band-pass
filtered QRS-complex and used
for signal matching.

```
                        D E T E C T O R
        +       -     +       -     +       -     +       -     +       -
```

R E F +	32663	34	11513	19	10874	9	11438	19	10161	35
−	27	−	17	−	16	−	14	−	6	−

```
        XYZ           I-III         aVL-F          V1-3          V4-6
```

Table 2.

Evaluation of the QRS detector of the Modular ECG Interpretation System (Talmon, 1983) with 1908 VCGs/ECGs as an independent testing population.

3.3. Detection of atrial activity

A similar, though more intricate, strategy can be followed for the location of P-waves. They are small as compared to the QRS-complex and about 100 µV or less, and of the order of magnitude of the noise in the bandwidth of 0.10 to 150 Hz, that can vary from 10 µV to even 100 µV or more. The frequency spectrum of such P-waves, however, lies far below this 150 Hz: roughly in between 0.10 and 8 Hz. Other prior information that can be built into the algorithms is that such P's can be coupled to QRS-complexes or not, and do most of the time occur with a repetition rate of less than 200 per minute. The duration of the P-wave is about 60 to 100 msec., its shape may vary from person to person and from lead to lead. If the P-wave is coupled to the QRS, the range of the PR-interval distribution is less than 30 msec.
The processing of P-waves may require much computer time unless we use data reduction methods and optimized algorithms to speed up the processing. Often we have to look for a compromise between what is theoretically (from the standpoint of signal processing) desirable and practically (from the standpoint of program size and processing time) feasible. P-wave detection is an illustrative example in this respect.

First of all, we discriminate between "coupled" and "non-coupled" P-waves. This is of importance, since regular rhythms are most commonly seen (in more than 90% of all patients). For that reason the detector has first of all to ascertain whether such coupling is present or not. The detection of "non-coupled" P-waves is much more cumbersome and requires considerable computational effort. For both approaches we will discuss the processing stages mentioned earlier (for illustration purposes we follow the lines of thought published by Hengeveld (1976)).

● preprocessing of coupled P's

In order to enhance the probabilities of finding coupled P-waves, the preprocessing is only done in a window before the onset of a QRS-complex, by filtering each ECG signal in a proper bandwidth (0.10-8 Hz) to increase the SNR of the P-wave. Since the upper frequency has been decreased it is allowed to diminish the sampling rate in this interval as well (e.g. to 100 Hz).

● features and classification of coupled P's

The parameters on which the decision is based whether the P-waves are coupled to the QRS-complexes are computed as follows. The instants of maximal and minimal amplitude within the window are determined and the differences are computed between these instants and the estimated QRS-onset. This yields per ECG-lead 2 intervals (for 3 leads, of course, 6 intervals). For the entire recording the ranges of the interval distributions are computed and if only one of these is small enough (i.e. < 30 msec.), for at least 80% of all QRS-complexes present, the decision of coupled P-waves is made.
If the P-waves cannot be classified as coupled to the following QRS, it still remains to be investigated whether P's are yet present and at what instants. For that reason, the entire processing is started once more, now by using shape information. We will follow the stages in this second approach as well.

● preprocessing of non-coupled P's

First of all the search window is enlarged from the end of the preceding T-wave until the onset of the next QRS-complex. Filtering and sampling rate reduction as well as computation of the derivatives of the signals is done in the same way as discussed before. The derivative itself is computed after having cut away the QRS-complex (see Figure 6a) in order to diminish the effect of the high-amplitude QRS on the filter output.
Next, the signal is rectified and two thresholds are applied, at 75% and 50% of the extreme value within the search area. By combining the outputs of the two threshold detectors we construct a ternary signal (Figure 6e), which is a highly reduced version of the original signal and most of the time of zero amplitude.
In practice, only the instants of level crossing are stored and used for further processing as will be made clear in the following.

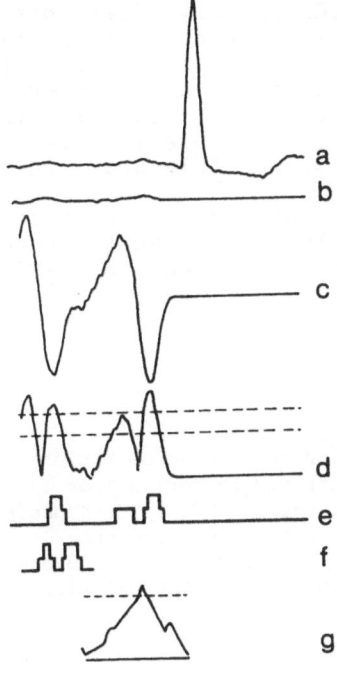

Figure 6.

Steps in the recognition of non-coupled
P-waves. In the original signal (a), the
QRS is cut away (b), in order to diminish
the response of the high-amplitude QRS in
the band-pass filtered output as seen in
(c). The latter signal is rectified (d)
and thresholds are applied to derive a
ternary signal (e) is crosscorrelated
with a template (f) that has been computed from a training population of P-waves.
The matching function is seen in (g).
Again a level is applied to detect the
presence of P-waves.

● features and classification of non-coupled P's

In the next stage we compute the cross-correlation between the
ternary signal and a template, previously computed from a
learning set of P-waves, preprocessed in the same manner (and
not from the individual ECG recording, as in QRS detection).
In this template (Figure 6f) the information about the set of
P-waves is condensed - albeit in a rather crude way for
reasons of processing speed. Of course it would in some
instances be better to use the prior information about the
P-wave shapes of the individual ECG, but, as written in par.
3.1, this is not always feasible so that in such cases the
statistical properties of a population of signals is used
instead. So, the parameters that are used for recognition are
the instants of the different level crossings, which can be
visualized as a ternary signal. In practice, this
cross-correlation or matching again does not imply any
multiplication, since it can be proven that the entire
correlation can be carried out by simple additions and
subtractions of intervals, to be computed only at the instants
of level crossings. An example of the correlation as a
function of time is shown in Figure 6g. If the correlation
reaches a maximum above 0.80, the presence of a P-wave is
assumed. The procedure is carried out for each individual lead
available and for all TQ-intervals.

Most interpretation systems for ECGs do only offer overall evaluation results. The available literature in this field gives only seldom the reasons for ECG-misclassification, which might have happened anywhere during the various steps and stages of processing. For many reasons it is of utmost importance to trace the shortcomings of all intermediate steps involved in the interpretation, so that possible weak links in the chain of steps can be improved.

For the two different approaches to P-wave detection this has been done by Plokker (1978). Evaluation results from a population of about 1900 patients can be seen in Table 3, after Talmon (1983).

	DETECTOR	
	+	−
+	27942	48
−	106	−

REF.

Table 3.

Evaluation of the P-wave detection method, described in par. 3 (for coupled P-waves in VCGs). The numbers are derived from 27,990 P-waves (XYZ-leads) from 1908 ECG recordings. 48 P's are missed and 106 falsely detected.

We will not conclude this paragraph on detection without mentioning that in processing biological signals such as ECGs, the finding of other events is just as important to avoid wrong (FP) detections. This regards the detection of 'spikes' (sometimes with similar shapes as the QRS) resulting from electrical disturbances in the environment of the patient; the measurement and correction of 60 Hz (50 Hz) main voltage; the effect of electrode polarization causing wandering baselines or even amplifier saturation.

Furthermore, there is the disturbance of biological origin: patient movements and their effects on the ECG like baseline fluctuations, electromyographic signals and the modulation of the signal (up to a modulation depth of 50%) caused by respiration. In order to obtain a reliable interpretation of the ECG with a minimum of FP and FN, all steps (the detectors, parameter estimators and classifiers) have to reckon with these disturbances. In many systems special detectors and pattern recognition algorithms have been built-in to find baseline drifts, spikes, EMG and so on. Especially in cases where a superposition of signal and non-stationary disturbances exists, discrimination is very complicated or even impractical, given the finite amount of time allowed for an ECG computer interpretation, e.g., because of economic implications.

4. TYPIFICATION

Morphologic classification of signals such as in ECG interpretation, as we will report in this chapter, is done at 3 different steps: we treated already the detection of the QRS, where a ternary template is employed for a rough indication of waveshapes; in ·this paragraph the morphologic classification is called typification, intended to find the normal or modal beat by labelling all waveshapes; in the diagnostic classification it is directed towards a discrimination between (degrees or combinations of) disease patterns.

● preprocessing

In this step we depart from the original signal(s), given the fiducial points found by the detection. As in all pattern recognition applications, also here the question rises what set of features to search for typification. We repeat that as much a priori information should be utilized as is known and available. For illustration we discuss again one specific development (Van Bemmel, 1973). We know that the duration of a QRS-complex is on the average not longer than 100 msec. and that most signal power is found in the bandwidth between about 8 to 40 Hz. For these reasons, the QRS is filtered by a digital convolution procedure around the reference point and the sampling rate is reduced to 100 Hz, in such a way, that the instantaneous amplitudes (or, in VCG, vectors) are located in an area around and phase-locked with the fiducial point, at 10 msec. distance apart, where most of the signal power is located. In practice, this could mean e.g. 3 or 6 parameters before and resp. 7 or 4 parameters after the reference point. The location of the window of instantaneous amplitudes is therefore dependent on QRS morphology. From this set of 10 filtered, instantaneous amplitudes per QRS-complex, the features are computed for typification or labelling.

● features and classification

The parameters that are used for the discrimination between different types of QRS-shapes within one ECG, are based on signal power computed by means of the variance-covariance matrix. Let, for one or more leads k the set of 10 instantaneous amplitudes be represented by the vectors $\underline{v}_k$. The series of K consecutive QRS-complexes can be represented by the set $\{\underline{v}_k\}$. For these vectors $\underline{v}$ we determine the variance-covariance matrix by

$$\text{cov}(j,k) = \underline{v}_j^T \cdot \underline{v}_k \quad \text{(T for transposed)} \qquad (7)$$

of which the instantaneous power can be written as $P(k) = \text{cov}(k,k)$.
The cross-correlation matrix can be written as

$$\rho(j,k) = \text{cov}(j,k) \, [\text{cov}(j,j)\,\text{cov}(k,k)]^{-\frac{1}{2}}. \qquad (8)$$

Both the ρ's and the instantaneous power $P(k)$ are used as features for typification. Two complexes with indices j and k are said to be identical if

$$\text{"}P(k)/w < P(j) < w.P(k)\text{" AND "}\rho(j,k) > \lambda_\rho\text{"} \qquad (9)$$

in which w is a weighting coefficient and λ_ρ a threshold, still to be determined from a learning population. In Figure 7 we see the effect of λ_ρ on the typification. Based on such studies, suitable values for w and λ_ρ are: w = 2 and λ_ρ = 0.80. This means that in 10-dimensional feature space two complexes are called identical if they fall within a cone with a spatial angle determined by λ and within two spherical shells determined by w.
To speed up the computation time, for an ECG of, say, 20 beats, not the entire matrix of 20 x 20 terms is computed, but in practice a sequential method is employed which only needs a small part of the matrix. Starting with the first complex, the first row of the matrix (i.e., the covariances with all other complexes) is computed. Next, only those rows are computed for which the conditions of similarity were not fulfilled, which brings the number of computations back to about 10%. For all leads available this procedure is repeated. If more than one lead is available, again a syntactic majority rule is applied which is optimized by a learning population. Also the determination of the dominant beat is done by such rules, making use of intervals between the different types of complexes. Table 4, taken from Talmon (1983), presents a result of the algorithm for QRS-typification. The typification of ST-T waves is done in similar ways, also based on instantaneous amplitudes, falling however in a much lower frequency bandwidth. The combined results of QRS- and ST-T labelling finally gives the dominant complexes that can be used for diagnostic shape classification.

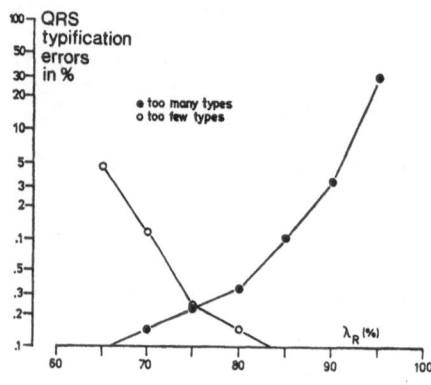

Figure 7.

Effect of the typification threshold on the number of correctly labelled QRS-complexes. If the level is too high, all complexes are called identical and vice versa. In case of parallel leads, combinatory rules are applied for the optimization of typification.

		T Y P E							
	1	2	3	4	5	1	2	3	4
1	31914	8	0	0	0	43107	51	0	0
2	2	271	0	1	0	11	352	3	0
REF. 3	0	0	24	1	0	1	1	21	0
4	0	0	0	2	1	0	0	0	2
5	0	0	0	0	1				
		V C G				E C G			

Table 4.

Decision matrix for QRS typification. In 1908 records (all leads) 75,774
QRS-complexes were seen, with up to 5 different waveshapes. The overall
result was an error rate of less than 0.03% for the VCG and 0.15% for the
ECG.

● supervised learning

Thus far we have restricted ourselves to the labelling of
QRS-waves from ECG recordings of rather short (e.g., 5-15
sec.) duration. If this problem has to be solved for very long
recordings, as in a coronary care unit or for ambulatory ECG
monitoring, slightly different techniques can be used (Swenne,
1973; Ripley, 1975; Feldman, 1977). Especially in the first
situation, all operations have to be executed in real-time or
even faster. If the time is allowed, in such circumstances
interactive pattern recognition may offer great advantages
(Kanal, 1972). Several systems, therefore, make use for
waveform recognition of man-machine interaction (Swenne,
1973). As soon as the computer (e.g. by using the same methods
as explained before) finds an unknown QRS-shape, the user
(nurse, physician) is requested to indicate whether he wants
to label this wave as normal or, e.g., as a PVC or wants to
ignore it. The computer stores the patterns belonging to the
indicated beats in memory for future comparison. In this way
two goals are served: the user determines the labelling for
the individual patient himself and he is alarmed as soon as
waves of strange or abnormal shape suddenly occur. During
training (supervised learning) and thereafter, the computer
determines the gravity points of the cluster ϕ_k, belonging to
type k as follows:

$$\underline{m}_k = \sum_{i=1}^{n_k} \underline{v}_i / n_k \tag{10}$$

$\underline{v}_i$ being the (10-dimensional) feature vector for complex i and
n_k being the number of times the complex of type k has been
observed. The dispersion of the cluster is determined in the
usual way:

$$s_k^2 = \sum_{i=1}^{n_k} (\underline{v}_i - \underline{m}_k)^2 / (n_k - 1). \tag{11}$$

The distance from some new vector $\underline{w}_j$ to the clusters $\{\phi_k\}$ is computed by the normalized Euclidean distance:

$$d_{jk}^2 = (\underline{w}_j - \underline{m}_k)^2/s_k^2. \qquad . \qquad (12)$$

$\underline{w}_j$ is allocated to ϕ_k instead of ϕ_l if

$$"d_{jk} < \lambda_d \cdot d_{jl}" \text{ AND } "d_{jk} < \lambda_k". \qquad (13)$$

Proper measures for the thresholds are: $\lambda_d = 5$ and $\lambda_k = 3$ or 4. In order to allow a gradual change in waveshapes (letting the cluster ϕ_k slowly float in feature space), we may use recursive formulae as soon as $n_k > \lambda_n$ (during the training $\lambda_n = n_k$):

$$\underline{m}_k(n_k + 1) = \frac{\lambda_n \cdot \underline{m}_k(n_k) + \underline{v}_k}{\lambda_n + 1}. \qquad (14)$$

A suitable value for λ_n lies in the order of 20.
Operational systems do make use of these and similar algorithms for the labelling of waveforms (as reported e.g. in Nolle, 1977, Van Bemmel and Willems, 1977 or Thomas, 1979).

5. BOUNDARY RECOGNITION

After detection and wave labelling it is necessary to determine those parts in the signal that are of significance for diagnostic classification. In (biological) signals and patterns such parts are searched by segmentation methods or boundary detection. Once we know already approximately the location of the waves of interest in the ECG (P, QRS, ST-T), we have to locate as exactly as possible their boudaries; 5 points for one ECG beat.
We will discuss a few methods, as found in the literature and also indicate possible advantages and inaccuracies: straightforward threshold detection; matching with a signal part; cross-correlation with an amplitude-time template (e.g. Pipberger, 1972; Van Bemmel, 1973).

The detection signal used for boundary recognition is commonly one of the functions $d(i)$ as mentioned in par. 3 (a spatial velocity or vector magnitude or a combination of both). For illustration purposes we will restrict ourselves to $d(i)$, as computed with

$$T = |AR_N(X_k(i))| \qquad (15)$$

where AR_N is an autoregressive digital filter, computing some bandpass filtered version of the ECG $X_k(i)$, intended to obtain the derivative (while increasing the SNR) and based on $\pm N$ sample points around i.

● thresholds

Threshold detection is done by applying a fixed or relative amplitude level in d(i) within a window where the wave boundary has to be expected. In some cases, feedback is built in the method in such a way that the threshold may be adaptively increased if too many level crossings are seen within the window.

● signal matching

The second method that has been reported, is the use of a standard waveform around the point where the boundary is expected. This standard waveform s(k) is computed from a learning set of functions d(k) with known boundaries, indicated by human observers. The method then searches for the minimum of the estimator $e_s(i)$ within a given time window:

$$\text{MIN}_i \left\{ e_s(i) = \sum_{k=-N}^{M} (d(i+k) - s(k))^2 / w^2(k) \right\} \qquad (16)$$

with N and M points before resp. after the boundary.
For the weighting factor w(k), the dispersion of s(k) at point k is usually taken, so that e_s is the weighted mean squares difference between d and s. The minimum of $e_s(i)$ yields the boundary at $i = i_0$.
A disadvantage of this method is, that it is rather sensitive to noise, since in such circumstances the function d(i) may remain at relatively high amplitude levels.

● template matching

Two-dimensional (i.e., time and amplitude) templates have been developed for waveform boundary recognition as well. In such applications a signal part is considered as a pattern in 2-dimensional space, to be matched with another 2-D template, constructed from a learning set. We will briefly explain the method.
Here again we start from the set of L functions $\{d^\ell(i)\}$, reviewed by human observers (boundaries were indicated in the original signals $X_k(i)$). Around the boundaries, windows are applied (see Figure 8), to be used later on in the cross-correlation.

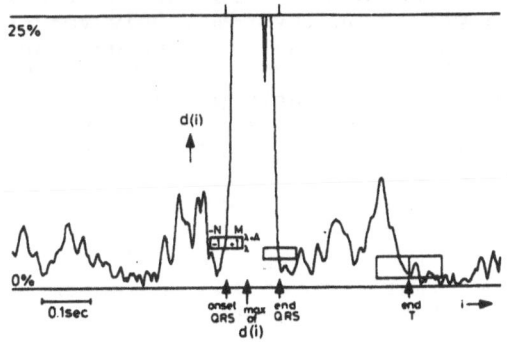

Figure 8.

Example of the windows that are applied in the detection function d(i) for the recogni- tion of wave boundaries. Within these windows a template is matched to a function computed from d(i).

Within the window area we determine a multi-level threshold function f as:

$$f_\lambda^\ell(i) = \text{sign } \{d^\ell(i) - \lambda\}. \tag{17}$$

i is the sample number, ℓ one of the L functions d^ℓ and λ the applied threshold; "sign" takes the sign of the expression in between brackets. So, the area where the function d(i) is larger than λ, is given the value +1, otherwise the value -1. As a matter of fact, see above, this is the most simple boundary detector, yielding a response only at the place where d(i) crosses λ.

We now define a template $T_\lambda(i)$ in which the statistical properties of all f^ℓ are comprised:

$$T_\lambda(i) = \frac{1}{L} \sum_{\ell=1}^{L} f_\lambda^\ell(i). \tag{18}$$

It can be shown that T_λ is a linear function of the cumulative density distributions of the functions d^ℓ at points i. Once the template T_λ is obtained, it is cross-correlated with all individual threshold functions f^ℓ of the learning population. This yields in general new boundary points at maximum correlation, which can form the basis for the construction of a new template T_λ. This process of convergence may be repeated a few times until a stable template results, no longer influenced by the observer variation in the training set.

In order to speed up the processing time, again a compromise is made between theoretical and practical requirements. This is acquired by simplifying the template T_λ, that may contain any value in between +1 and -1, to only the values +1, 0 and -1. This is done by applying a threshold λ_T, to obtain the simplified template W_λ:

$$W_\lambda(i) = \begin{cases} \text{sign}(T_\lambda(i)) & \text{for} \quad |T_\lambda(i)| > \lambda_T \\ 0 & \text{for} \quad |T_\lambda(i)| \leq \lambda_T \end{cases} \tag{19}$$

A suitable value for λ_T lies somewhere around 0.30. The advantage of W_λ instead of T_λ is that in this case again only additions and subtractions are computed and no multiplications are involved.

Methods such as the ones described here are in routine use for a wide variety of ECG interpretation systems. Only very few reports appeared in the literature giving evaluation results of the algorithms on well-documented ECGs. Yet, these boundaries form the basis for all diagnostic procedures.

The inaccuracies that are still allowable for P-, QRS- and ST-T boundaries are in the order of 15, 5 and 30 msec. resp. at both sides of the onsets or endpoints.

Some interpretation programs for ECGs adopt the boundary detection to each complex separately and apply next a majority rule to determine the most probable locations of the wave edges (e.g. by the determination of the median of the measured distribution of recognized boundaries). Other programs apply the edge detection only after coherent averaging of the dominant beats found by the typification step. The outcomes of both approaches are essentially different, because of the different influence of disturbances on both methods.

Promising wave parsing methods, also applied to ECGs have been reported by Stockman (1976) and Horowitz (1977), that are essentially syntactic approaches to this problem.

After many years of research in the wide field of Pattern Recognition for general edge or boundary detection methods, still no general method is as yet available. The only common factor between all reported techniques is that they at least strive at the maximization of the likelihood of the same phenomenon and one can only hope that they converge to identical solutions.

Problems which involve the segmentation of ECGs (in general: signals) have much in common with the boundary recognition methods as treated here. Again, it fully depends on the signal characteristics and the ultimate goal of the user what strategy is followed.

6. FEATURE SELECTION AND CLASSIFICATION

The proper selection of features is the basis for all pattern and signal classification. As soon as we have determined in earlier steps the signal parts to be classified, the question arises: which features?

This question is also a main issue for ECG interpretation. Some investigators supposed that those parameters by which the original ECG can be reconstructed (e.g. an orthonormal basis such as the Nyquist samples, Fourier, Karhunen-Loève or Chebyshev components) are a sufficient basis for a feature space (e.g. Young, 1963). This, however, is only seldom true, since these parameters are ideal for a syntactic shape reconstruction, but do not necessarily have a semantic information content.

Features that have diagnostic discriminatory power are very often computed from non-linear combinations of the syntactic basic components, such as products, ratios, squares or time intervals, that may be related to biological events and phenomena. Such parameters will hardly ever automatically arise, even not by non-linear mapping techniques. For that reason only sound theoretical reasoning based on fundamental knowledge of the biological process - see also par. 1.2 - is the ideal way to obtain relevant features.

In many cases, however, the significance of the features is only a posteriori demonstrated by means of operations on well-documented populations of ECGs, often referred to as heuristic feature selection.

● logical vs. statistical

In ECG interpretation in general two approaches are followed to solve the waveshape classification problem (as is usually also done for other problems): logical methods (tables, trees, syntactic rules) and statistical techniques (linear, non-linear, fuzzy, Bayes' rule) or combinations; all of them essentially multi-parameter methods. Logical decision trees are the most widely used, being better associated with human reasoning than multivariate statistical methods, although the optimization of the latter techniques can be more easily done than for logical trees or tables (see e.g. Cornfield, 1973; Wartak, 1969; Wolf, 1972; Van Bemmel and Willems, 1977). A final answer to the optimum strategy to be followed in ECG interpretation is certainly hampered by the fact that not always a one-to-one relationship can be established between the ECG and the heart disease involved; consequently, many different criteria exist for identical diseases. Further complicating factors are the inter-individual variability; the fact that a disease can appear in varying degrees; and the combination of diseases at different stages of severity. If one realizes the huge amount of degrees of freedom in combinations of, say, only 7 or 8 a main groups of ECG-shape abnormalities (left or right ventricular hypertrophy, anterior, posterior/diaphragmatic, inferior and lateral myocardial infarction, and right- or left ventricular conduction defects) for almost all possible ages and races and for both sexes, almost no training population of ECGs would be sufficiently large to solve the classification problem in a definite way. Here again, the use of clinical information and knowledge is of utmost importance, to be built into the classification rules. For these reasons it is not surprising that most practical solutions of ECG interpretation make use of logical reasoning and binary trees.

● classification of contours

Although classification results for wave contours have not in general been reported for biological signal interpretation systems, they have been published for almost all existing ECG programs. Except for the study by Bailey almost no objective evaluation study has been published based on the same populations (Bailey, 1974). Classification results, of course, differ widely from one application area to the other (e.g. in screening or in a heart clinic). Some programs (Pipberger, 1975) are primarily based on independent, i.e. non-ECG information (history, catheterization data, autopsy reports etc.) instead of on the diagnosis by cardiologists based on ECG morphology. This approach to ECG diagnosis, however, has not received the expected interest from the medical community. If the final diagnosis based on the ECG itself and obtained from a team of cardiologists is used for reference purposes (e.g. Bonner, 1972), the best results reported thus far claim a percentage of > 95% of correctly classified waveforms.

Although the proper choice of features primarily determines the results of the classification and the model that is being used for discrimination can only reveal the requested performance on the basis of these properly chosen feature vectors, the statistical approach - at least from a theoretical point - offers some advantages over a logical reasoning. An advantage is, e.g., the fact that in a multivariate approach we may easily and anlytically take into account prior probabilities for the different diseases and cost and utility factors. The aposteriori propability of having a disease k out of K, given the prior probabilities p(k) and the feature (symptom) vectors $\underline{x}$ with their conditional probabilities p($\underline{x}$/k), can be expressed with Bayes as:

$$p(k/\underline{x}) = p(\underline{x},k) \left[\sum_{j=1}^{K} p(\underline{x}/j) \, p(j) \right]^{-1} \tag{20}$$

The classification of vector $\underline{x}$ to a certain class is determined by the minimum of p(k/$\underline{x}$), if desired beforehand weighted with a matrix of cost factors. In case the vectors $\underline{x}$ have normal distributions for all diseases k and assuming identical variance-covariance matrices D for all distributions $\underline{x}$/k, with $\underline{m}_{jk} = \underline{m}_j - \underline{m}_k$ ($\underline{m}_k$ the mean of class k), we may write for the aposteriori probabilities:

$$p(k/\underline{x}) = \left[1 + \sum_{j=1,\neq k} \exp(\underline{x}^T D^{-1} \underline{m}_{jk} - \tfrac{1}{2} \underline{m}_{jk}^T D^{-1} \underline{m}_{jk}) \, p(j)/p(k) \right]^{-1} \tag{21}$$

Cornfield (1973) has shown the influence of the prior probabilities in such models if used in clinical practice (see also Pipberger, 1975). If too many disease classes (age, race, sex etc.) in different degrees and combinations have to be discerned, such statistical models require an impractically large population for training the parameters. In such cases it appeared to be wise to combine the advantages of the purely statistical approach with that of the heuristic and logical solution to the classification problem.

● classification of rhythms

Rhythm diagnosis is based on the measured PP, RR and PR intervals as well as P-wave and QRS-morphology, found by the detection and typification or waveform labelling steps. If no detailed diagnosis is given of complicated rhythms, but just categories of larger groups of certain arrhythmias, many programs claim a percentage of correctly diagnosed ECGs well above 95%, being very acceptable in clinical practice or for screening purposes (see Willems, 1972; Gustafson, 1978; Plokker, 1978).

- serial electrocardiography

During the last years many programs for ECG classification
have incorporated algorithms for serial analysis of ECGs, e.g.
Macfarlane, 1975; Pipberger, 1977. Improvement in the final
classification is claimed, which is not surprising because
differences in morphology as compared to an earlier recording
can be taken into account. This requires, however, very
standardized locations of the electrodes, since especially in
the chest leads a minor misplacement may cause large changes
in QRS-shape.
Present research in contour classification is, besides the
further investigation of serial electrocardiography, primarily
done into the derivation of features from multiple leads
(Kornreich, 1973); the stability of classifiers (Willems,
1977; Bailey, 1976); the use of fuzzy set theory (Zadeh, 1965)
and syntactic approaches to classification (Pavlidis, 1979).

- features for exercise ECGs

Processing of ECGs acquired during physical ,exercise bears
elements of the interpretation of short-lasting routine ECGs
and of the analysis of ambulatory ECGs. Usually, a few special
exercise leads are taken and analyzed as short epochs during
increasing stress, at maximal stress and during recovery. The
noise problem is solved by coherent averaging techniques.
Further, the choice of relevant complexes (detection and
typification) and the recognition of boundaries is similar to
ECG analysis at rest. References to specific methods,
parameters, systems, and evaluation results can be found in
Simoons (1975) and Sheffield (1977).

7. DATA REDUCTION

Electrocardiograms offer different possibilities for a
considerable data reduction, required for digital
transmission, compact recording as in ambulatory monitoring or
long-term storage for serial comparison of waveforms. We
mentioned already, that the ECG, if only consisting of not too
many different waveshapes, can be represented by a combination
of point processes and wave contours. In practice, however, we
never know beforehand what waveform is to be expected.
Still, several 'silent' epochs are present in the ECG (the TP
and PR intervals) and the different waves have a significantly
distinct frequency spectrum. These properties may be used for
data reduction. Cox (1968) was one of the first who used these
characteristics of the ECG to develop an algorithm to obtain a
tenfold data reduction. Especially in patient monitoring this
and similar techniques are being used. Essentially, such
methods replace a signal by samples at unequal time intervals,
only measured if a certain threshold of the first or second
difference is crossed. Bertrand (1977) applied this and other
algorithms in a system for transmission.

Other techniques for ECG compression make use of a series of
orthogonal basic functions for the reconstruction of the
waveforms. Well-known is the Karhunen-Loève expansion (see
Young, 1963) or a Chebyshev transform. The first method,
yielding the eigenvectors, was evaluated by Womble (1977)
together with reduction by spectral techniques. As has been
observed already, such methods do not take into account the
semantic information comprised in the ECG. For that reason,
they are most helpful in detecting trends in intervals or
sudden changes in waveshapes in individual patients; for
contour classification they are rather inefficient, since e.g.
tiny Q-waves may be missed by the fact that their signal power
is less than the distortions allowed, if integrated over the
duration of the wave. This is the reason why most long-term
storage systems either store the samples of the dominant beat
or even the entire recording, eventually sampled at 250 Hz.
Another reason is the fact that the technical means for
inexpensive storage and retrieval have gradually diminished
the need for data reduction algorithms, that are always more
or less increasing the signal entropy.

8. DISCUSSION

Electrocardiology, started with Einthoven, was greatly
stimulated during the last decades by the advent of the
digital computer. Still, although most problems in the
recognition and detection or waves have principally been
solved, no definite solution has come in sight for the
classification problem. The major reasons are (1) the lead
selection, different form center to center, (2) the lacking of
generally accepted diagnostic criteria, based on non-ECG
information and - related to this - (3) the non-existence of a
well-documented data base of representive ECGs for the
development of algorithms and criteria and for evaluation of
existing programs. It is to be expected that in the 1980's
substantial progress will be made in all these areas, because
of cooperation between research centers involved in this area
and because of the fact that non-ECG information is now more
readily available in most centers than in the past.
Standardization of this patient information and signals is a
prerequisite for the advancement of the research in this
field.
The progress of methods and techniques for ECG interpretation
can be considered to be a model for all kinds of other signal
processing systems. Especially the use of pattern recognition
(L & T populations, feature selection, classification) is very
suited for biological signal processing.

REFERENCES

J.J. Bailey, S.B. Itscoitz, J.W. Hirsfeld, L.E. Grauer and M.R. Horton, "A method for evaluating computer programs for electrocardiographic interpretation", Circulation, vol. 50, parts I, II and III, pp. 73-93, 1974.

J.J. Bailey, M. Horton and S.B. Itscoitz, "The importance of reproducibility testing of computer programs for electrocardiographic interpretation", Comput. and Biomed. Res., vol. 9, pp. 307-316, 1976.

M. Bertrand, R. Guardo, F.A. Roberge and P. Blondeau, "Microprocessor application for numerical ECG encoding and transmission", Proc. IEEE, vol. 65, pp. 714-722, 1977.

R.E. Bonner, L. Crevasse, M.I. Ferrer and J.L. Greenfield, "A new computer program for analysis of scalar electrocardiograms", Comput. and Biomed. Res., vol. 5, pp. 629-653, 1972.

J. Cornfield, R.A. Dunn, C.D. Batchlor and H.V. Pipberger, "Multigroup diagnosis of electrocardiograms", Comput. and Biomed. Res., vol. 6, pp. 97-120, 1973.

J.R. Cox, F.M. Nolle, H.A. Fozzard and G.C. Oliver, "AZTEC, a preprocessing program for real time ECG rhythm analysis", IEEE Trans. Biomed. Eng., vol. BME-15, pp. 128-129, 1968.

J.R. Cox, F.M. Nolle and R.M. Arthur, "Digital analysis of the electroencephalogram, the blood pressure wave and the electrocardiogram", Proc. IEEE, vol. 60, pp. 1137-1164, 1972.

C.L. Feldman, "Trends in computer ECG monitoring", in: Trends in Computer-processed Electrocardiograms, J.H. van Bemmel and J.L. Willems, eds., Amsterdam: North-Holland Publ. Comp., pp. 3-10, 1977.

D.E. Gustafson, A.S. Wilsky, J. Wang, M.C. Lancaster and J.H. Triebwasser, "ECG/VCG rhythm diagnosis using statistical signal analysis", IEEE Trans. Biomed. Eng., vol. BME-25, pp. 344-361, 1978.

S.J. Hengeveld and J.H. van Bemmel, "Computer detection of P-waves", Comput. and Biomed. Res., vol. 9, pp. 125-132, 1976.

S.L. Horowitz, "Peak recognition in waveforms", in: Syntactic Pattern Recognition Applications, K.S. Fu, ed., New York: Springer, pp. 31-49, 1977.

L.N. Kanal, "Interactive pattern analysis and classification systems: a survey and commentary", Proc. IEEE, vol. 60, pp. 1200-1215, 1972.

L.N. Kanal, "Patterns in pattern recognition", IEEE Trans. Inform. Theory, vol. IT-20, pp. 697-722, 1974.

P.W. Macfarlane, H.T. Cawood, T.D.V. Lawrie, "A basis for computer interpretation of serial electrocardiograms", Comput. and Biomed. Res., vol. 8, pp. 189-200, 1975.

F.M. Nolle, "The ARGUS monitoring system: a reappraisal", in: Trends in Computer-processes Electrocardiograms, J.H. van Bemmel and J.L. Willems, eds., Amsterdam: North-Holland Publ. Comp., pp. 11-19, 1977.

T. Plavidis, "Methodologies for shape analysis", in: Biomedical Pattern Recognition and Image Processing, K.S. Fu and T. Plavidis, eds., Berlin: Dahlem Konferenzen 1979, Verlag Chemie, pp. 131-151, 1979.

H.V. Pipberger, J. Cornfield and R.A. Dunn, "Diagnosis of the electrocardiogram", in: Computer Diagnosis and Diagnostic Methods", J. Jacquez and C.C. Thomas, eds., Springfield: C.C. Thomas, pp. 355-373, 1972.

H.V. Pipberger, D. McCaughan, D. Littman, H.A. Pipberger, J. Cornfield, R.A. Dunn, C.D. Batchlor and A.S. Berson, "Clinical application of a second generation electrocardiographic computer program", Am. J. Cardiol., vol. 35, pp. 597-608, 1975.

H.V. Pipberger, S.C. Sabharwal and H.A. Pipberger, "Computer analysis of sequential electrocardiograms", in: Trends in Computer-processed Electrocardiograms, J.H. van Bemmel and J.L. Willems, eds., Amsterdam: North-Holland Publ. Comp., pp. 303-308, 1977.

H.W.M. Plokker, Cardiac Rhythm Diagnosis by Digital Computer, Thesis, Free University Amsterdam, 188 pp., 1978.

K.L. Ripley and R.M. Arthur, "Evaluation and comparison of automatic arrhythmia detectors", in: Computers in Cardiology, IEEE Comp. Soc., pp. 27-32, 1975.

L.T. Sheffield, "Survey of exercise ECG analysis methods", in: Trends in Computer-processed Electrocardiograms, J.H. van Bemmel and J.L. Willems, eds, Amsterdam: North-Holland Publ. Comp., pp. 373-382, 1977.

M.L. Simoons, H.B.K. Boom and E. Smallenburg, "On-line processing of orthogonal exercise electrocardiograms", Comput. and Biomed. Res., vol. 8, pp. 105-117, 1975. G. Stockman, L.N. Kanal and M.C. Kyle, "Structural pattern recognition of carotid pulse waves using a general waveform parsing system", Comm. ACM, vol. 19, pp. 688-695, 1976.

C.A. Swenne, J.H. van Bemmel, S.J. Hengeveld and M. Hermans, "Pattern recognition for ECG monitoring, an interactive method for the recognition of ventricular complexes", Comput. and Biomed. Res., vol. 5, pp. 150-160, 1973.

J.L. Talmon and J.H. van Bemmel, "Modular software for computer-assisted ECG/VCG interpretation", in: MEDINFO-74, J. Anderson and J.M. Forsythe, eds., Amsterdam: North-Holland Publ. Comp., pp. 653-658, 1974.

J.L. Talmon, Pattern Recognition of the ECG, Thesis, Free University Amsterdam, 1983.

L.J. Thomas, K.W. Clark, C.N. Mead, K.L. Ripley, B.F. Spenner and G.C. Oliver, "Automated cardiac dysrhythmia analysis", Proc. IEEE, vol. 67, pp. 1322-1337, 1979.

J.H. van Bemmel, J.L. Talmon, J.S. Duisterhout and S.J. Hengeveld, "Template waveform recognition applied to ECG/VCG analysis", Comput. and Biomed. Res., vol. 6, pp. 430-441, 1973.

J.H. van Bemmel and S.J. Hengeveld, "Clustering algorithm for QRS and ST-T waveform typing", Comput. and Biomed. Res., vol. 6, pp. 442-456, 1973.

J.H. van Bemmel and J.L. Willems, eds., Trends in Computer-processed Electrocardiograms, Amsterdam: North-Holland Publ. Comp., 437 pp., 1977.

J.H. van Bemmel, "Strategies and challenges in biomedical pattern recognition", in: Biomedical Pattern Recognition and Image Processing, K.S. Fu and T. Plavidis, eds., Berlin: Dahlem Konferenzen 1979, Verlag Chemie, pp. 13-26, 1979.

J.H. van Bemmel, "Recognition of electocardiographic patterns", in: Handbook of Statistics, vol. II, P.R. Krishnaiah and L.N. Kanal, eds., Amsterdam: North-Holland Publ. Comp., pp. 501-526, 1982.

J. Wartak and J.A. Milliken, "Logical approach to diagnosing electrocardiograms", J. Electrocardiol., vol. 2, pp. 253-260, 1969.

J.L. Willems and H.V. Pipberger, "Arrhythmia detection by digital computer", Comput. and Biomed. Res., vol. 5, pp. 263-278, 1972.

J.L. Willems and J. Pardaens, "Differences in measurement results obtained by four different ECG computer programs", in: Computers in Cardiology, IEEE Comp. Soc., pp. 115-121, 1977.

H.K. Wolf, P.J. Macinnis, S. Stock, R.K. Helppi, P.M. Rautaharju, "Computer analysis of rest and exercise electrocardiograms", Comput. and Biomed. Res., vol. 5, pp. 329-346, 1972.

M.E. Womble, J.S. Halliday, S.K. Mitter, M.C. Lancaster and J.H. Triebwasser, "Data compression for storing and transmitting ECGs/VCGs", Proc. IEEE, vol. 65, pp. 702-706, 1977.

T.Y. Young and W.H. Huggins, "Intrinsic component theory of electrocardiograms", IEEE Trans. Biomed. Eng., pp. 214-221, 1963.

L.A. Zadeh, "Fuzzy sets", Inform. and Control, vol. 8, pp. 338-353, 1965.

ALGORITHMS FOR WAVE FORM CLASSIFICATION

Chr. Zywietz

Arbeitsbereich Biosignalverarbeitung
im Zentrum Biometrie, Medizinische Informatik und Medizintechnik
Medizinische Hochschule Hannover
3000 Hannover 61, Bundesrepublik Deutschland

ABSTRACT

Algorithms for wave form classification serve two main purposes:
a) signal typing and b) diagnostic allocation of signal forms to diagnostic groups.
Wave form typing algorithms can be designed for interactive (supervised) learning or for self adaptive operation. Interactive learning procedures can be applied effectively in cases where only a few signal types occour and where a large number of forms has to be classified, i.e. in Holter ECGs or in monitoring. The performance of classification algorithms can often be improved by use of multidimensional feature vectors and transformed variables using their inner interdependence to enlarge the inter-group distance. For diagnostic allocation algorithms decision three type or multivariate. classificators, i.e. the Bayes-formula are available. While morphology classification of signal forms can be done in a pure syntactical way, the development of diagnostic allocation algorithms needs, that the groups into which the signal shall be classified have to be defined by signal independent criteria from outside.

MORPHOLOGY CLASSIFICATION AND DIAGNOSTIC ALLOCATION

Algorithms for wave form classification can serve two main purposes:

1. classification of signal morphology

   + (pattern recognition)

   + separation of desired signals from noise

   + separation of signal forms, i.e. complex typing in ECG analysis

2. diagnostic allocation

   + allocation of (a set of) independent variables to a set of dependend variables (i.e. diagnostic groups).

For both types of classification feature extraction procedures preced the classification process. There is however a basic difference in the validation of the classification results. The performance evaluation of signal morphology classification procedures is done simply as reclassification procedure of signal forms of a test collective, which has been built in the same way as the learning population. The evaluation of diagnostic allocation algorithms requires the analysis of classification results of a test collective, which has been defined from independent outside information. The composition of a test collective for performance analysis of signal morphology classification algorithms is on the other hand determined by the same information and the same criteria as used for the learning population. Now further outside information or criteria are available. The following discussion will deal with both types of classification algorithms but no pattern recognition problems i.e. detection of waveforms will be treated. It is assumed, that any type of feature extraction has been performed before and that for the classification procedures parameter vectors are available.

CLASSIFICATION ALGORITHMS FOR WAVE FORM TYPING

Interactive wave form clustering

A very effective method for signal classification is the combined use of human pattern recognition capabilities with the algorithmic calculation power of a computer. A method for interactive typing or clustering of ECG complexes, which is in fact a method of supervised learning, has been described in 1973 by Swenne et al.

Fig. 1 depicts how the method works:

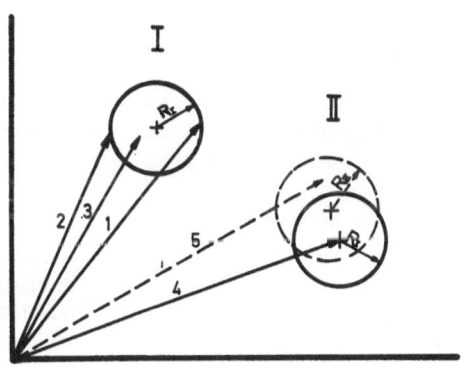

Fig. 1 interactive clustering

Let $\vec{V}_1$, $\vec{V}_2$ be vectors derived from two given wave forms which have been defined as wave form type I by a human observer. By a certain procedure the computer defines the cluster center I with radius R_1 (i.e. mean and distance of the vectors). From the next wave form $\vec{V}_3$ is obtained and automatically allocated to type I because it falls within the cluster type I.

The 4th wave form deviates somewhat from the other wave forms and therefore the human observer allocates vector $\vec{V}_4$ to a cluster type II. The computer defines preliminary cluster center two by means of vector $\vec{V}_4$ and uses the radius of cluster 1 for the preliminary cluster II.

Vector $\vec{V}_5$ may be again allocated to the wave form type II and now the cluster center 2 is calculated, i.e. as mean between vector $\vec{V}_4$ and $\vec{V}_5$ and the cluster radius is defined on the basis of the distance of these two vectors. All wave form vectors falling into cluster I or II are now automatically allocated to these two clusters until either a new vector falls outside of these two clusters and forms a new 3rd cluster or which may be neglected if one wishes only to select and keep those vectors which fall into cluster I or II alone.

It takes a couple of minutes of operator interaction to train such an algorithm.

The method can be effectively applied where a large number of wave forms has to be typed and where the number of deviating wave types is limited, i.e. in ECG monitoring recordings in coronary units or in Holter ECGs.

<u>Self learning algorithms</u>

For routine short term ECG recordings an interactive complex typing procedure for economical reasons cannot be applied. In this case a self adaptive procedure may be helpful. Fig. 2 and 3 depict the principle of the method.

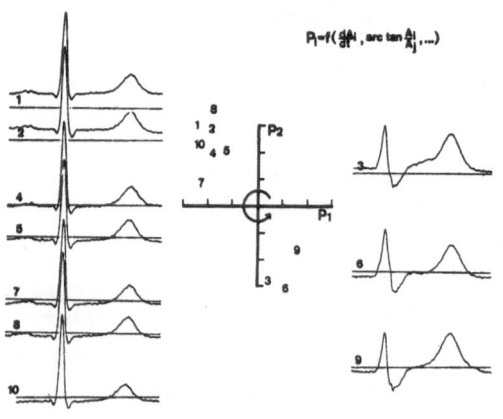

Parameters p_1, p_2 derived from the ECG complexes 1...10 represent the ECG complexes in the p_1-p_2-plane.

Fig. 2 ECG-complex representation

For each QRS-complex two parameters, i.e. a first derivative of the ab-
stroking part and a transformed quotient of positive and negative peak-
amplitudes are calculated and "recorded" in the p1, p2 plane. As can be
seen from fig. 2 the normal complexes are located in the left upper quadrant,
while the deviating complexes 3, 6, 9 are located in the right lower quadrant.

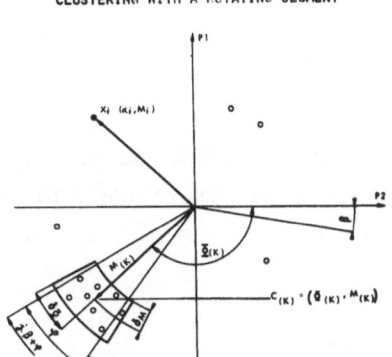

CLUSTERING WITH A ROTATING SEGMENT

Fig. 3

The plane is than scanned with a
stepwise rotating sector. The
frequency of complexes matching
with each sector step is determined and where its maximum oc-
cours a cluster of complexes is
assumed. The cluster is then calculated from the mean vector and
the standard deviation and vector length. The procedure is repeated until all complexes of the
record have been typed.

β = scanning steps

M_K = mean length of "cluster
vector" for cluster K

ϕ_K = mean angle of "cluster
vector" for cluster K

δ_M, δ_ϕ = measures for cluster
width

By this method in routine ECG recordings about 95% of the complexes can be
correctly typed. The final decision is made in a subsequent cross correlation procedure. The advantage of the method is its "self-adaptive" behaviour
to different ECG wave forms, which occur in different patients. The frequency of complexes and RR-interval analysis determines which is - in the
pretyping phase - the dominant beat. Another advantage is fast computing as
compared to cross correlation procedures.

Overlapping distribution and transformation of classification variables

The two methods described above work succesfully if the classification
parameters do not overlap each other.
While in fig. 2 each of the two parameters itself could separate the two
complex types in many situations the frequency distribution of either one

of the classification parameters overlap each other as shown in fig. 4.
The two classification parameters x1 and x2 for group A and group B show
a strong overlap and it can be easily verified that neither by a clustering method using the procedure by Swenne nor by the method with the rotating sector the group separation would be possible.
In this situation a transformation of the variables which decreases the
intra-group distance and increases the intergroup distance may be a helpful tool. This can be achieved by discriminant function analysis.
Let us assume, we find a function,

$$Y = b_1 : x_1 + b_2 \cdot x_2$$

on which the points, characterizing the groups A and B in our $x_1 - x_2$ plane
can be projected in such a way that the overlap becomes minimal. To calculate the coefficients b of the discriminant function a goal function is
defined

$$\lambda = \frac{(\bar{Y}_A - \bar{Y}_B)^2}{\sum_{i=1}^{I_A} (Y_{iA} - \bar{Y}_A)^2 + \sum_{i=1}^{I_B} (Y_{iB} - \bar{Y}_B)^2} \rightarrow \text{Max!} \qquad (3)$$

where:

$\bar{Y}_k$ = mean of the discriminant value for group k (k = A, B)

Y_{ik} = discriminant value for measurement of case i for group k

I_k = number of measurements in group k.

These discriminant coefficients have to be determined in such a way that
the ratio of the squared distance of the discriminant mean values of the
two groups and of the squared disctance values within the groups becomes
a maximum. For detailed explanations see Lachenbruch, 1975. The results of
this operation can be seen on fig. 5. Projection of the $x_1 - x_2$ measurements on the discriminant function shows now for the two groups nearly complete separation with only two cases falling into the other group.
Without further detailed explanations we conclude from this observation
that
a) the use of more than one variable

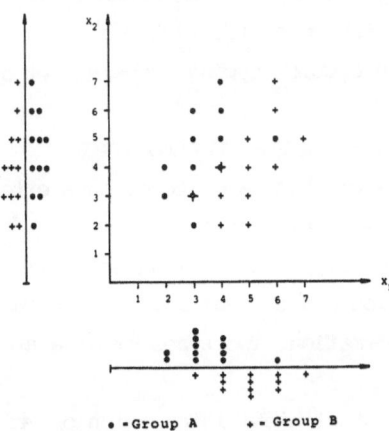

GROUPS WITH OVERLAPING DISTRIBUTION
OF VARIABLES

Fig. 4 For each group A,B two parameters x_1 and x_2 are known. Separate
analysis of each of the parameters does not allow to identify
the group they belong to.

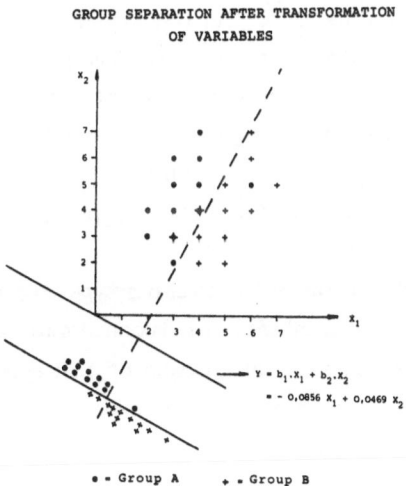

GROUP SEPARATION AFTER TRANSFORMATION
OF VARIABLES

Fig. 5 The "simultaneous" analysis of both variables (using their interdependence) allows to separate the groups almost completely.

and b) any transformation procedure may be helpful for improved group
separation and signal classification.

In view of Holter ECG analysis the consequence of this observation is, that
two channel analysis is by far superior as compared to single channel analysis not only because of the more effective use of available data but also
of improved reliability in complex typing (Zywietz et al 1981).

CLASSIFICATION ALGORITHMS FOR DIAGNOSTIC ALLOCATION

It is not the purpose of this paper to discuss extensively classification algorithms for diagnostic allocation.

The basic difference for development of diagnostic allocation algorithms
is that the group definition and the validation procedure has to be based
on signal independent information. Two types of data are necessary and have
to be matched:

ECG data and ECG independent clinical information on which group definition
can be based. For example besides the ECGs, data from cath lab on coronaro-
graphy, ventricle wall motility, ventricle wall thickness, and/or cardio-
scintigraphic data have to be collected and analyzed. Groups formed out of
these signal independent data can be Normals, Myocardial Infarction,
Right Ventricular Hypertrophy, Left Ventricular Hypertrophy and so on.
Characteristic parameters for these groups have to be found within the signal used for classification i.e. the ECG. One has first to find out on which
parameters the various desease groups are "imaged". Again the method to
find these parameters can be the discriminant function analysis, mentioned
before. Once the characterizing parameters are found two basic strategies
for classification procedures are possible:

a) so called "logistic" or decision three type algorithms and
b) statistical procedures.

The advantage of logistic or decision three type algorithms is, that one can
obtain for example differentiation between Normal and LVH by using an ECG
amplitude criterium which exceeds in case of LVH a certain threshold. The
problem is, however, that in decision three type algorithms only single variables can be evaluated and that functional interdependence between several
variables cannot be considered adequately.

The "prototype" for statistical classification algorithm is the Bayes
classification:

$$p(Ai \mid B) = \frac{p(Ai) \cdot p(B \mid Ai)}{\sum\limits_{1}^{j} p(Ai) \cdot p(B \mid Ai)}$$

where:

Ai, i = 1 ... j desease group

$p(A_i|B)$ = posterior probability that the case under the condition of measurement B belongs to group Ai

$p(A_i)$ = a priori probability for the desease group Ai

$p(B|A_i)$ = conditional probability for measurement B under desease group Ai.

For clarification let us assume the following example:

hospital population

2000 patients	a-priori-probability
A_1 = 600 Normals	$p(A_1) = 600/2000 = 0.30$
A_2 = 900 Infarctions	$p(A_2) = 900/2000 = 0.45$
A_3 = 500 Left Ventr. Hypertr.	$p(A_3) = 500/2000 = 0.25$

For a given measurement vector (i.e. Q–duration, J–point amplitude, T–amplitude – "B" –)the conditional probabilities to belong to group A_i shall be:

$$P(B|A_1) = 0.02; \quad P(B|A_2) = 0.05; \quad P(B|A_3) = 0.01$$

Consideration of the composition of the total hospital population results for the conditional posterior probability for allocation of the measurement vector "B" to each of the groups in:

$$p\,(A_1|B) = \frac{0.30 \cdot 0.02}{0.30 \cdot 0.02 + 0.45 \cdot 0.05 + 0.25 \cdot 0.01} = 0.193$$

$$p\,(A_2|B) = \frac{0.45 \cdot 0.05}{0.30 \cdot 0.02 + 0.45 \cdot 0.05 + 0.25 \cdot 0.01} = 0.726$$

$$p\,(A_3|B) = \frac{0.25 \cdot 0.01}{0.30 \cdot 0.02 + 0.45 \cdot 0.05 + 0,25 \cdot 0.01} = 0.081$$

For the given measurement vector "B" the classification probability is therefore:

$$\text{Normal} = 19.3\%$$
$$\text{Infarction} = 72.6\%$$
$$\text{Left Ventr. Hypertr.} = 8.1\%$$

312

Although this statistical method can give quite impressive results, there
are a few problems in designing an apropriate model and in interpreting
the results.

1. The first problem is that the model should include all possible desease
   groups which cannot be realized practically.
2. The groups are mutual exclusive.
3. A normal distribution of the variables is assumed.
4. Equal covariance matrixes are assumed.
5. Double diagnosis or non model cases are unpredictable allocated. Because
   of the mutual exclusive groups, in the presence of two deseases the
   posterior probabilities for these two deseases can be in the best case
   50%. This not very well accepted by the clinical user. More over, the
   posterior probabilities are often misunderstood as degree of certainty
   although they only express the relative distance of the classified measurement vector to the groups within the model. The problems mentioned
   have led to the development of another type of multivariate classification algorithms published by Klusmeier 1978 and Zywietz 1977.

The basic idea is to use multivariate two group tests and to combine the
results in a validation logic.

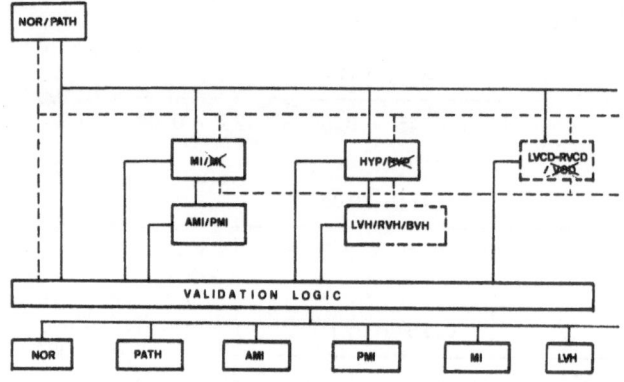

In MAK1 in a first
test all cases are
checked whether their
distance to group
NORMAL is smaller
than to (all) patho-
logical cases. This
information is stored
and in further tests
the distances to spe-
cific pathological
groups are also cal-
culated. Within the
validation logic the
test results are com-
bined and a conclusive
statement is derived.

Fig. 6 Multivariate Alternative Classification MAK1

Fig. 6 and fig. 7 show the structure of these classification algorithms
which have been called Multivariate Alternative Classification MAK1 and
MAK2. The basic idea is to take advantage of multivariate tests but to separate the groups individually by particular tests and to simulate in this
way a non linear discriminant function behaviour.

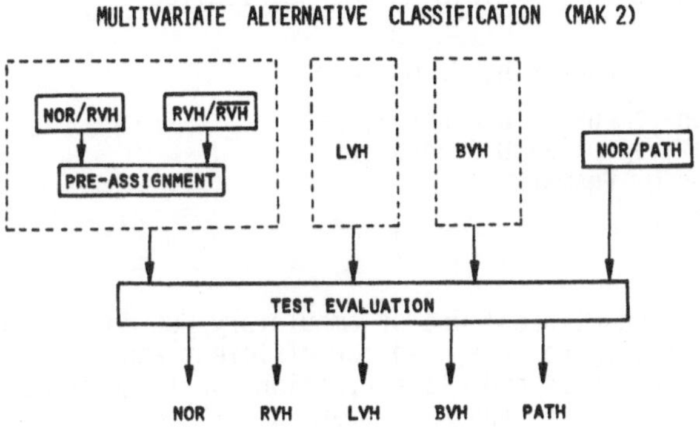

MULTIVARIATE ALTERNATIVE CLASSIFICATION (MAK 2)

In MAK2 the relative distance between NOR and RVH, LVH and BVH and the distance between the specific and all other pathological groups is tested. The Test Evaluation Logic combines the test results to conclusive statements.

Fig. 7

The advantages of this of Multivariate Alternative Classification are that,

a) individual sets of variables for each group can be selected,

b) the number of variables (and therefore the number of cases) for each desease group can be relatively small,

c) the expansibility of the classification logic.

The main difference between MAK1 and MAK2 is, that in MAK2 which has been developed for classification of pediatric VCGs for the latter a large collective of Normals for various age groups was available and that only two or three major desease groups can be expected. Therefore the normal group was for all tests the reference group and the algorithm determines independently for each of the groups LVH, RVH and BVH the posterior probability whether the case belongs to the group Normal or to one of the pathological groups.

REFERENCES

Klusmeier, S. et al. 1978. Multivariate Alternativklassifikation, ein Versuch zur Überwindung einiger Nachteile der Bayes Klassifikation. Inf. Syst. i.d. Med. Versorg., 729-736, Schatthauser Verlag Stuttgart, New York 1978, Reichertz, Schwarz Edits.

Lachenbruch, P.A. 1975. Discriminant Analysis, Hafner Press, A Division of Macmillan Publ. Co., Inc. New York, N.Y.10022

Swenne, C.A. et al. 1973. Adaption of Parameters for Interactive Coronary Care, Digest of the Xth Int. Conf. on Med. and biolog. Engin. Dresden 1973, p37

Zywietz, Chr. et al. 1977. A New VCG Analysis Program for Children with multivariate Diagn. Classification. Computers in Cardiology 1977, 95-99, IEEE CATAL. Nr. 77CH1254-2C

Zywietz, Chr. et al. 1981. HES LKG, a New Program for Computer Assisted Analysis of Holter Electrocardiograms. Computers in Cardiology 1981, 169-172, ISSN No. 0276-6574

ALGORITHMS FOR ECG WAVEFORM ANALYSIS AND CLASSIFICATION

J. Damgaard Andersen, E. Gymoese
Medical Department B, Rigshospitalet
Blegdamsvej 9, 2100 Copenhagen Ø
Denmark

ABSTRACT

An important problem in the clinical use of ambulatory ECG monitoring is the analysis of recordings. There is a need for efficient and reliable algorithms for ECG waveform analysis and classification for large computer systems used at research laboratories and at commercial ECG scanning services. Furthermore, efficient algorithms are required in portable solid state recorders for preprocessing the ECG due to the limited storage capacity. A systematic comparison of efficiency and clinical utility of the most widely publicized algorithms has not yet been performed and it is unknown which principle for classification is most well suited for practical use, with noise and artefact-filled recordings. Such comparative evaluations of algorithms will be required before they are used in microprocessor-based portable equipment.

INTRODUCTION

The development of very large scale integrated (VLSI) circuits in the next years will create new opportunities for clinical use of microelectronics. Microprocessors are becoming increasingly more powerful and the storage capacity of semiconductor memories is growing rapidly. Therefore it will become possible to develop small portable ambulatory recorders (solid state recorders) which can be used instead of the present-day tape recorders. In the future recording circuits may also be incorporated in pacemakers for implantation (Bhatt and Schober, 1982). The advantage of solid state recorders is that they have no mechanical parts, which means that they are much more reliable and that they consume less power than conventional mechanical tape recorders. But even if the capacity of solid state recorders increases in the next years, it cannot match the large amount of data produced in a standard long-term recording. Twenty-four hours of two channel ECG recording, at 100 samples per second with 8 bits resolution, which is a typical state-of-the-art system (Gymoese, Andersen and Sandøe, 1977), represents 17.28 megabytes. The largest memory chip available today, a 256-kbit dynamic RAM (Bursky, 1983) can store only approximately five minutes of single channel ECG with similar resolution without data compression (Fig. 1). Even if memory chips could contain more data, effective analysis algorithms are required to ease the job of analy-

lyzing the recording and identifying episodes of interest. Moreover, reliable event detection programmes (e.g. able to identify the beginning of
an episode of tachycardia) could trigger solid state storage of the episode
including its prehistory. Present day tape-based recorders have severe limitations in their ability of faithfully reproducing ST-segment changes
(Bragg-Remschel 1982). This problem could also be solved by solid state
recording and algorithm-based real time analysis of the ST-segment.

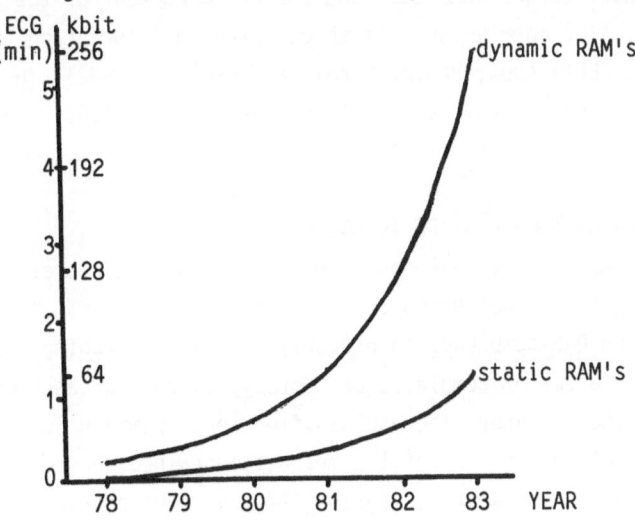

Fig. 1. Evolution of storage capacity of memory chips during
the last five years.

The most important problem in systems designed to analyze ambulatory ECG
recordings is long turnaround time and varying quality of the delivered
report (Wenger, Mock and Ringquist, 1982). Results from both custom-engi-
neered large computer analysis systems and from commercial scanning services require an ongoing quality control procedure in order to maintain
reasonable standards. This is because presently used classification
algorithms do not work satisfactorily when the recording is noisy or
contains artefacts. Unfortunately, it is impossible to avoid noise and
artefacts in ambulatory recordings both from sources within the body
(respiration and muscle movements) and from external sources. External
noise arises from patient-electrode interface sites, external AC-fields
and polarisation of electrodes (Andersen et al, 1977; Wenger, 1982).
Simultaneous recording of more than one lead reduces this problem
(Andersen et al, 1977) but until now only few algorithms for analysis of
simultaneous leads have been presented.

QRS DETECTION AND DELINEATION

The first important step in any ECG analysis algorithm is the proper detection and delineation of the QRS complex (Thomas et al, 1979). This is usually performed by searching for one or more slopes exceeding preset values within certain predefined time windows. Most often the threshold values are adjusted dynamically, based on some maximum values in the previously detected QRS complexes and the noise content of the ECG ('Gymoese et al, 1979). Also more advanced methods based on information theory has been employed (Börjesson, Pahlm, Sörnmo and Nygårds, 1982). The article by Pahlm and Sörnmo in this volume (Pahlm and Sörnmo, 1983) contains a thorough discission of algorithmic approaches to QRS detection.

TEMPLATE MATCHING (CORRELATION TECHNIQUE)

Once the QRS complex has been detected, it must be classified as either normal or abnormal or belonging to a certain class. The simplest approach for recognizing QRS-complexes is probably "template matching" (Fu, 1968). In this method a set of templates or prototypes, one for each QRS class, is stored in the computer. The unclassified input pattern is compared with the templates of each class until a match is obtained, based on some prede-fined matching or similarity criterion. If the input pattern matches the template of a particular pattern class better than it matches any other template, then the input is classified as belonging to this class.

The template matching method is used in many systems for analysis of ambulatory recordings. In our computer-based system RAMSES (Gymoese, An-dersen and Sandøe, 1978) QRS complexes are sequentially compared to as many as 200 templates. Although the computational load can be reduced by opti-mization of correlation coefficient calculations (Collins and Aerzbacher, 1981) as well as by microprogramming the correlation algorithm as done in this system, there are inherent disadvantages in the template matching method. One is that it can be difficult to select a good (representative) template from each pattern class and to define a proper matching criterion. This problem has been reduced in our system by letting the system define its own templates on a minimum distance criterion and let a cardiologist merge system templates to clinically meaningful classes after an automatic classification procedure. Still, as pointed out by Cox (1972) correlation technique can cause problems because of the difficulty of temporally align-ing waveforms with respect to a common reproducible point. This is coped

by starting correlation from a "centroid point" or center of gravity
of detected peak configuration (Gymoese, Andersen and Sandøe, 1978)
and shifting templates with respect to each other in order to check if
a better match can be obtained.

FEATURE EXTRACTION

Another approach is a classification based on a set of selected
measurements extracted from the input pattern (Fu, 1968). These selected
measurements, called "features", are supposed to be invariant or less
sensitive to commonly encountered variations and distortions, and also to
contain less redundancy. Ideally all features should be independent, with
each QRS represented as a point in an orthogonal N-space. If this approach
is used, the classification problem can be divided into two subproblems.
The first is to define what measurements should be taken from the input
signal. The second is classification of the pattern based on measurements
taken from selected features. This way of handling the classification is
frequently employed. If N features are used to characterize a wave and
the measurements are represented as a point in the N-dimensional space,
this space can be divided into regions for the purpose of classification.
If a point representing a QRS belongs to a particular region, the QRS is
member of the corresponding class. Both time domain and frequency domain
as well as combined features have been used. In the ARGUS system (Mead,
1976) QRS height, duration, offset (displacement with respect to baseline)
and area were used as features. QRS complexes were grouped in families
according to the similarity of the four features. These features are pure
temporal features. The method was later extended to include the following
frequency domain features: the first spectral moment (the center of gravity
of the amplitude or power spectrum from 5 to 25 Herz) combined with the
5 Herz and 10 Herz phase angles. The latter features were found to be useful adjuncts to the time domain features (Mead, 1978). Many methods for
partitioning the feature space have been described (Fu, 1968). Most often
linear discriminant functions are used (Fu, 1968; Murthy and Rangaraj, 1979;
Kugler, 1982). A classifier can even be implemented as a training or learning classifier (Ahmed and Rao, 1975).

OTHER CLASSIFICATION METHODS

Other classification methods have been based on expansion of the ECG-signal in orthogonal functions followed by classification (Ahmed and Rao, 1975). Several authors have tried discrete Karhunen-Loève expansion, intrinsic components, principal factors or principal components, all synonyms (Womble, Halliday, Mitter, Lancaster and Trienwasser, 1977). Karhunen-Loève expansion and subsequent classification by discriminant analysis has been described recently (Kugler, 1982). The principle of intrinsic components has also been used to design an ECG-filter (Hambley, Moruzzi, and Feldman, 1974). Since discrete Karhunen-Loève expansion requires the determination of eigenvectors of large matrices, a considerable amount of computation is involved. By using the most significant components much simplification can be obtained. This method has been used for classification at Södersjukhuset, Stockholm, where the QRST-complex is first represented as the weighted sum of four approximately orthonormal basis signals and subsequently classified (Nygårds and Hulting, 1979).

In recent years there has also been a trend characterized by inclusion of additional high-level information such as exclusion of electrophysiologically unrealizable patterns. For this purpose the use of syntactic pattern recognition has been attempted (Fu, 1974; Horowitz, 1980).

CONCLUSION

As may be apparent from the preceding overview, quite a number of different approaches have been employed to solve the ECG waveform and classification problem. As stated by Thomas (1979): "The wide variety of algorithmic approaches to ECG analysis testifies to the extreme difficulty of defining a single strategy which can deal succesfully with the broad range of ECG signals commonly encountered". From a clinical viewpoint many of the algorithms used in the daily routine now may differ only marginally. Each algorithm seems to have its own "problem" ECG's, which it has difficulty of coping with. A systematic mapping of the deficiencies of these commomly used algorithms has, however, not been performed. Only through such a systematic exploration can the algorithms be improved. This requires extensive testing, using available databases, but also in clinical environments and presupposes free dissemination of information, ideas and algorithms.

REFERENCES

Andersen,J.D, Gymoese, E. and Sandøe, E. 1977. Interactive analysis techniques with RAMSES (Random Access Mass Storage ECG-analysis System).
In: Computers in Cardiology (Eds. P.G. Hugenholtz and J.R. Cox)
(IEEE Computer Society, Long Beach, California, No 77CH1254-2C).
pp. 417-420.

Ahmed, N. and Rao, K.R. 1975. Orthogonal transforms for digital signal
processing. (Springer Verlag, Berlin).

Bhatt, S. and Schober, R.C. 1982. Holter monitoring using implanted pacemakers. In: The third decade of cardiac oacing (Eds. S.S. Barold and
J. Mugica).(Futura Publishing Company, New York). pp. 333-343.

Bragg-Remschel, D.A., Anderson C.M. and Winkle R.A. Frequency response
characteristics of ambulatory ECG monitoring systems and their implication for ST segmant analysis. A. Heart J.;1982:103,20-31.

Buffet, J. Gautier, J.-P., and Jacquet J.-P. The software pacemaker -
feasibility of recording pacemakers. In: The third decade of cardiac
pacing (Eds. S.S. Barold and J. Mugica)(Futura Publishing Company,
New York, 1982).

Bursky, D. Digital LSI: 1983 forecast. 1983. Electronic Design 31,102-128.

Börjesson, P.O., Pahlm, O., Sörnmo, L., and Nygårds, M.-E. Adaptive
QRS detection based on maximum a posteriori estimation. IEEE Trans.
Biomed. Engn. 1982.29,341-351.

Cox, J.R., Nolle, F.M., and Arthur, R.M. 1972. Digital analysis of the
encephalogram, the blood pressure wave and the electrocardiogram.
Proc. IEEE 60, 1137-1164.

Fu, K.S. 1968. Sequential methods in pattern recognition and machine
learning. (Academic Press, New York).

Fu, K.S. 1974. Syntactic methods in pattern recognition. (Academic Press,
New York).

Gymoese, E., Andersen, J.D., and Sandøe, E. Random access mass storage
ECG-analysis system (RAMSES): a new system for quantitative analysis
of long-term ECG's. In: Computers in Cardiology (Eds. J.R. Cox and
P.G. Hugenholtz)(IEEE Computer Society, Long Beach, California, 1978).
(No. 78C1391-2C).pp. 221-224.

Hambley, A.R., Moruzzi, R.L., and feldman, C.L. 1974. The use of intrinsic
components in an ECG filter. IEEE Trans. Biomed. Engn. 21,469-473.

Horowitz, S.L. 1975. A syntactic algorithm for peak detection in waveforms
with application to electrocardiography. Comm. A.C.M. 18,281-285.

Horowitz, S.L. 1980. Classifying of ECG waveforms. In: Optimization of
computer ECG processing (Eds. H.K. Wolf and P.W. Macfarlane).
(North-Holland Publishing Company, Amsterdam).pp. 155-157.

Kugler, J. 1982. ECG classification based on Karhunen-Loève expansion
and discriminant analysis. In: 2. Int. Pattern Recognition Conf.,
Berlin (IEEE Computer Society, Long Beach, California).(No. 82CH
1801-0).

Mead, C.N., Clark, K.W., Oliver, C.G., et al. 1976. Progress toward fully
automated processing of ambulatory ECG's. In: Computers in Cardiology
(J.R. Cox and P.G. Hugenholtz, eds.).(IEEE Computer Society, Long
Beach, California, Cat. no. 76CH1160-1C).pp. 183-188.

Mead, C.N., Moore, S.N., Spenner, B.F., et al. 1978. Detection of multiform PVC's using a combination of time domain and frequency domain
information. In: Computers in Cardiology (Eds. J.R. Cox and P.G.
Hugenholtz). pp. 343-346.

Nygårds, M.-E. and Hulting, J. 1979. An automated system for ECG monitoring.
Comp. Biomed. Res. 12, 181-202.

Pahlm, O. and Sörnmo, L. 1983. Algorithmic approaches to QRS detection. In this volume.

Collins, S.M. and Arzbaecker, R.C. 1981. An efficient algorithm for waveform analysis using the correlation coefficient. Comp. Biomed. Res. 14,381-389.

Thomas, L.J., Clark, K.W., Mead, C.N., Ripley, K.L., Spenner, B.C., and Oliver, G.C. 1979. Automated dysrhythmia analysis. Proc. IEEE 67, 1322-1337.

Wenger, N.K., Mock, M.B., and Ringquist, I. 1982. Ambulatory ECG recording: clinical perspectives. In: Ambulatory electrocardiographic recording (Eds. N.K. Wenger, M.B. Mock and I. Ringquist).(Year Book Medical Publishers, Chicago).pp. 425- 441.

Womble, M.E., Halliday, J.S., Mitter S.K., Lancaster, M.C., and Triebwasser, J.H. Data compression for storing and transmitting ECG's/VCG's. Proc. IEEE 1977,65,702-706.

DISCUSSION

Chairman: B. McA Sayers

3.4 – Algorithms for the classification of biological signal waveforms.

CERUTTI: One of the major problems in dealing with the statistical models
is the case in which the variance of the noise is very high. So my
question is: do you have some opinion of what is the change of the
descriminant function analysis in presence of high variance in the noise?
ZYWIETZ: First of all, before going to a classification algorithm, you have
a feature selections procedure, and you have tried to handle the noise
before: various types of signal noise and even some part of biological
noise which may be inerent in an ECG recorder. So you try to reduce this
type of noise by signal pre-processing, this is the first point. Secondly
if you take noise in a broader sense as variations from individal to
individal, what you arrive at depends on the number of groups you are
considering. Classifications accuracy is today in the range of 85% to
90%,in diagnostic classification. If you want to improve that, it would
take a tremendous amount of work,   and I don't know if we can improve by 2
or 3%.

TOPIC: 3.5

Portable real time processors versus playback systems

AMBULATORY MONITORING: REAL-TIME ANALYSIS VERSUS TAPE SCANNING SYSTEMS

Roger G. Mark* and Kenneth L. Ripley**

*Biomedical Engineering Center for
Clinical Instrumentation
Massachusetts Institute of Technology
Cambridge, MA 02139 USA
**Thoraxcentrum
Erasmus University
Rotterdam, The Netherlands

INTRODUCTION

Long term ambulatory monitoring has become an important diagnostic technique, particularly in cardiology. The monitoring of electrocardiographic data has found many important applications, as discussed previously by others in this workshop. The technique is used to evaluate patients with known ventricular ectopic activity who may be at risk for sudden death, to monitor patients after myocardial infarction, to evaluate patients with intermittent symptoms possibly due to cardiac arrhythmias, to document the effectiveness of antiarrhythmic drug therapy, and to check the function of implanted cardiac pacemakers (1-9).

There are two major technical approaches to ambulatory monitoring (Fig. 1). The first is to tape-record continuous electrocardiographic data from two or more leads for a period of 24-48 hours, and to comprehensively analyze it at a later time. The second approach, made possible by modern microprocessor technology, is to analyze the electrocardiogram in real-time with a battery-operated, portable computer, storing summary statistics and selected exerpts of ECG data, which may be reviewed and edited at a later time (10). The amount of data stored in a real-time analysis system is limited primarily by the memory technology employed.

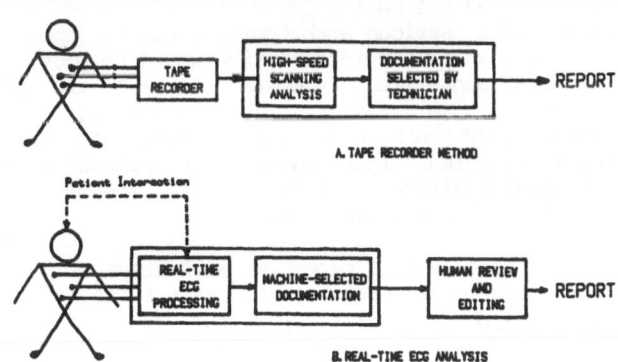

Figure 1. Two Technical Approaches for Ambulatory Monitoring

Tape recording systems have become well established over the past 15 years. Early tape scanners relied heavily on well trained technicians interacting with rather simple scanning equipment. Contemporary tape scanning systems have become quite complex, employing sophisticated computers to assist the operator, and to produce more quantitative and consistent reports. However, to achieve optimal results, even the most advanced scanning systems require intelligent human supervision. Tape systems have the advantage of preserving all of the data from the monitoring period, and they utilize moderately priced recording instruments. A disadvantage of tape systems is the significant delay between starting the recording and obtaining the completed analysis. In addition, the usual scanning systems still rely heavily on technician performance, and their accuracy and precision are subject to human error and fatigue. Error rates in quantitating ventricular couplets and ventricular tachycardia may be significant (20%) in even "research grade" scans. More typical "clinical" scans may show even higher error rates (11). Unfortunately, the physician-user of ambulatory monitoring, whether tape-based or real-time, is almost never in a position to assess the false negative errors in the procedure.

Real-time systems have now begun to move from the research laboratory into clinical use. A few commercial systems have been available for several years, and others are under advanced development. In general these systems continuously analyze the ECG in real time using sophisticated computer algorithms with capabilities quite comparable to those in the best computer-based tape scanning systems. As pointed out in Figure 1, real-time analysis systems also require intelligent human editing and review in order to achieve optimal results. The major limitation of most real-time arrhythmia monitors is the fact that much of the ECG data is not stored for later review. Only selected "significant" rhythm strips are preserved. (In theory, of course, it is possible to overcome this limitation by expanding the memory capacity sufficiently using tape, miniature disks, or other technologies.) A second limitation of real-time systems is the fact that the portable monitors are quite sophisticated, and at least at the present time tend to be more expensive than tape recorders. (It is reasonable, however, to expect these costs to decrease with advances in technology.)

Real-time systems permit more rapid access to the processed data. It could be available even during the monitoring period if needed, using telephonic data transmission. Thus, serious arrhythmias could be reported immediately, and more timely therapeutic intervention would be possible. Real-time systems have the added capability of interacting with the patient during the monitoring process. This feature may be used to more completely document patient behavior, symptoms, emotional states, and the relation of these to cardiac arrhythmias. Intelligent use of patient-interactive devices can avoid creating additional patient anxiety, and may even provide the possibility for therapeutic interventions.

In the remaining sections of this paper, we will attempt to summarize currently available commercial systems, to present the major features of a typical real-time arrhythmia analysis algorithm, to compare the performance of real-time and tape systems as they now exist, and to speculate on future trends.

REVIEW OF CURRENTLY AVAILABLE COMMERCIAL SYSTEMS

Advances in technology, primarily circuit integration techniques, have led to the miniaturization of computer processors and associated hardware to an extent that permits their use in applications requiring totally portable systems. The possibilities for applying this technology to ambulatory monitoring have now been realized through the efforts of a number of academic and commercial organizations. Our purpose here is to acquaint the reader with those systems which are available commercially. The information which follows has been obtained both by reviewing published literature and by conversations with the manufacturers, mostly by telephone. Although the authors have made every effort to collect this data accurately, errors may have inadvertently crept in. If so, we apologize to the vendors and the readers alike.

By the Summer of 1983, six manufacturers will be marketing systems designed for real-time ambulatory monitoring. These systems will be available from: COM Medical Systems, Ltd.; Datamedix, Inc.; International Medical Corporation; Medical Concepts, Inc.; Medicomp, Inc.; and Survival Technology, Inc. A feature-by-feature comparison of the systems offered by these manufacturers is presented in Table 1. The comparison is divided into sections: general data, ambulatory monitoring unit (AMU), strips, report generator (RPG), statistics, patient interaction, diagnostics, warranty and price. Data unknown to the person contacted is indicated with a "?". Criteria which are not applicable to a specific system are indicated with a "-". Data unavailable for proprietary reasons is shown as "PROPR". Because of obvious space limitations, the information is somewhat cryptic but hopefully should be interpretable.

Some comments might be useful first with respect to the portable analyzer data. Analyzers which are fully digital do all signal processing using a microprocessor after conversion of the analog signal to digital data. Hybrid approaches use analog analysis of the signal in addition to digital processing. One approach is not necessarily better than the other; performance is dependent on each individual implementation. A comparison of processing power is beyond the scope of this paper. However, two rough indices which are commonly used are the word-width of the processor and the program memory size. Since all microprocessors in these devices probably have eight-bit words, program memory size becomes a major indicator of the sophistication of the individual analyzer. As a result, some manufacturers are clearly reluctant to reveal where they rank on this criterion. The type of program memory has relevance to the end-user. ROM memory is set at the factory and cannot be changed unless memory chips are exchanged. RAM memory is volatile and has to be reloaded with each power-up of the memory. In these devices, ROM has the advantage that initialization of the ambulatory monitor is quick, requiring only the insertion of batteries; RAM memory must be loaded for each patient and this takes time. However, RAM has the advantage that program changes are easy to make, but this is relevant only if the RPG unit has removable-media mass storage so that the manufacturer can provide updates easily.

Concerning arrhythmia detector performance, it is extremely difficult to make comparisons between systems in this regard, even when detailed evaluations have been performed (vide infra). However, a very rough index of how hard the manufacturer is "trying" in this regard might be to look at program memory size and the number of analysis channels. Sophisticated analysis algorithms require more memory than simple ones. Furthermore, there is a higher likelihood of good performance when more ECG channels are analyzed. The simplest approach is of course one continuous channel. Next in sophistication is analysis of one channel but to switch back and forth between two available channels when needed because of noise. The next is two continuous channels and finally three continuous channels. All are

TABLE 1 (See text for explanation)

Comparison Criteria	COM Medical	Datamdx Inc.	Int'l Medical	Medical Concpts	Mediamp Inc.	Survivl Tech.
First offered	1983	1981	1976	1981	1983	1983
AMU volume (cc)	1235	640	1177	520	549	645
Weight (g)	950	555	862	980	424	680
Power source	6xAA	2x9V	4xAA	5xAA	2x9V	5AA+merc
Configuration	DIGITAL	DIGITAL	HYBRID	HYBRID	DIGITAL	DIGITAL
Processor type	8-BIT	8-BIT	PROPR	8-BIT	PROPR	PROPR
Program memory (type)	ROM	ROM	ROM	ROM	RAM	ROM
Program memory (kb)	PROPR	32K	PROPR	16K	PROPR	PROPR
Analog response	0.1-40	.05-100	?	.037-58	.05-100	.05-35
Digital filtering	YES	40Hz LP	YES	NO	NO	YES
Sampling rate (sps)	256	250	256	125	250	200
Sample size (bits)	8	8	?	10	8	?
Channels analyzed	3.CONT	1.CONT	1.CONT	1.SWIT	2.CONT	3.CONT
ST analysis	YES	YES	YES	YES	YES	YES
Pacer detect	YES	YES	YES	NO	NO	YES
Monitor lead impedance	YES	YES	NO	HOOKUP	NO	YES
Max period (hrs)	24	24	72	24	24	25
Strip memory	DG.TAPE	RAM	AN.TAPE	DG.TAPE	RAM	RAM
Strip memory size (kb)	-	32	-	-	?	PROPR
No. channels/strip	1,2,3	1,2	2	2	2	1,2,3
Strip length (sec)	12	8.2	10	6,9,12	4-15	8
Strip memry (chan*mins)	360	4.4	240	48	8	**
RPG processor	16-BIT	8-BIT	PROPR	8-BIT	16-BIT	PROPR
Program memory (type)	RAM	ROM	ROM	ROM	RAM	?
Program memory (kb)	64	256	PROPR	96	1000	?
Mass storage	YES	NO	YES	NO	YES	YES
CRT/ECG Display	YES	YES	YES	NO	YES	?
Max report (pages)	16	26	ROLL,Z	ROLL	46	20
Print report (mins/pgs)	9/16	5/26	20	15-20	15/35	10
Strips within report	NO	YES	NO	NO	YES	YES
Printer technology	DOT.MTX	DOT.MTX	DOT.MTX	EL.STAT	EL.STAT	DOT.MTX
Printer type	EPSON	CUSTOM	EPSON	?	VERSTEC	CUSTOM
Turn-key/interactive	BOTH	INTER	T-KEY	T-KEY	BOTH	T-KEY
Report editing	YES	YES	YES	NO	YES	YES
Store protocols	NO	YES	YES	NO	YES	YES
Statistics memory	RAM+TAP	RAM	AN.TAPE	DG.TAPE	RAM	RAM
Stat data resolution	15 SEC	30 MIN	?	15 MIN	10 MIN	DYNAMIC
PVC morphology data	NO	YES	?	NO	YES	YES
Pt. Interaction Ev btn	YES	YES	YES	YES	YES	YES
Fdback-loose electrode	NO	NO	NO	NO	NO	YES
Fdback-battery failure	YES	NO	NO	NO	NO	YES
Fdback-arrhythmic event	YES	NO	NO	NO	YES	YES
Ask-patient activities	NO	NO	NO	NO	YES	NO
Ask-patient symptoms	NO	NO	NO	NO	YES	NO
Diagnostics Intrnl AMU	YES	YES	YES	NO	YES	YES
Intrnl RPG	YES	YES	YES	NO	YES	YES
Analog loopback test	NO	YES	YES	YES	YES	NO
US Warranty (mths)	12	12	6	12	<12	12
US Domestic Price						
RPG+Ptr+2xAMU (x$1000)	42	39.5	25-88	25	50	44
AMU (x$1000)	5.0	4.0	4.2	5.0	5.0	4.5
Reference	12	13	14	15	16	17

found among the six offerings. However, since most manufacturers are very secretive about the size of their analysis programs, no conclusions can be drawn.

The memory for ECG strips in these devices currently comes in three types: RAM, digital tape and analog tape. Assuming that the user wants an ambulatory monitor of roughly the same size as a conventional ambulatory tape recorder, then RAM has the lowest weight and power requirement per unit volume but also the lowest capacity. Digital tape has the same weight-power requirements as analog tape but storage, although providing more accuracy, is less efficient. Survival Technology has found a mechanism for providing the best of both worlds by incorporating a telephone modem that allows the patient to dump a full RAM memory to the doctor over the phone line, although this does require additional involvement from the patient. COM has provided a unique and potentially very useful feature to aid the user in the selection of clinically relevant strips from the AMU's potential maximum of 1800. In addition to the strips, every RR interval and associated beat type found during the 24 hour analysis period is also saved. This data can later be used for plots and also to allow the user to localize areas of interest so that time-indexed searches of the stored strips can be performed.

The same considerations mentioned above concerning processing power of the ambulatory units applies to the report generator unit as well: word-length times memory size is a rough index to power. All processors here probably have eight bits except COM and Medicomp, which have sixteen. The presence of removable-media mass storage in the RPG is an additional factor which increases the overall power and flexibiity of the instrument because this allows patient data storage and later retrieval for editing or report modification. It also permits storage of report and analyzer programs, making system updates easier. International Medical and Medical Concepts are special cases because patient data is stored on tape so it can be retrieved more than once. However, this approach does not truly qualify as a mass storage device. Several systems allow the user to tailor the contents of the report to the individual physician-user. The presence of mass-storage makes this tailoring easier by allowing multiple individual report protocols to be stored and retrieved without re-entering the protocol each time. Although the Datamedix system has no mass storage, it provides this capability by storing protocols in volatile memory.

Because the patient is carrying an intelligent monitoring device, the possibilities for patient interaction are greatly increased. The simplest interactive mechanism available is the patient event button which all systems provide. The next step beyond this is to provide the patient with system status information such as loose electrodes, battery failure or, in the case of Survival Technology, full memory. An arrhythmia status might also be fed back in the form of a "check in with your doctor" message which might also subsume the other statuses mentioned above. Arrhythmia feedback is controversial because of the potential for upsetting the patient at a time when serious arrhythmias are present. All of these types of feedback generally involve a beep to the patient and possibly a code on a simple display device. Medicomp goes a level beyond this with an optional "peripheral" which connects to the ambulatory monitor. This device has a text display and speech synthesis circuitry both for the periodic audio and visual presentation of questions concerning activities and for questions about symptoms when a event button is pressed or when certain arrhythmias are detected.

System pricing is relatively straight-forward with the exception of the price for a typical International Medical system. The range of prices shown in Table 1 indicates that from this manufacturer there are several different RPG configurations available with different report formats and different speeds. For comparison purposes, the price of a Trendsetter system from Avionics with arrhythmia detector, printer and two 447 recorders is about $80,000.

REAL-TIME ARRHYTHMIA ALGORITHMS AND THEIR EVALUATION

Real-time ambulatory monitoring systems generally employ quite sophisticated arrhythmia detection programs. They are on a par with the more advanced coronary care unit monitoring systems, and are similar in many cases to the minicomputer-based systems which perform high speed analysis of ECG tapes. We were unable to obtain detailed algorithm information from present manufacturers of real-time monitors, who tend to protect such information as proprietary. However, we can present the general features of a real-time arrhythmia analysis algorithm currently under development at the Biomedical Engineering Center for Clinical Instrumentation at the Massachusetts Institute of Technology (18). This program has been designed to run in a real-time ambulatory monitor and should be representative of the current state-of-the-art. It is known as ARISTOTLE (Ambulatory Real-time Interactive System for Testing On Two-Lead ECG's). The emphasis during the development of ARISTOTLE has been to achieve high accuracy in identifying ventricular arrhythmias. However, ARISTOTLE includes features which permit identification of certain supraventricular arrhythmias and ST-segment changes as well. In outline, ARISTOTLE's analysis of the two-lead ECG may be described in terms of the following stages (Fig. 2).

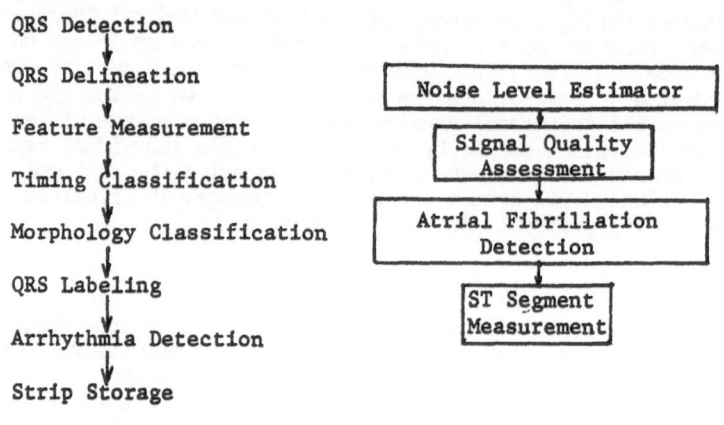

Figure 2.

(1) QRS Detection: ARISTOTLE's QRS detector uses a digital matched filter (19), dynamic threshold adjustment, and a look-back procedure to reduce false negatives in the presence of sporadic low amplitude QRS complexes. It is basically a single-channel detector which is capable of switching channels if signal quality deteriorates or if an unusually lengthy pause is noted. It is considered to be of sufficient accuracy that no further artifact rejection logic is required.

(2) Noise Level Estimation: A simple estimate of noise level is made for each channel by measuring the mean absolute error with respect to the observed ECG of a linear interpolation between two points on the baseline.

(3) QRS Delineation: A search is conducted backward from the R-wave peak for a "flat region" of the signal which locates the baseline for each channel. The noise estimate derived in the previous stage determines the criterion for flatness. The PQ junction and J point are found using a criterion which tests both flatness and proximity to the measured baseline. The PQ junction and J point measurements are taken on only one lead (the one used by the QRS detector).

(4) Feature Measurement: Seven heuristic features are measured on each lead. The features are offset, amplitude, and absolute area as used in ARGUS (20); a T-wave measure as described by Lovelace et al. (21); signed area; an estimate of width derived from the absolute area and the amplitude; and a weighted mean of the onset-to-peak and onset-to-nadir intervals. All features other than the T-wave measure are computed over the interval between the PQ junction and the J point as determined in the previous stage.

(5) Signal Quality Assessment: A linear discriminant function of four variables (the noise level and signal-to-noise ratio for each lead) is evaluated (22). The signal-to-noise ratios are estimated from the QRS amplitudes and the noise estimate derived above. If the discriminate function indicates a substantial difference in signal quality between the two leads, the remainder of the processing stages will perform a single-lead analysis on the better lead. Otherwise, data from both leads will be used.

(6) Timing Classification: Each QRS is categorized as premature, on-time, or late, in accordance with a comparison of the preceding RR interval against an expected interval. (The expected interval is calculated in step 9 below, once it is known which beats are normal.)

(7) Morphology Classification: A clustering algorithm which uses a Mahalanobis distance approximation (ignoring off-diagonal elements of the covariance matrix) constructs clusters of similar QRS complexes in a seven-dimensional feature space. If single-lead analysis has been selected by the signal quality assessment above, the seven dimensions of the feature space are simply the seven features measured on the selected lead. If two-lead analysis is selected, three features are taken from each lead, and a seventh is taken from the lead used by the QRS detector.

(8) QRS Labeling: Clusters are labeled "supraventricular" or "ventricular" by an algorithm which incorporates heuristics based on frequency of occurrence, mean prematurity of beats, and similarity to previously recognized clusters. Each beat is given a label according to its prematurity and the label of its cluster. The possible labels are normal, SVPB, PVC, ventricular escape, and unknown.

(9) Derivation of Expected RR Intervals: The mean and estimated standard deviation of normal-to-normal QRS intervals are calculated. Using this information and knowledge of the interval sequence, it is possible to detect atrial fibrillation in many cases.

(10) ST Segment Measurement: Using the point of maximum response to the QRS matched filter as a fiducial reference, ST-segment elevation/depression is measured at two points for each normal QRS. (These points are 120 and 140 msec after the fiducial.) An incremental averaging technique is used to smooth these measurements over time (23).

(11) Detection of the Arrhythmias: Once the sequence of beat types and RR intervals is known, it is relatively straightforward to identify arrhythmias such as couplets, runs of ventricular tachycardia, idioventricular rhythm, bigeminy, trigeminy, atrial couplets, SVT, and sudden rate changes.

When any of these conditions is detected, a two-lead ECG strip with beat labels, centered on the event of interest, may be saved. This may also happen if an asystolic pause is found by the QRS detector, if atrial fibrillation is detected in step 9, or if a significant change in ST level or slope is noted in step 10. The decision to save a strip depends on the past history of arrhythmias and on the amount of memory remaining for strip storage. Replacement of previously stored strips by higher priority events is permitted.

Although ARISTOTLE represents a typical arrhythmia analysis program, there are enormous numbers of possible variations. For each of the major program modules many different approaches have been described in the literature. In fact, the task of morphology classification alone may be realized in virtually hundreds of ways (24). Several excellent reviews have been published which document a wide variety of arrhythmia algorithms (25-28). There appears to be no significant difference in sophistication between programs running in contemporary real-time ambulatory monitoring systems, and those running in either modern coronary care unit arrhythmia monitors or in sophisticated, high-speed, Holter tape analysis systems. However, retrospective analysis of an entire 24-hours of data, possible only with tape-based systems, offers one theoretical advantage not available to real-time systems. Morphologic and timing features of more than 100,000 QRS complexes may be examined at one time. This extensive feature space may be more optimally divided into clusters of similar morphology than is possible with the more restricted features spaces of typical real-time systems. Not all tape scanning systems take advantage of this technique of course, and it does demand large disk storage capacity.

How well do automated arrhythmia analysis systems work? The problems associated with answering this question have long been recognized (26,29-31), yet there is still no universally accepted evaluation methodology for arrhythmia detectors. An important step forward has been achieved in the past few years with the development and distribution of annotated arrhythmia databases. Two such databases are publicly available now (32-35), and numerous others probably exist within individual university and industrial laboratories. Beat-by-beat algorithm evaluations using these annotated databases is certainly one important dimension of the evaluation process for arrhythmia detectors. Beat-by-beat trials using annotated databases, however, do not provide a complete evaluation. Long-term trials using a wide variety of actual patient data must also be conducted both in the laboratory and in the clinic. Only in this way may total system performance be thoroughly investigated under conditions approaching those of real life.

In preparing for this workshop, we made an effort to obtain quantitative evaluation data on the arrhythmia detector performance of several commercial systems. We spoke to manufacturers of both real-time and tape-based systems. Unfortunately, it was not possible to find completely satisfying answers to our questions. On the other hand, we obtained some information which may reveal "ball-park" estimates of performance.

At present there is no uniform standard for reporting the results of database evaluations. Some precedents exist in the literature (36-39), but have yet to become generally accepted by the user community. In general, beat-by-beat evaluations are conducted as follows. The data, in either digital or analog form, is presented to the program under test, which processes the signals and attaches an annotation to each detected beat (see Figure 3).

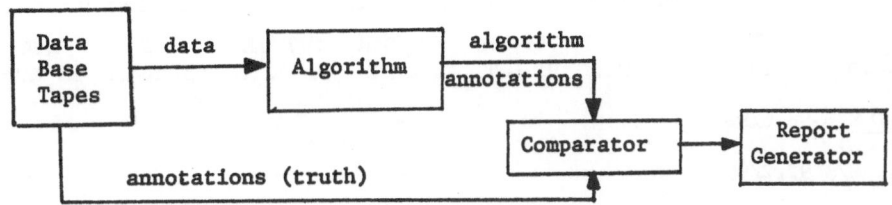

Figure 3. Scheme for Beat-by-Beat Evaluations

The algorithm's annotations are then compared to the database "truth" annotations using a suitable mapping policy. Widely used measures of algorithm
performance have been the sensitivity and positive predictive accuracy for
detecting QRS complexes and PVCs. Some groups have reported similar measures for other clinically important events such as ventricular couplets,
ventricular tachycardia, and supraventricular tachycardia. Table 2 shows
the evaluation data which we were able to obtain for selected real-time and
tape-scanning algorithms. The table identifies the system or algorithm
tested, the database used, and representative performance figures. The
numbers are not directly comparable since the databases were generally not
identical. The trial of the Medical Concepts systems reported by Kennedy
(40) is not quite a beat-by-beat evaluation, but it is the most exhaustive
clinical trial of a real-time system to be reported to date.

In evaluating high-speed tape scanning systems, it is important to use data
which reflects the algorithm's performance in the absence of human editing.
The figures for ARGUS/2H and the Marquette systems are for such unsupervised operation. Some commercial systems have been designed in such a way
as to require human supervision, and hence performance figures from them
are not comparable to unsupervised algorithms. Feldman (43) has reported
excellent performance of his Cardiodata system, but since it was run in a
supervised mode, the results cannot be compared to the others in Table 2.

Although the data within Table 2 is also not strictly comparable, one can
draw some general conclusions. First, all algorithms appear to do extremely well in detecting QRS complexes, with sensitivities and positive
predictive accuracies of better than 99.8%. The sensitivity for detecting
PVC's is also very good—ranging from 92 to 99%, suggesting considerable
improvement in the technology over the past decade (29). This sensitivity
is significantly better than that obtainable using traditional Holter scanning systems which rely on skilled technician vigilance (44,45). (In these
systems, PVC sensitivity is seldom better than 85-90%, and tends to degrade
considerably as tape complexity increases.) It is of interest to note that
the performance of real-time algorithms does not appear to be very different from that of tape scanning systems. It seems reasonable to expect
therefore that such systems will be as capable of detecting clinically significant arrhythmias as the more costly tape-scanning computers.

TABLE 2 (See text for explanation)

Data-base	COM MEDICAL	MARQUETTE ELEC INC.	MEDICAL CONCPTS	MEDICOMP INC.	MIT ARISTOTLE	MIT ARISTOTLE	WASH. U. ARGUS/2H
	AHA 22 TAPES	MIT/BIH 48 TAPES	799 HRS PT DAT	MIT/BIH 42 TAPES	MIT/BIH 48 TAPES	AHA 55 TAPES	AHA 15 TAPES
Typ S/S	98.6/96.7	-	-	-	-	-	-
PTP S/S	92.2/99.9	-	-	-	-	-	-
PAT S/S	96.0/99.7	-	-	-	-	-	-
QRS S/P	-	99.8/99.8	-	99.9/99.9	99.8/99.8	99.9/99.9	99.8/100
PVC S/P	-	97/92-95	92/92	-	93.3/86.0	97.2/93.6	99.2/100
Cup S/P	-	-	80/97	-	87.3/69.0	96.4/91.1	-
VT S/P	-	-	81/92	-	84.8/36.4	96.4/87.5	-
Atp S/P	-	-	-	97.9/98.2	-	-	-
Ref	12	40	41	16	22	22	42

Typ = Typical   Atp = Atypical
PTP = Premature Typical   PAT = Premature Atypical
Cup = Couplet
S/S = Sensitivity/Specificity
S/P = Sensitivity/Positive Predictive Accuracy

COMPARISON OF REAL-TIME ANALYZERS AND TAPE SCANNING SYSTEMS

When assessing the relative merits of state-of-the-art systems for real-time and tape-based ambulatory ECG analysis, several features deserve consideration:

Tape systems have the advantage of recording all the ECG data, so repeat scans are possible if questions arise. Although it is very rare that tapes are re-scanned in their entirety after the physician report is prepared, it is quite common for the scanning technician to review sections of tape which are difficult. New disk-based scanning systems facilitate the rapid and efficient manipulation of the data for human editing.
Tape systems permit human review and editing of all data, while real-time systems provide the human editor with only a subset of the data. False positive errors are correctable in real-time systems, but all false negative errors are permanent and non-correctable. The number of "rhythm strips" is quite variable in different commercial real-time systems. Design trade-offs have generally resulted in a moderate number of strips. Those systems utilizing solid state memory generally store 36-90 rhythm strips, while those systems relying on tape memory systems typically store several hundred strips. The percent of rhythm strips which are false positive may range from 15% to 60% depending on data. If the false positive

strip rate gets excessive, user confidence deteriorates—even if detection sensitivities remain very high. (There is therefore a danger that designers may sacrifice sensitivity for low false positive rates to increase apparent customer satisfaction.)

Real-time systems distribute investment differently. The portable units are relatively expensive ($4-5,000) compared to tapes ($1500-2500). On the other hand, the scanner/report generator is significantly less expensive, and transtelephonic remote analysis from the doctor's office is also feasible for real-time systems. Thus, for small physician groups, there may be economic advantages in using real-time systems.

Both real-time and tape systems require technician involvement in reviewing, editing and preparing reports. There may be slightly less time required for real-time report preparation, but not much. The set-up procedure for real-time systems is sometimes more complex than for tape recorders.

Real-time systems have the unique advantage of providing for patient interaction. This capability may provide for increased safety of drug trials, more effective correlation of symptoms and activities with cardiac rhythm changes, and the possibility for therapeutic intervention using either medications or behavioral techniques. Although these theoretical advantages are clear, the actual clinical utility of patient interaction remains to be established. This feature is offered at present by only one manufacturer (Medicomp).

FUTURE TRENDS

Over the past decade, we have witnessed remarkable advances in technology which have made possible the realization of practical devices for real-time ambulatory ECG analysis, which in 1975 was only a dream. Major improvements in automated arrhythmia analysis have occurred, and present day algorithm performance may very well exceed standard Holter scanning technology. As computational power available to portable systems continues to increase, algorithm performance will also improve. In the coming decade, we believe that automated analysis of the ECG will yield information which is not obtainable by manual methods. Some of this information may well be of prognostic value to patients (46-48), and it will be essential to have the data analyzed in real-time in order to manage the patient on a timely basis. It is conceivable that tightly coupled diagnostic-therapeutic loops will become feasible to manage arrhythmias with either drugs or by electrical means. The importance of life style and life stress situations will become increasingly recognized. Real time arrhythmia analysis will permit us to better document these situations, and also to help patients modify their behavior appropriately.

With the increasing complexity of implantable cardiac pacemakers, functional analysis of these devices becomes more and more difficult for anyone without detailed knowledge of the individual pacer type, its myriad parameters and intimate familiarity with its theory of operation. More likely for the future is pacemaker functional diagnosis by computer. Real-time ambulatory monitors are excellent vehicles for accomplishing this since they can analyse pacer function during normal patient activities. Because diagnosis of the new DDD pacers requires specific knowledge of the individual pacer, pacemaker manufacturers are investing in technology which will allow external interrogation of the functioning device. This same technology is likely to be incorporated into real-time ambulatory monitors so that these devices can communicate with the pacer during ambulation, with simultaneous analysis of the ECG and pacer spikes. The availability of the unfiltered ECG signal to the analyzer enhances the reliability of this approach. The results of ECG analysis correlated with pacer parameter settings would then become the basis of an automated functional diagnosis of pacer operation.

The capabilities of individual real-time ambulatory monitoring systems are likely to expand to include more than just the basic analysis protocol for the multi-channel surface ECG. Assuming that the monitoring device contains RAM memory rather than ROM, there is no reason that these devices could not also control and report on exercise tests, monitor arrhythmias using a surface lead and an esophageal lead, monitor specific parameters with higher than normal resolution (eg, heart rate for sleep apnea studies, heart-rate/ST-segment correlation studies, etc). Furthermore, since the RPG is likely to be a general-purpose computer system, we can expect to see functions included which are beyond those concerned with generating ambulatory ECG reports. Examples might be medical office management, inventory control, order entry systems, word processing, patient information systems, etc. Personal computer systems already offer these functions along with multi-user multi-tasking operating systems so it would not be suprising to find such functions included with future RPGs.

The economics of the technology favor real-time analysis systems. More powerful processors, denser memories, and the possibility of building algorithms into specialized VLSI circuits will all make possible lower cost, lower power, and smaller portable systems with increased storage capacity. These same technical movements will decrease the costs of computer-based tape scanning systems as well, although, because of their need for large mass storage devices, perhaps not to the same extent. Based on conversations with the real-time equipment manufacturers, the findings of their marketing analyses indicate that the current size of the ambulatory equipment sales market for the U.S. is $60 to $65 million and, for the world, about $90 million. At this point in time, equipment purchases for scanning services account for about 50% of this total while 30% to 35% is for in-house processing equipment. The remainder of the market, 15% to 20%, is already claimed by real-time equipment manufacturers. The overall sales of scanning services are about $160 million world-wide. If current growth continues, this figure could reach $450 million by 1987. Looking to the future, however, market analysts project that by 1985, 50% of ambulatory equipment sales will be for real-time equipment. A major ingredient in this optimism is the fact that the ambulatory equipment market has yet to stabilize. Based on these projections, the likelihood is very high that considerable development effort will be invested in this particular technological application and that more manufacturers will enter the "real-time" arena. Assuming that third party payers reimburse equally for both procedures, it is likely that the next decade will see an increase in the use of real time systems—particularly by small group practices and perhaps even individual cardiologists. However, it is unlikely that they will ever completely replace tape systems.

REFERENCES

1. Corday, E., Bazika, V., Lang, T., et al. 1965. Detection of phantom arrhythmias and evanescent electrocardiographic abnormalities: use of prolonged direct electrocardiorecording. JAMA 193:417.
2. Lown, B., Calvert, A., Armington, M., et al. 1975. Monitoring for serious arrhythmias and high risk of sudden death, Circulation, 52:suppl. III, 189-98.
3. Crawford, M., O'Rourke, R., et al. 1974. Comparative effectiveness of exercise testing and Holter monitoring for detecting arrhythmias in patients with previous myocardial infarction, Amer. J. Cardiol. 33:132.
4. Harrison, D.C., Fitzgerald, J.W. and Winkle, R.A. 1976. Ambulatory electrocardiography for diagnosis and treatment of cardiac arrhythmias. New Engl. J. Med. 294:373.
5. Kennedy, H.L. and Caralis, D.G. 1977. Ambulatory electrocardiography, a clinical perspective. Ann. Intern. Med. 87:729.
6. Famularo, M.A. and Kennedy, H.L. 1982. Ambulatory electrocardiography in the assessment of pacemaker function. Am. Heart J. 104:1086-94.
7. Vismara, L.A., Vera, Z., Foerster, J.M., et al. 1977. Identification of sudden death risk factors in acute and chronic coronary artery disease. Am. J. Cardiol. 821:39.
8. Michelson, E.L. and Morganroth, J. 1980. Spontaneous variability of complex ventricular arrhythmias detected by long-term electrocardiographic recording. Circulation 61:690.
9. Harrison, D.C., Fitzgerald, J.W. and Winkle, R.A. 1978. Contribution of ambulatory electrocardiographic monitoring to antiarrhythmic management. Am. J. Cardiol. 41:996.
10. Mark, R.G., Moody, G.B., Olson, W.H., et al. 1981. Event recorders and future systems. In "Ambulatory Electrocardiographic Recording" (Eds. N.K. Wenger, M.B. Mock, L. Ringqvist). (Yearbook Medical Publishers, Chicago). pp. 113-132.
11. Salerno, D., Hodges, M., Granrud, G., et al. 1983. Inaccuracy of commercial 24-hour ECG analyzers for quantitation of simple and complex ventricular arrhythmia. J. Am. Coll. Cardiol. 1(2):597.
12. Personal Communication from Mr. Dan Winterstein, COM Medical Systems, Inc., P.O. Box 222, Tirat Hacarmel 30251, Isreal.
13. Personal Communication from Mr. Michael Zack, Datamedix, Inc., Route One, Sharon, MA 02067, USA.
14. Personal Communication from Mr. Jens Muller, International Medical Corporation, 64 Inverness Drive East, Englewood, CO 80112, USA.
15. Personal Communication from Dr. Peter Balnave, Medical Concepts, Inc., 137 Gaither Drive, Mt. Laurel, NJ 08054, USA.
16. Personal Communication from Mr. Douglas Hoag, Medicomp, Inc., 1250 West NASA Blvd., Melbourne, FL 32901, USA.
17. Personal Communication from Mr. Herb Reinhold, Survival Technology, Inc., 7801 Woodmont Avenue, Bethesda, MD 20814, USA.
18. Mark, R.G., Moody, G.B., Olson, W.H., et al. 1979. Real-time ambulatory arrhythmia analysis with a microcomputer. In "Computers in Cardiology" (IEEE Computer Society, Los Alamitos, CA). pp. 57-62.
19. Arnold, J. 1972. Time-domain filtering of electrocardiograms. S.B. Thesis, Massachusetts Institute of Technology, Dept. of Electrical Engineering, Cambridge, Mass., U.S.A.
20. Nolle, F.M. 1972. ARGUS, a clinical computer system for monitoring electrocardiographic rhythms, D.Sc. Dissertation, Washington University, St. Louis, Missouri, U.S.A.

21. Lovelace, D.E., Knoebel, S.B. and Zipes, D.P. 1976. Recognition of ventricular extrasystoles in sedentary vs. ambulatory populations. In "Computers in Cardiology" (IEEE Computer Society, Los Alamitos, CA). pp. 9-12.

22. Moody, G.B. and Mark, R.G. 1982. Development and evaluation of a 2-lead ECG analysis program. In "Computers in Cardiology" (IEEE Computer Society, Los Alamitos, CA). pp. 39-44.

23. Watanabe, K., et al. 1980. Computer analysis of the exercise ECG: a review. Prog. Cardiovasc. Dis. 22:423.

24. Rappaport, S., Gillick, L., Moody, G., et al. 1982. QRS morphology classification: quantitative evaluation of different strategies. In "Computers in Cardiology" (IEEE Computer Society, Los Alamitos, CA). pp. 33-38.

25. Ripley, K.L. and Murray, A. 1980. Introduction to automated arrhythmia detection. IEEE Computer Society, Los Alamitos, CA.

26. Thomas, L.J., Clark, K.W., Mead, C.N., et al. 1979. Automated cardiac dysrhythmia analysis. Proc. IEEE, 67:309-324.

27. Oliver, G.C., Ripley, K.L., Miller, J.P., et al. 1977. A critical review of computer arrhythmia detection. In "Computer Electrocardiography: Current Status and Criterion" (Ed. L. Pordy). (Futura Publishing Co., Mt. Kisco, NY). pp. 319-360.

28. Cox, J.R., Nolle, F.M. and Arthur, R.M. 1972. Digital analysis of the electroencephalogram, the blood pressure wave, and the electrocardiogram. Proc. IEEE, 60:1137-1164.

29. Ripley, K.L. and Arthur, R.M. 1975. Evaluation and comparison of automatic arrhythmia detectors. In "Computers in Cardiology" (IEEE Computer Society, Los Alamitos, CA). pp. 27-32.

30. Feldman, C.L. 1974. Evaluation of arrhythmia detectors. In "Computers in Cardiology" (IEEE Computer Society, Los Alamitos, CA). pp. 21-27.

31. Cox, J.R., Hermes, R.E. and Ripley, K.L. 1981. Evaluation of performance. In "Ambulatory Electrocardiographic Recording." (Eds. N.K. Wenger, M.B. Mock, and I. Ringqvist). (Yearbook Medical Publishers, Chicago). pp 183-198.

32. Hermes, R.E. and Oliver, G.C. 1981. Use of the American Heart Association database. In "Ambulatory Electrocardiographic Recording." (Eds. N.K. Wenger, M.B. Mock, and I. Ringqvist). (Yearbook Medical Publishers, Chicago). pp 165-181.

33. Hermes, R.E., Geselowitz, D.B. and Oliver, G.C. 1980. Development, distribution and use of the American Heart Association database for ventricular arrhythmia detector evaluation. In "Computers in Cardiology" (IEEE Computer Society, Los Alamitos, CA). pp. 263-266.

34. Schluter, P.S., Peterson, S.K., Siegel, L.C., et al. 1978. A database for arrhythmia detector evaluation. Proceedings of the 31st ACEMB.

35. MIT-BIH Arrhythmia Database: Tape directory and format specification. 1980. Biomedical Engineering Center for Clinical Instrumentation, Technical Report No. 010, MIT Cambridge, MA 02139.

36. Schluter, P., Mark, R., Moody, G., et al. 1980. Performance measures for arrhythmia detectors. In "Computers in Cardiology" (IEEE Computer Society, Los Alamitos, CA). pp. 267-270.

37. Zeelenberg, C. and Meij, S.H. 1981. Evaluation and optimization of an existing arrhythmia detection system by using an annotated ECG database. In "Computers in Cardiology" (IEEE Computer Society, Los Alamitos, CA). pp. 103-108.

38. Wang, J.Y., Shaya, M.N., Helfenbein, E.D., et al. 1982. The design and evaluation of a real-time arrhythmia monitoring algorithm. In "Computers in Cardiology" (IEEE Computer Society, Los Alamitos, CA). pp. 363-366.

39. Mark, R.G., Schluter, P.S., Moody, G., et al. 1982. An annotated ECG database for evaluating arrhythmia detectors. In "Frontiers of Engineering in Health Care-1982." Proc. of 4th Annual IEEE EMBS Soc. Conf.
40. Kennedy, H.L., Sprague, M.K., Shriver, K.K., et al. 1982. Real-time analysis Holter ECG - a new approach. Circulation, 66 (supp. II):74.
41. Mead, C.N., Pull, H.R., Clark, K.W., et al. 1982. Expanded frequency-domain ECG waveform processing: Integration into a new version of Argus/2H. In "Computers in Cardiology" (IEEE Computer Society, Los Alamitos, CA). pp. 205-209.
42. Personal communication from Dr. Paul Schluter of Marquette Electronics, Inc., Milwaukee, Wisconsin. Data refer to developmental version of system operating in Spring 1982.
43. Feldman, C.L. 1981. How should Holter monitoring analysis be performed? In "The evaluation of new antiarrhythmia drugs." (Eds. J. Morganroth and E.N. Moore). (Martinus Nijhoff Publishers, The Hague, The Netherlands).
44. Stein, I.M., Plunkett, J. and Troy, M. 1980. Comparison of techniques for examining long-term ECG recordings. Medical Instrumentation, 14:69-72.
45. Thomas, L.J., Clark, K.W., Mead, C.N., et al. 1981. Supraventricular arrhythmias: strategies for detection. In "Ambulatory Electrocardiographic Recording." (Eds. N.K. Wenger, M.B. Mock, and I. Ringqvist). (Yearbook Medical Publishers, Chicago), pp. 213-232.
46. Lovelace, D.E. and Knoebel, S.B. 1982. Time series analysis in predicting ventricular arrhythmias. In "Computers in Cardiology" (IEEE Computer Society, Los Alamitos, CA). pp. 45-48.
47. Adam, D.R., Powell, A.O., Gordon, H., et al. 1982. Ventricular fibrillation and fluctuations in the amplitude of the repolarization vector. In "Computers in Cardiology" (IEEE Computer Society, Los Alamitos, CA). pp. 241-244.
48. Akselrod, S., Gordon, D., Ubel, F.A., et al. 1981. Power spectrum analysis of heart rate fluctuation: a quantitative probe of beat-to-beat cardiovascular control. Science, Vol. 213:220-222.

TOPIC: 3.6

Evaluation of ambulatory monitoring systems:
experiences and perspectives

EVALUATION OF AUTOMATED ARRHYTHMIA MONITORS

USING AN ANNOTATED ECG DATABASE

R.G. Mark and G. B. Moody

Biomedical Engineering Center for Clinical Instrumentation
Harvard-MIT Division of Health Sciences and Technology
Massachusetts Institute of Technology
Cambridge, Massachusetts 02139

ABSTRACT

This paper documents the design and development of the MIT/BIH arrhythmia database. This two-channel, digital database which contains a wide variety of ventricular and supraventricular arrhythmias is suitable for algorithm evaluation and development. Procedures are suggested for its use, and examples of a variety of output formats are presented.

INTRODUCTION

Automated arrhythmia monitors are complex instruments which are called

upon to perform very important and sometimes critical roles in patient care.

The design and improvement of such systems has been a major focus of engi-

neering effort for at least two decades. Although much creative energy has

been expended in algorithm development, the quantitative evaluation of ar-

rhythmia detectors remains a difficult and controversial problem. Repro-

ducible testing of arrhythmia systems, using a universally accepted "yard-

stick" is a need widely recognized by system designers and prospective

users (Ripley et al., 1977; Schluter et al., 1980; Hermes et al., 1980).

In response to this need, at least two annotated arrhythmia databases have

recently been developed and are now generally available. One, developed

under the auspices of the American Heart Association (Ripley et al.,1978),

is distributed by the Emergency Care Research Institute in Plymouth Meet-

ing, Pennsylvania. The second was developed by us at Massachusetts Insti-

tute of Technology and Beth Israel Hospital in Boston, Massachusetts
(Mark et al., 1982). These databases are important evaluation tools
which permit detailed and quantitative beat-by-beat algorithm testing.
In this paper we will review the development of our database, and propose
methodology and policies for its use in algorithm evaluation and development. It should be stated at the outset, however, that a beat-by-beat
evaluation using annotated databases, while a necessary part of completely assessing an arrhythmia analyzer, is not sufficient. Evaluation of performance must also be done using long-term data (8-10
hours or more) and clinical trials.

DEVELOPMENT AND SPECIFICATION OF THE MIT/BIH DATABASE

The database consists of 48, half-hour, two-channel ECG records
containing a wide variety of ventricular and supraventricular arrhythmias,
conduction abnormalities, and artifact. Pacemaker rhythms are included
as well. The records were selected from a library of over 4,000, 24-hour
ambulatory ECG recordings obtained by the Arrhythmia Laboratory at Beth
Israel Hospital in Boston, Massachusetts from both in-patients (60%)
and out-patients (40%). Original tape-recordings were made on Avionics
Model 445 2-channel recorders using modified Lead II and modified Lead
V_1 configurations.

Twenty-three of the database records (the "100 series") were selected randomly from the library to provide a typical cross-section of ECG
waveforms and artifact. A table of random numbers was used to select
particular tapes and half-hour segments. Data was used so long as at
least one of the two channels was interpretable.

The remaining twenty-five ECG records (the "200 series") were selec-
tively chosen to represent more rarely occurring but clinically important

arrhythmias. Episodes of ventricular tachycardia, flutter, and other complex rhythms were included in this set. Several records were specifically selected on the basis of their expected difficulty for computer analysis due to background rhythm, QRS morphology variation, or artifact.

The two-channel analog tape epochs were digitized at a sampling rate of 360 Hz with 11-bit resolution over a 5 mV range. The samples were stored as 8-bit signed differences. The overall bandwidth was 0.1 Hz to 100 Hz, which was considered adequate for testing arrhythmia analysis programs.

The digitized data was next annotated by a simple QRS detector program which arbitrarily labeled each beat as "normal". This preliminary label was used only as an aid in the human annotation protocol.

Each ECG record was then edited, beat-by-beat, by two independent experts. They were each given 30-minute, 2-channel strip chart recordings of the data, where each beat recognized by the simple QRS detector had been labeled "N". All beats that were missed by the QRS detector, or falsely detected, or not NORMAL were relabeled appropriately by the human annotators. They also identified the underlying cardiac rhythm and its changes, and episodes of artifact and noise.

The revised annotations of each reader were separately incorporated into the digitized database with the help of a displaying waveform editor. The database format allowed up to eight independent annotation channels to be preserved.

The annotations of the two independent observers were next automatically compared by a program that identified all disagreements. A

third strip chart recording was made to document them. The disagreements were resolved by a third reader, and final corrections were incorporated into the database to produce a set of "consensus annotations".
The fiducial location of each beat annotation was not strictly controlled,
except that it was within the QRS complex in all cases, and usually near
the maximum peak.

The consensus annotation channel was then checked by an "auditor"
program that verified the logical relationship between QRS complex labels
and rhythm labels. For example, all complexes within a run of ventricular tachycardia were examined to see if they had a "PVC" label.
Omitted beats were detected by listing the longest R-R intervals and
their times of occurrence. After the consensus annotation channel was
audited and corrected, it became the final "truth" annotation channel.

The completed ECG database was recorded on 9-track magnetic tape
in a format compatible with the American Heart Association database
for ventricular arrhythmias. The additional annotation codes provided
by our database have been added as a superset to specify atrial arrhythmias, conduction defects, changes in predominant rhythm, and episodes
of noisy data. A detailed list of annotation codes is given in Table 1
together with AHA equivalents. Table 2 lists the rhythm onset annotations.

TABLE 1: MIT-BIH Database Annotation Codes
(Showing AHA Database Equivalents)

Mnemonic	MITBIH Code	AHA	Description
NORMAL	01	N	normal QRS
LBBB	02	N	left bundle branch block
RBBB	03	N	right bundle branch block
ABERR	04	N	aberrantly conducted beat
PVC	05	V	ventricular Premature Beat
FUSION	06	F	fusion beat ****
NPC	07	N	nodal premature beat
APC	08	N	atrial premature beat
SVPB	09	N	nodal or Atrial premature beat
VESC	10	E	ventricular escape beat
NESC	11	N	nodal escape beat
PACE	12	P	paced beat
UNKNOWN	13	Q	cannot identify, QRS like event.
NOISE	14	O,U	beginning of NOISE *
QUIET	15	O	end of NOISE *
SPIKE	16	O	single QRS-like artifact
P	17	O	P-wave **
Q	18	O	Q-wave **
R	19	O	R-wave **
S	20	O	S-wave **
T	21	O	T-wave **
COMMENT	22	O	comment (text) annotation ***
FIRST	23	O	first annotation (optional) **
LAST	24	O	last annotation (optional) **
BBB	25	N	left or right bundle branch block beat
PACESP	26	O	pacemaker spike without capture
AXIS	27	O	axis shift
ONSET	28	O	rhythm onset (text) annotation ***
OFFSET	29	O	offset comment **
LEARN	30	O	learning **
FLWAV	31	O	ventricular flutter wave
VFON	32	[	onset of ventricular flutter/fibrillation
VFOFF	33	]	end of ventricular flutter/fibrillation
AEB	34	N	atrial ectopic beat
NEB	35	N	nodal ectopic beat
MISSB	36	O	missed beat
BLAPB	37	O	blocked APB
AXLMX	38	O	legal codes are < AXLMX **

* Annotation codes 14 and 15 are used in pairs. If the subtype <1>, no beats are labeled until the next code 15.

** These codes are reserved for future use, and should be ignored.

*** This annotation has a text string, terminated by a null <0>.

**** In the context of paced rhythm (tapes 102, 104, 107, and 217, annotation code 6 is used for pacemaker fusion beats.

TABLE 2: Rhythm Onset Annotations

Rhythm onset annotation (MIT-BIH annotation code 28) include an ASCII string which begins with a "(":

(AB	atrial bigeminy
(AFIB	atrial fibrillation
(AFL	atrial flutter
(AT	atrial tachycardia
(B	ventricular bigeminy
(BI	first degree heart block
(BII	second degree heart block
(BIII	third degree heart block
(IVR	idioventricular rhythm
(N	normal sinus rhythm
(NOD	nodal (A-V junctional) rhythm
(PAT	paroxsysmal atrial tachycardia
(PREX	pre-excitation (WPW)
(SBR	sinus bradycardia
(SVTA	supraventricular tachyarrhythmia
(T	ventricular trigeminy
(VFIB	ventricular fibrillation
(VFL	ventricular flutter
(VT	ventricular tachycardia

The rhythm annotations make it possible to evaluate algorithm performance in the presence of different underlying rhythms. For example, regions of atrial fibrillation and flutter are indicated on the database, permitting automatic evaluation of atrial fibrillation detectors or evaluation of PVC detectors in the presence of atrial fibrillation.

Table 3 presents a condensed summary of the database showing a rough breakdown of QRS types and rhythm episodes. Because of the complex arrhythmias, changing QRS morphologies, noise and artifact included in the database, we consider it a relatively difficult challenge for automated arrhythmia detectors. A more complete description of the database is available in the tape directory (MIT/BIH, 1980).

TABLE 3 : <u>A Condensed Summary of the Database</u>

a. QRS Types (some sub-types combined)

<u>QRS Type</u>	<u>Number</u>	<u>Percent</u>
Normal	78,591	71.6
Bundle Branch Block	11,804	10.7
SVPB	2,542	2.3
Aberrated SVPB	150	0.14
Other Supraventricular	328	0.30
Paced	7,029	6.4
PVC	7,127	6.5
Fusion/Paced	982	0.89
Fusion/PVC	803	.73
Total	109,790	

b. Rhythm Annotations (partial list)

<u>Rhythm Episode</u>	Records Containing <u>Examples</u>
NSR (incl. Tachy, brady)	45
Paced	4
Bundle Branch Block	8
Atrial Flutter/Fibrillation	7
SVTA	6
Junctional Rhythm	3
2° Heart Block	1
WPW	1
Idioventricular Rhythm	2
VT/V Flutter	13

An analog form of the database has also been prepared, using 4-channel FM tape. The primary reason for this format is economic, since the cost of equipment to play back digital tapes is prohibitive to some users. The analog data is recorded on two of the four FM channels, and the remaining two channels contain annotation data and five second time ticks encoded as EIA RS-232 bit-serial voltage levels compatible with most computers.

The database has been made generally available. To date it has been distributed to approximately 30 industrial and university groups in the United States and abroad.

USE OF THE DATABASE IN ALGORITHM EVALUATION

Creation of Annotation Files

A beat-by-beat evaluation requires that the digital database records be used as input to a version of the arrhythmia algorithm which can produce its own beat-by-beat annotations. To evaluate arrhythmia analysis software running on the same machine that supports the database, it is a fairly simple matter to replace the usual data acquisition routine with a call to a database utility subroutine which reads a sample. Similarly, it is not difficult to arrange for each beat label from the algorithm and its time of occurrence to be recorded by calling a utility routine which writes an annotation file. The result of the process is a file of algorithm annotations in the same format as the reference "truth" annotation file supplied with the database. The two annotation files can then be compared as discussed in the next section.

Frequently the arrhythmia monitor under test is physically separate from the computer managing the database. In this case, the database machine can transmit serial digital data or can be programmed to generate analog ECG output from the digital records. The arrhythmia monitor must be modified to return annotations and their times of occurrence to the database machine which can then produce an annotation file as above. Alternatively, the ECG and fiducial markers (from channel 4) may be obtained from the FM analog tape format of the database.

Comparison of Annotation Files

This stage of the evaluation is of critical importance, since all later results depend upon the proper execution of the comparison. The implementation of an annotation comparator requires resolution of several issues:

1. Annotation mapping: the conversion of one annotation alpha-

bet into another.

2. Beat matching: finding pairs of annotations, one from each annotation file, which are considered to refer to the same QRS complex.

3. Run matching: finding pairs of runs of PVC's, one from each annotation file, which are considered to refer to the same run.

4. Choosing output formats.

The MIT/BIH annotation alphabet allows differentiation of 19 QRS types, and includes a variety of non-QRS labels. The AHA annotation alphabet can easily be mapped into the MIT/BIH code without loss of information, although the reverse is not so, since the AHA code lacks rhythm labels and does not differentiate supraventricular ectopic beats from normals.

For many purposes, however, a much smaller annotation set is adequate. In evaluating PVC detection, we have used a set consisting of $\overline{PVC}$ (sometimes we use the N symbol for this group), PVC, Fusion PVC, and $\overline{QRS}$. In this mapping, PVC's, R-on-T PVC's, ventricular flutter waves, and ventricular escape beats are considered PVC's. Fusion beats in non-paced records are considered fusion PVC's; and all other beat types are classed as $\overline{PVC}$'s.

The beat matching algorithm is based on the notion of a "match acceptance window". Since, in general, it is unreasonable to expect precise simultaneity of database annotations and algorithm annotations, the beat matching algorithm selects pairs of annotations, which are separated by a time interval no greater than the match acceptance window. If an annotation has no match in the other file within the match acceptance window, it is paired with a (dummy) "not QRS" annotation. (This would correspond to either a missed beat or a false QRS detec-

tion, depending on which file contained the extra annotation.) If two
or more annotations in either file lie within the match acceptance
window of an annotation in the other file, the closest match is accepted. (See Figure 1.) If there are 'no annotations in the other file
to correspond with the extras, they are paired with dummy "not QRS"
annotations. Thus all beat annotations in both files are paired, and
the output of the beat matching algorithm is a stream of paired annotations.

In our experience, a suitable match acceptance window has been 150
milliseconds. This permits a substantial annotation misalignment, as
may occur if one annotator labels the peak, and the other the nadir of a
PVC, for example. Since the closest matches are always counted, no problems of ambiguity arise.

The clinical importance of ventricular couplets and runs prompted us
to develop a run matching algorithm. Throughout the following discussion,
isolated PVC's and ventricular couplets are regarded as "runs" with lengths
of 1 and 2 beats respectively. The run matching algorithm takes as input

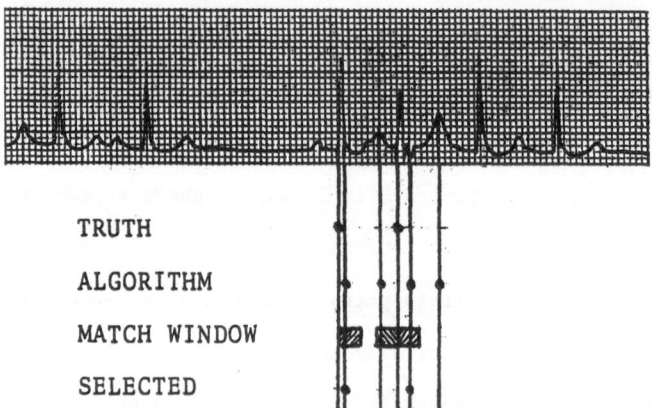

TRUTH

ALGORITHM

MATCH WINDOW

SELECTED

Fig.1: Match Acceptance Window

the stream of paired annotations produced by the beat matching algorithm.
The lengths of each run in each file are noted. Whenever a pair of non-
PVC's is received from the beat matching routine, any pending runs are
compared by length. The result of the comparison is entered into the
run-by-run confusion matrix. If two or more runs occur on either
channel before a pair of non-PVC's is found, only the longest will be
used in the comparison. Thus, the basic criterion for matching runs
depends on finding runs which overlap without requiring beat-by-beat
agreement for each beat in the run. (See Fig. 2.) We adopted this
approach based on the belief that a device capable of recognizing consecutive PVC's, at a time when consecutive PVC's are occurring is performing the most important function of an arrhythmia monitor properly,
and the details of beat-by-beat comparisons are less important (and may
in any case be determined from other outputs of the comparator). We
have arbitrarily declared an annotation pair containing a fusion PVC to
be a pair of non-PVC's (i.e. a run terminator). Thus, a monitor is
neither penalized nor rewarded for its treatment of fusion PVC's in this
context.

Fig.2: Run Length Comparison Algorithm

Beat Sequence

Truth: xxVxxVVxxVVVVVVxxVVVVVVVxxxVxxxxxx xx
Algorithm: xxVxxVVxxVVVVxxxxVVVxVVVVxxxxxVVxxVxx

Run Length

Truth	1	2	6	7	1	0	0
Algorithm	1	2	4	4	0	2	1

Output Formats

In presenting evaluation results it is important to indicate exactly what data was excluded from the evaluation if any. We have usually adopted the following policies:

1. Learning beats associated with algorithm start-up are excluded.

2. Regions of ventricular flutter and fibrillation are excluded. All other background rhythms and noisy areas are included.

3. Fusion PVC's are excluded when calculating PVC detector performance.

Lumped results for an entire database may be presented in matrix form. Figure 3 shows evaluation results for a two-channel analysis algorithm (ARISTOTLE) on the MIT/BIH and the AHA databases (Moody et al., 1982). From such matrices it is a simple matter to calculate several commonly used measures of algorithm performance:

		A l g o r i t h m						A l g o r i t h m		
		$\overline{\text{PVC}}$	PVC	$\overline{\text{QRS}}$				$\overline{\text{PVC}}$	PVC	$\overline{\text{QRS}}$
T	$\overline{\text{PVC}}$	98,067	935	142		T	$\overline{\text{PVC}}$	120,372	664	91
R	PVC	400	6,632	79		R	PVC	299	11,963	45
U	FSN	402	387	5		U	FSN	614	137	Ø
T						T				
H	$\overline{\text{QRS}}$	118	140			H	$\overline{\text{QRS}}$	33	156	–

MIT/BIH Database   AHA Database (55 tapes)

Fig. 3: Evaluation of ARISTOTLE Using
two Annotated Databases

$$\text{QRS sensitivity} = \frac{\text{\# true QRS's detected}}{\text{\# true QRS's}}$$

$$\text{QRS positive predictive accuracy} = \frac{\text{\# true QRS's detected}}{\text{total \# detected events}}$$

$$\text{PVC sensitivity} = \frac{\text{\# true PVC's detected}}{\text{\# true PVC's}}$$

$$\text{PVC positive predictive accuracy} = \frac{\text{\# true PVC's detected}}{\text{total \# events called PVC's}}$$

The calculated values for these parameters for both databases are shown for ARISTOTLE in Table 4. The detector parameter α described by Cox et al.,(1981), is also shown, together with their "average detection probability", $\bar{p}$. Table 5 presents the sensitivity and positive predictive accuracies for couplets, short (3-5 beat) runs of ventricular tachycardia, and long (greater than 5 beat) runs.

TABLE 4 : Lumped Results for ARISTOTLE

	MIT/BIH	AHA Database
QRS Sens.	99.79	99.90
QRS Pos. Pred. Acc.	99.76	99.86
PVC Sens.	93.26	97.20
PVC Pos. Pred.	86.05	93.59
Alpha	10.0	25.45
Average detection Prob, $\bar{p}$	90.9%	96.2%
Total QRS's	107,049	134,185
Total PVC's	7,111	12,307

TABLE 5: Couplet and Run Detection

	MIT/BIH	AHA Database
Couplet Sens.	87.26	96.43
Couplet Pos.Pred.Acc.	69.07	91.12
Short Run Sens.	84.85	96.42
Short Run Pos. Pred. Acc.	36.36	87.47
Long Run Sens.	88.24	83.33
Long Run Pos. Pred.Acc.	46.88	46.88

Lumped results do not reflect the substantial variability in algorithm performance on different patient records within the database. Results for individual records may show PVC sensitivities which range from 0% to 100% - an observation not conveyed in the lumped results. Individual tape results may be expressed in tabular form as in Table 6. While this format is quite complete, it is quite awkward. Cumulative distributions of detector sensitivities provide information on individual variability, and have suggested by Cox et al., (1981). An example of such a cumulative distribution is shown in Figure 4, using data from an evaluation of a single patient bedside arrhythmia monitor (Schluter, 1981). In this particular distribution each patient record is weighted by the number of PVC's. The resulting "gross detection ratio" of 84.1% reflects the probability of correctly identifying a PVC from the universe of all beats in the database. Another aggregate sensitivity measure is the "average detection ratio" in which results from each patient record are weighted equally, independent of the number of PVC's involved. The cumulative distribution of sensitivities for the bedside monitor is shown in Figure 5. The average detection ratio of 67.8% is considerably less than the gross sensi-

TABLE 6

Summary of evaluation results for aristotle [truth/aristotle]

Tape	N/N	V/N	F/N	-/N	N/V	V/V	F/V	-/V	N/-	V/-	F/-	QRS Se	QRS +P	PVC Se	PVC +P
100 2221	0	0	0	0	1	0	0	0	0	0	0	100.00	100.00	100.00	100.00
101 1804	0	0	1	9	0	0	3	1	0	0	0	99.94	99.78	-	0.00
102 2125	1	0	0	7	3	0	0	0	0	0	0	100.00	100.00	75.00	30.00
103 2002	0	0	0	30	0	0	0	0	1	0	0	99.95	100.00	-	0.00
104 2175	1	0	12	0	0	0	0	6	2	1	0	99.86	99.18	0.00	0.00
105 2397	2	0	23	83	36	0	44	3	0	0	0	99.88	97.41	94.74	22.09
106 1432	4	0	0	26	514	0	0	0	1	0	0	99.95	100.00	99.04	95.19
107 2027	2	0	0	0	51	0	0	0	0	6	0	99.71	100.00	86.44	100.00
108 1651	4	1	36	35	10	1	9	13	0	0	0	99.24	97.42	71.43	18.52
109 2435	2	1	0	7	36	0	0	0	0	0	0	100.00	100.00	94.74	83.72
111 2069	0	0	0	2	1	0	0	1	0	0	0	99.95	100.00	100.00	33.33
112 2488	0	0	0	0	0	0	0	0	0	0	0	100.00	100.00	-	-
113 1733	0	0	0	12	0	0	0	0	0	0	0	100.00	100.00	-	0.00
114 1774	0	0	0	7	43	4	0	1	0	0	0	99.95	100.00	100.00	86.00
115 1899	0	0	0	3	0	0	0	0	0	0	0	100.00	100.00	-	0.00
116 2211	0	0	2	19	108	0	1	23	1	0	0	98.98	99.87	99.08	84.38
117 1474	0	0	0	10	0	0	0	0	0	0	0	100.00	100.00	-	0.00
118 2205	0	0	0	7	15	0	0	0	0	0	0	100.00	100.00	100.00	68.18
119 1503	0	0	1	2	431	0	0	0	0	0	0	100.00	99.95	100.00	99.54
121 1808	0	0	0	2	1	0	0	1	0	0	0	99.94	100.00	100.00	33.33
122 2425	0	0	0	0	0	0	1	0	0	0	0	100.00	99.96	-	0.00
123 1446	0	0	0	18	0	0	0	0	0	3	0	99.80	100.00	0.00	0.00
124 1507	2	4	0	9	44	1	0	0	1	0	0	99.94	100.00	93.62	83.02
200 1720	31	1	0	18	773	0	1	0	6	0	1	99.73	99.96	95.43	97.60
201 1607	1	2	0	64	197	0	0	41	0	0	0	97.86	100.00	99.49	75.48
202 2042	0	1	0	20	18	0	0	4	0	0	0	99.81	100.00	100.00	47.37
203 2332	42	0	28	147	381	1	51	11	17	0	0	99.04	97.35	86.59	65.80
205 2521	1	9	0	1	69	2	0	1	1	0	0	99.92	100.00	97.18	98.57
207 1536	72	0	0	85	119	0	5	3	5	0	0	99.56	99.72	60.71	56.94
208 1500	78	117	7	44	886	247	2	9	6	2	0	99.41	99.69	91.34	95.06
209 2938	0	0	1	14	1	0	1	0	0	0	0	100.00	99.93	100.00	6.25
210 2359	3	2	1	32	169	5	3	4	19	2	0	99.04	99.84	88.48	82.84
212 2677	0	0	1	8	0	0	1	12	0	0	0	99.56	99.93	-	0.00
213 2593	69	259	0	25	150	103	0	0	1	0	0	99.97	100.00	68.18	85.71
214 1940	0	1	1	14	251	0	1	2	2	0	0	99.82	99.91	99.21	94.36
215 3137	1	0	0	13	159	1	0	0	1	0	0	99.97	100.00	98.76	92.44
217 1927	9	0	1	68	149	0	3	1	3	0	0	99.81	99.81	92.55	67.73
219 2028	0	0	1	10	61	1	1	1	2	0	0	99.86	99.90	96.83	84.72
220 1984	0	0	0	13	0	0	0	0	0	0	0	100.00	100.00	-	0.00
221 1983	0	0	0	6	386	0	0	0	1	0	0	99.96	100.00	99.74	98.47
222 2405	0	0	0	23	0	0	1	5	0	0	0	99.79	99.96	-	0.00
223 2062	63	3	0	6	408	11	0	0	1	0	0	99.96	100.00	86.44	98.55
228 1642	3	0	0	9	347	0	3	2	0	0	0	99.90	99.85	99.14	96.66
230 2194	0	0	0	10	1	0	0	0	0	0	0	100.00	100.00	100.00	9.09
231 1516	0	0	0	2	2	0	0	0	0	0	0	100.00	100.00	100.00	50.00
232 1726	0	0	2	4	0	0	3	0	0	0	0	100.00	99.71	-	0.00
233 2188	9	1	0	11	808	10	0	0	1	0	0	99.97	100.00	98.78	98.66
234 2699	0	0	0	0	3	0	0	0	0	0	0	100.00	100.00	100.00	100.00
Tot 98067	400	402	118	935	6632	387	140	142	79	5					

Total QRS: 107049   Gross detection ratios: 99.79   99.76   93.26   86.05
Total PVC: 7111   Average detection ratios: 99.79   99.77   88.46   54.03
alpha = 9.9995   Estimated detection ratio: 90.91

354

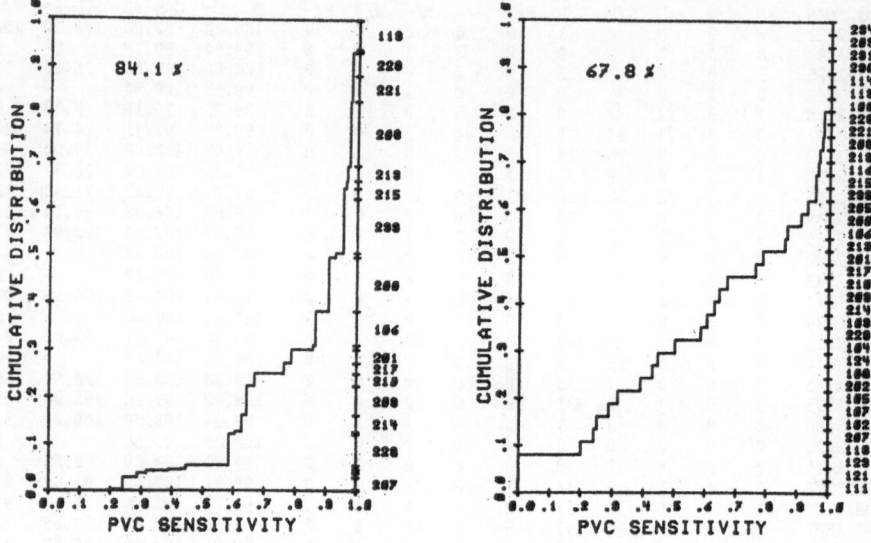

Fig.4: Records Weighted By
        PVC Count

Fig.5: Records Weighted Equally

tivity and is the expected value of PVC sensitivity for a single pa-

tient selected at random from a population comparable to the database.

Cox et al., (1981) have proposed a stochastic model for the PVC de-

tection process and have developed an alternative estimate of detector

performance by fitting the cumulative distribution with a degenerate

beta distribution of the form p^{α}. The "average detection probability"

then is given by $\overline{p} = \dfrac{\alpha}{1 + \alpha}$. While it appears that these measures

are not database independent, they may be useful is expressing algo-

rithm performance in a more robust manner. Table 4 includes calcu-

lations of the alpha parameter and the average detection probabilities

for ARISTOTLE.

DISCUSSION

Automated cardiac arrhythmia detectors are very complex systems
which are representative of a general trend toward stand-alone "intelligent" clinical instruments. Large amounts of physiologic
data are processed to provide the physician with highly "digested"
results. The task of evaluating such devices is enormous, very complex, and may be even more difficult and expensive than the initial
development of the instrument.

Annotated ECG databases are a critical ingredient of the evaluation
process, a fact recognized by many. The availability of universally
accepted databases will be of great benefit to both system developers
and potential users. The ability to make meaningful system comparisons
should enhance inter-institutional communication and should facilitate
progress in algorithm research.

The major limitation of annotated databases is their relatively
small size. It is not yet clear how many half hour ECG records are required to adequately represent the "universe". We have found that
48 records is a large enough set to make it difficult to "tune" an
algorithm successfully to the entire database, but it is a small enough
set that developers may be unreasonably swayed in their judgement by a
single record. The availability of the AHA database is a major addition
to our resources. Based on our experience, it would appear that the
MIT/BIH database is a bit more difficult than the AHA database for automated arrhythmia analyzers. The combination of the two databases provides developers and evaluators with a rather extensive and quite flexible resource. It is likely, however, that still more database development will be required to more adequately represent supraventricular arrhythmias and pacemaker rhythms.

Ideally, the evaluation of an algorithm should be done using a database different from that used during development. If the database were large enough, and a good enough sample of the "real world", this objection would be of less significance. The definition of "large enough" and "good enough" are at present elusive, however.

The correlation between laboratory evaluation using an annotated database and performance in the actual clinical setting remains to be established. Although database trials will be an important part of system evaluation, they are not in themselves a totally adequate measure of system performance. Evaluations using long term ECG data are of major importance. It appears, for example, that database records do not sufficiently represent the impact of noise and artifact on total system performance. While extensive laboratory testing of algorithms is a must, the success of a clinical instrument may depend equally upon such features as effective man-machine interfaces, and hardware and software robustness. Hence, careful multifacted clinical evaluations must supplement database trials.

REFERENCES

Cox, J.R., Hermes, R.E. and Ripley, K.L. 1981. Evaluation of performance. In "Ambulatory Electrocardiographic Recording". (Eds. N.K. Wenger, M.B. Mock and I. Ringqvist). (Yearbook Medical Publishers, Chicago). pp. 183-198.

Hermes, R. and Oliver, G. 1980. Use of the American Heart Association Database. In "Ambulatory Electrocardiographic Recording". (Eds. N.K.Wenger, M.B. Mock, and I. Ringqvist). (Yearbook Medical Publishers, Chicago). pp. 165-181.

Mark, R.G., Schluter, P.S., Moody, G.B. et al. 1982. An annotated ECG database for evaluating arrhythmia detectors. In "Frontiers of Engineering in Health Care - 1982". Proceedings of 4th Annual IEEE EMBS. pp. 205-210.

"MIT-BIH Arrhythmia Database: Tape Directory and Format Specifications". 1980. Biomedical Engineering Center for Clinical Instrumentation. Tech. Report No. 010. (MIT, Cambridge, Mass. 02139).

Moody, G.B. and Mark, R.G. 1982. Development and evaluation of a 2-lead ECG analysis program. Computers in Cardiology (in press).

Ripley, K. and Oliver, G.C. 1977. Development of an ECG database for arrhythmia detector evaluation. Computers in Cardiology. pp. 203-209.

Ripley, K.L., Geselowitz, D.B. and Oliver, G.C. 1978. The American Heart Association database: A progress report. Computers in Cardiology. pp. 47-54.

Schluter, P.S., Mark, R.G. and Moody, G.B. et al. 1980. Performance measures for arrhythmia detectors. Computers in Cardiology. pp. 267-270.

Schluter, P.S. 1981. "The Design and Evaluation of a Bedside Cardiac Arrhythmia Monitor". Ph.D. Thesis. Dept. of Electrical Engineering and Computer Science, (MIT, Cambridge, Mass. 02139).

CLINICAL EXPERIENCE WITH A SYSTEM BASED ON ANALYSIS
OF R-R INTERVAL PATTERNS

O. Pahlm

Department of Clinical Physiology
University Hospital, Lund, Sweden

ABSTRACT

Clinical experience with computer based analysis of long-term ECG recordings has been gained from about 6000 patients. The system is intended
for analysis of recordings from patients presenting with symptoms possibly
caused by cardiac arrhythmias. In such patients, elaborate analysis and
display of R-R interval patterns has been regarded as more important than
classification of QRS morphologies. With the aid of a comprehensive, yet
easily assimilated computer report of rhythm and efficient routines for retrieval and display of computer indicated episodes we have been able to limit the mean operator's time to about 10 minutes for a 24-hour recording.

INTRODUCTION

In the late 1970's we developed a system for rapid interactive analysis of long term ECG recordings (Pahlm et al., 1981). The system has also
been in use at the University Hospital, Linköping, Sweden, for about four
years. The two laboratories have gained clinical experience with the system
from the analysis of about 6000 recordings.

OUTLINE OF THE SYSTEM

Our concept of rapid and efficient analysis of long-term ECG recordings is based on four equally important features

1. Reliable QRS detection.
2. Graphic report of rhythm during recording, serving as a
   basis for computer-man interaction.
3. Rapid access of the original signal from the computer disk.
4. Convenient final report of relevant episodes found on the
   recording.

The QRS detector has been described elsewhere (Börjesson et al., 1982).
The computer report of a 24-hour recording covers two contiguous papers

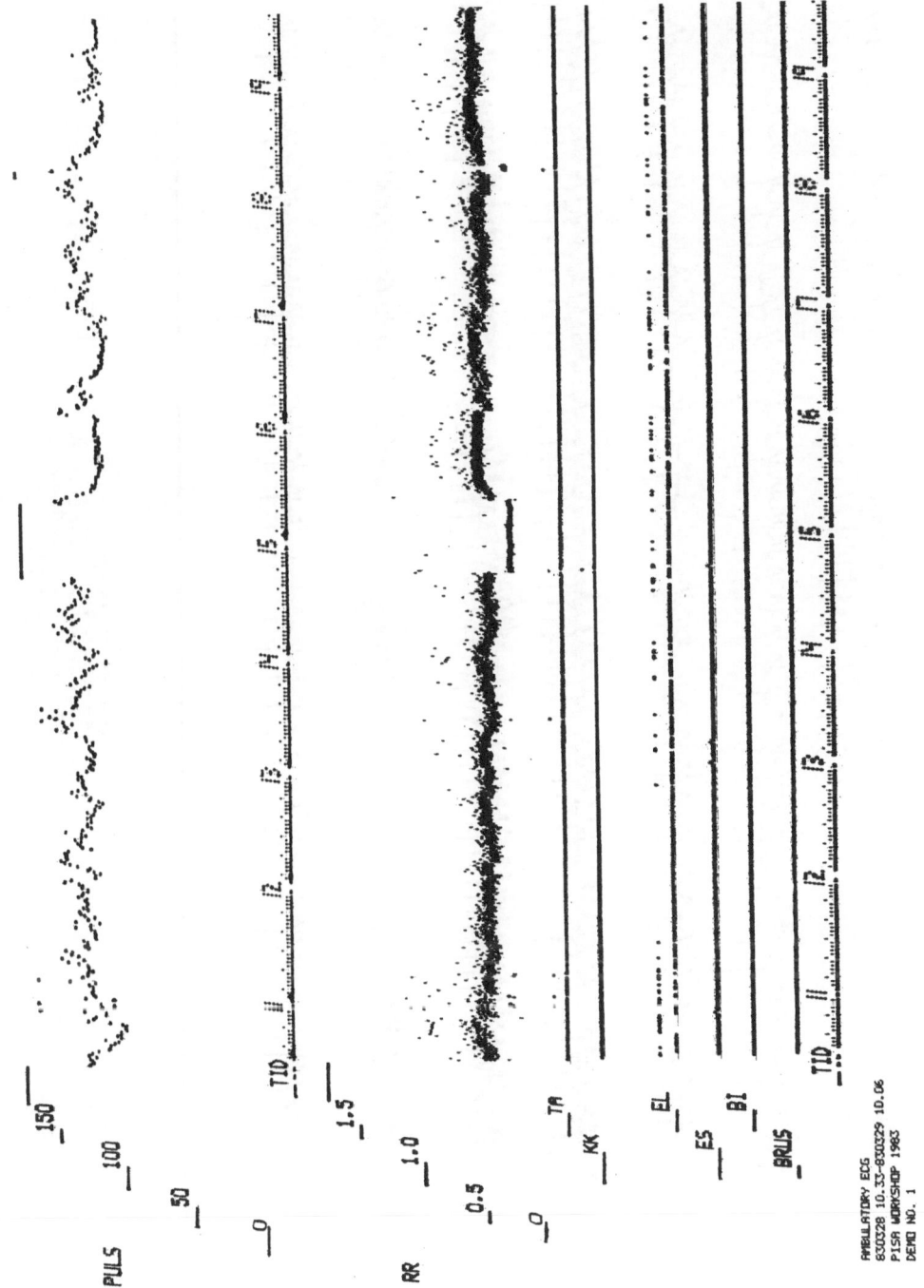

Figure 1. Part of computer report of 24-hour ECG recording. For details see text.

360

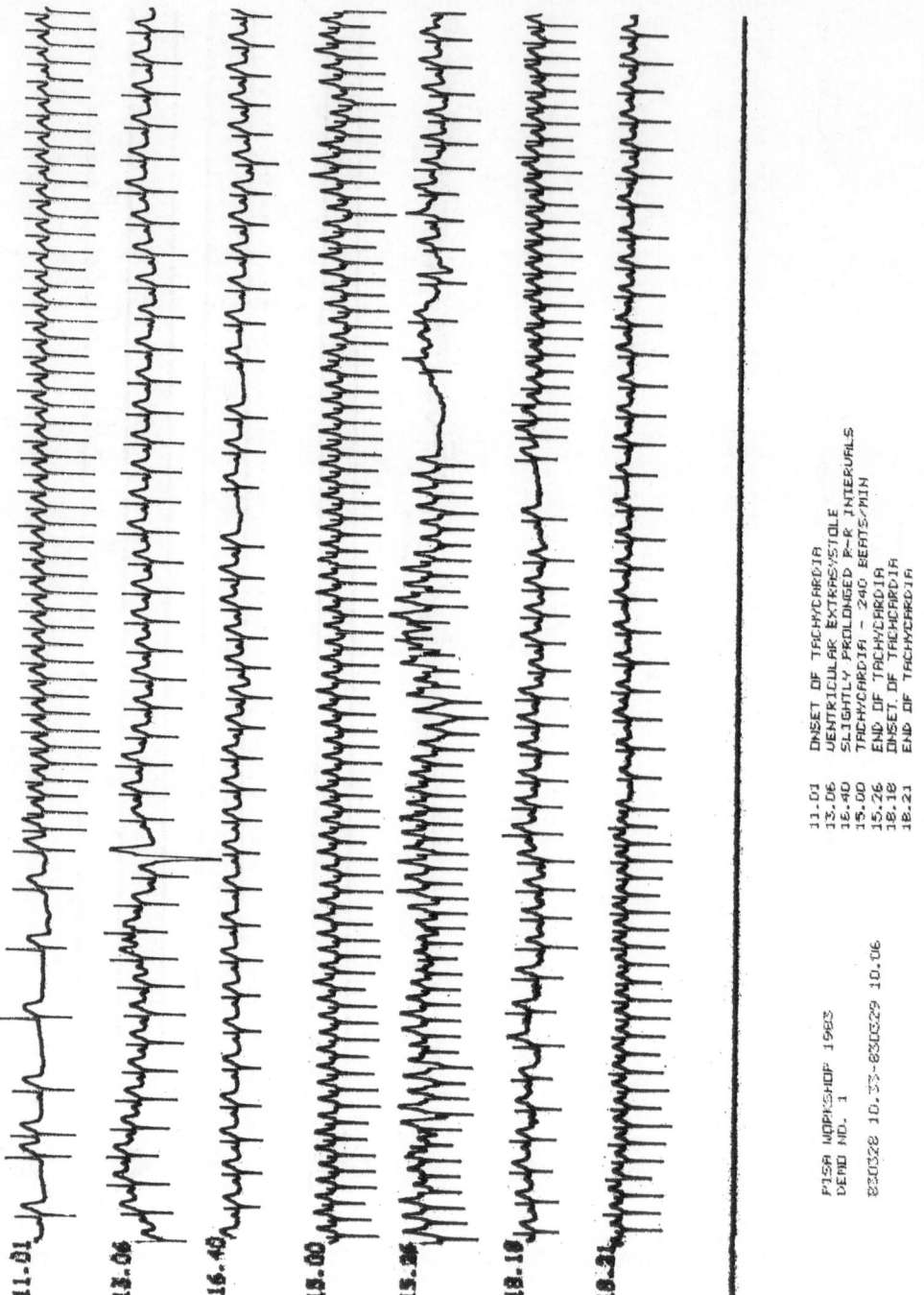

PISA WORKSHOP 1983
DEMO NO. 1
830328 10.33-830329 10.06

11.01   ONSET OF TACHYCARDIA
13.06   VENTRICULAR EXTRASYSTOLE
16.40   SLIGHTLY PROLONGED P-R INTERVALS
15.00   TACHYCARDIA - 240 BEATS/MIN
15.26   END OF TACHYCARDIA
18.18   ONSET OF TACHYCARDIA
18.21   END OF TACHYCARDIA

11.01
13.06
16.40
15.00
15.26
18.18
18.21

Figure 2. Lay-out of final report showing relevant episodes found during interactive analysis.

(size DINA4, 210x297 mm). Figure 1 shows an example of a computer report
taken from our clinical routine. The uppermost part of the report (marked
by "PULS") shows the heart rate versus time (range 0-175 beats/min). The
next part (marked by "RR") charts the distribution of R-R intervals; for
each minute, an array of dots shows the minimum, the 15th percentile, the
median, the 85th percentile and the maximum of the R-R interval distribution (range 0-1.75 sec.). The nature of the basic rhythm and changes in
rhythm are usually easily recognized from these plots.

The occurrence of typical sequences of R-R intervals is indicated by
dots adjacent to the lines denoted by TA (tachycardia), KK (couplets), EL
(prolonged R-R intervals), ES (extrasystoles) and BI (bigeminy). The occurrence of noise is indicated in the same way (BRUS). It is easily recognized
from figure 1 that the patient had a long episode of tachycardia starting
at about 14.50 (2.50 pm). The onset of the tachycardia is indicated on the
TA line; the stability of the R-R intervals is seen in the R-R interval
plot. The report also shows a few short episodes of tachycardia at other
instances, e.g. around 11 o'clock. The computer can find and display any
indicated event in a fraction of a second.

We usually attach print-outs of relevant ECG episodes to the final report. Figure 2 shows an example of a print-out from the patient discussed
above. Each page may contain up to eight 20-second ECG episodes. The page
is marked with the patient's number and name (though not in this example),
times for the beginning and the completion of recording and the time of day
when each episode occurred. Free text can be entered by the operator to describe the episodes.

DISCUSSION

The vast majority of 24-hour ECG recordings throughout the world are
probably still made on asymptomatic patients after myocardial infarction,
although there is no convincing evidence that treatment of asymptomatic
arrhythmias (such as frequent ventricular extrasystoles) will affect the
patient's prognosis.

There has been little interest in ambulatory monitoring of this group
of patients in Sweden. Emphasis has instead been on patients with symptoms
possibly caused by cardiac arrhythmias. Since such symptoms are invariably
accompanied by changes in the R-R interval pattern, we have in our system
emphasized reliable QRS detection and R-R interval analysis. The clinical

question at hand, the computer report and the patient's diary help the
operator to find the relevant information in the recording.

The detailed computer report, the efficient computer-man interaction
and the minimization of paper-handling have made our computer system an
effective tool in handling an increasing number of clinical long-term ECG
recordings. To date, about 6000 recordings have been analysed at the two
laboratories equipped with the system. The mean operator's time is only
about 10 minutes. Many recordings are handled in less than a minute, while
it may take up to 40 minutes for an occasional recording with poor technical quality and/or complicated arrhythmia.

REFERENCES

Börjesson, P.O., Pahlm, O., Sörnmo, L. and Nygårds, M.E. 1982. "Adaptive
    QRS detection based on maximum-a-posteriori estimation". IEEE Trans.
    Biomed. Eng., BME-29, pp. 341-351.
Pahlm, O., Jonson, B., Werner, O., Johansson, K. and Petersson, K. 1981.
    "Computer-aided visual analysis of long-term ECG recordings".
    Eur. Heart J. 2, pp. 487-498.

PILOT STUDY AND PRELIMINARY EXPERIENCES WITH A DATA BASE

FOR THE EVALUATION OF ALGORITHMS

FOR THE DETECTION OF ARRHYTHMIC AND ISCHEMIC EPISODES +

A. Taddei*, M. Varanini*, A. Macerata*, C. Marchesi* and C. Contini**,
A. Biagini*, M.G. Bongiorni*, M.G. Mazzei*, G.F. Mazzocca*, M. Baratto*

* Istituto di Fisiologia Clinica del CNR
** Istituto di Patologia Medica, Universita' degli Studi
via Savi, 8 - 56100 Pisa, Italia

ABSTRACT

The problem of the performance evaluation of algorithms for the analysis of the ECG signal is still unsolved in general terms; the most generally accepted solution to this problem is the comparison with an annotated ECG database. The preliminary experiences with a digital database for evaluating algorithms of analysis of arrhythmias and ST-T changes are described. At first the database has been applied for the QRS detector evaluation.

INTRODUCTION

The analysis of the long term ECG signal is generally performed by means of various systems with different degrees of automation; the automatic systems are more and more commonly used because the large amount of data makes a completely manual analysis difficult. Of course every technique of automatic analysis should be evaluated before its clinical application. However, there is a lack of information about the system performance and moreover the few available data are not useful for the comparison of different systems because there isn't a standard of evaluation. Thus the performance evaluation of the analysis algorithms is an unsolved problem. However, it is generally accepted that the best solution to this problem is the comparison with an annotated ECG database, representing the different clinical conditions. During the last years, many efforts have been performed to develop annotated ECG digital databases for the evaluation of arrhythmia detectors. The two well known databases are the AHA (Ripley, 1977; Hermes et al., 1981) and the MIT/BIH (Schluter et al., 1981). At our institute a database is under development for the evaluation of the algorithms for the analysis of the ambulatory ECG. This database includes the arrhythmic events as well as the ST-T

+ Partly supported by CNR Special Project on Biomedical and Clinical Engineering.

change episodes compatible with ischemia. Three hour ECG tracings are
selected out of 24 hour recordings from ambulatory patients and every QRS
complex is annotated in order to allow a beat by beat evaluation.

MATERIAL AND METHODS

The total amount of cases so far available are about 2000 patients
with arrhythmias and 200 patients with ST-T changes, which have been
monitored several times on about 1600 tapes. Twenty-four hour tapes have
been obtained by means of Avionics, Oxford Medilog 1 and Remco recording
units. From the tape set the most interesting cases are selected and a
three hour segment is individualized. Then the ECG signal of one lead is
sampled at the rate of 200 s.p.s. by means of a 12 bit A/D converter.
The digital data are input to a minicomputer (HP 1000F) and stored on a
magnetic tape. The 16 bit word is divided into two fields,respectively one
of 12 bits for storing the ECG sample code and the other of 4 bits
available for ECG event annotations (fig. 1).

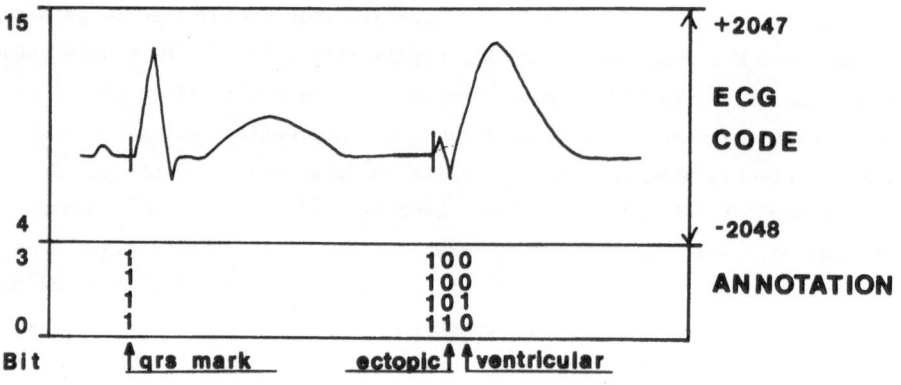

Fig.1   Codification of ECG samples and annotations.

ECG data are analyzed by a QRS detection program; every QRS complex is
identified and annotated with a code, which is stored in the database at
the QRS interval onset.   The ECG tracings of the database are hardcopied

by means of a graphic printer in a compact format, one page for two minutes, with the indication of the QRS complex onsets (fig. 2,4).

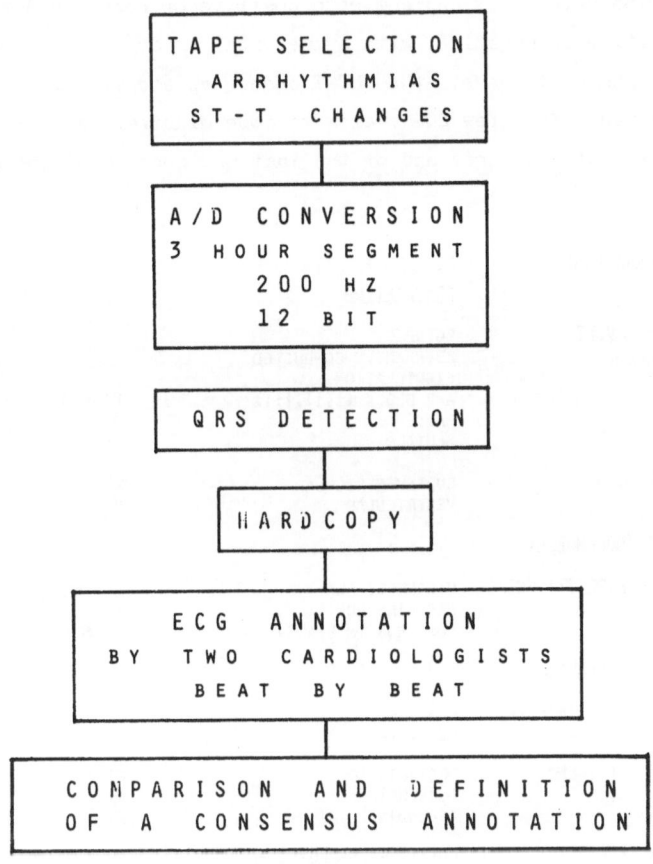

Fig.2 Database generation structure.

The ECG printout is submitted to two cardiologists of two different Institutes, that analyze independently beat by beat the same tracing in order to pick out the arrhythmic events and the ST-T change episodes.

A hierarchical classification scheme of the arrhythmias and of the ischemic changes has been proposed. According to this scheme the ECG events are divided in arrhythmic and ST-T changes. The arrhythmic beats are annotated by pointing out in a hierarchic order the type (ectopic, aberrantly conducted, fibrillation, etc...) (fig. 3), the origin of the excitation (supraventricular, ventricular), the morphology and the repetitiveness of the runs. The ST-T changes are annotated with the description of the morphology features of the ST-T interval. So the annotation indicates a ST segment with positive or negative deflection, a T wave, positive or negative, with symmetrical or asymmetrical morphology, or a two phase T wave; the ST-T change episodes, which have a time duration variable from few ECG cycles to some minutes, are identified by the annotation of the first and of the last QRS complex of the episode.

ARRHYTHMIAS

	DESCRIPTION	LABEL
1. EVENT	ECTOPIC	E
	ABERRANTLY CONDUCTED	C
	FIBRILLATION	F
	A-V BLOCK (I,II,III)	B1,2,3
	PAUSE	A
	FLUTTER	FL
2. SOURCE	SUPRAVENTRICULAR	S
	VENTRICULAR	V
3. MORPHOLOGY		1,2,...,15
4. REPETITIVENESS	N-COUPLET RUN	X + "N"
	N-GEMINY RUN	X - "N"
	LONG RUN (M BEATS)	X "M"

ST-T CHANGES

5. ST-T INTERVAL	POSITIVE	ST +
	NEGATIVE	ST -
6. ST TREND	RECTILINEAR	RT
	DESCENDING	DS
	ASCENDING	AS
7. T WAVE	POSITIVE SYMMETRICAL	PS
	ASYMMETRICAL	PA
	NEGATIVE SYMMETRICAL	NS
	ASYMMETRICAL	NA
	TWO PHASE	BF
8. MARKERS	ST-T CHANGE BEGINNING	IM
	END	FM

EXAMPLE: EV2 X-3
          ECTOPIC BEAT,VENTRICULAR,MORPH.2,TRIGEMINY
          ST+ PS IM
          BEGINNING OF ST-T ELEVATION EPISODE,T WAVE
          POSITIVE SYMMETRICAL.

Fig.3   Annotation scheme of the arrhythmias and ST-T changes.

The annotations are coded and stored in the database. The annotations of the two experts are compared and the differences are discussed in order to obtain a consensus annotation. The annotation codes of every beat are finally stored in the database and the editing of the incorrectly detected QRS complexes is carried out.

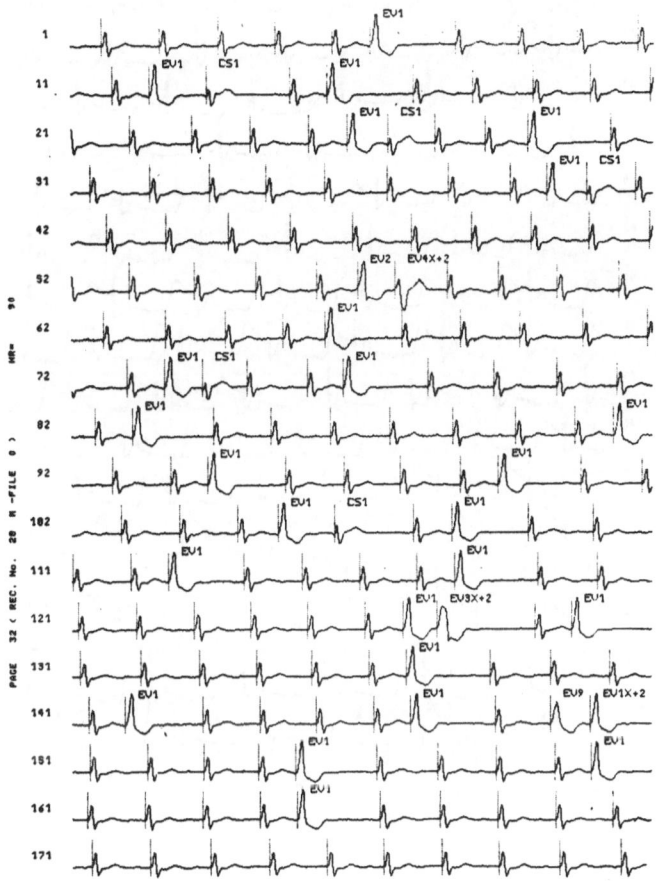

Fig.4   Hardcopy of two minute   ECG segment with ectopic beats and couplets.

Some examples of ECG tracings of the database are described in fig. 4,5,6.   Fig. 4 represents a two minute ECG segment of an arrhythmic tracing with ectopic beats (labelled EV1, EV2, etc...), aberrantly

368

conducted beats (CS1) and couplets (EV2–EV4 X+2,...).   Fig.   5
represents the onset of a ST segment elevation (ST+IM) and   fig.   6 a
complete one minute episode of T wave positive elevation.

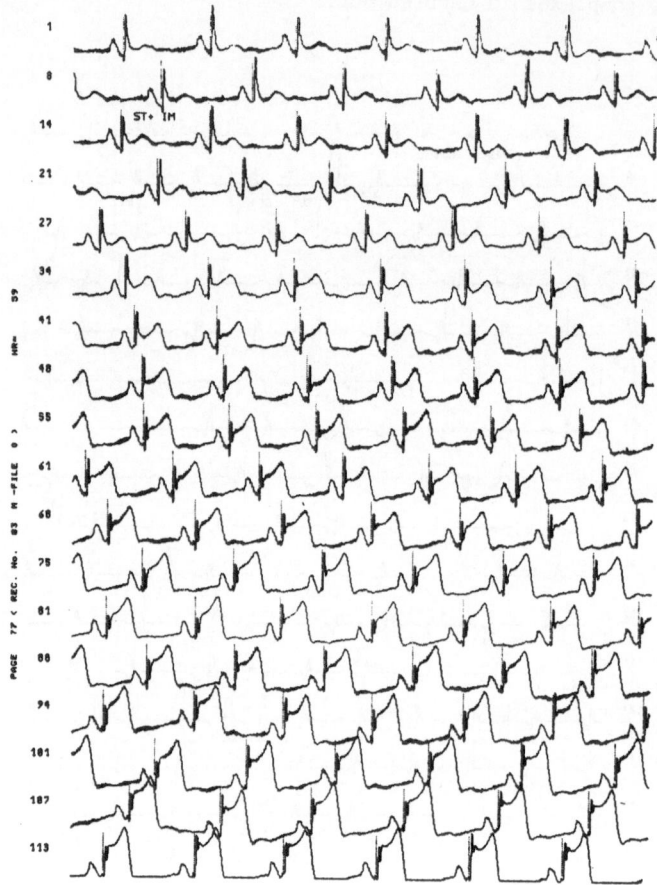

Fig.5   Onset of an episode of ST segment elevation.

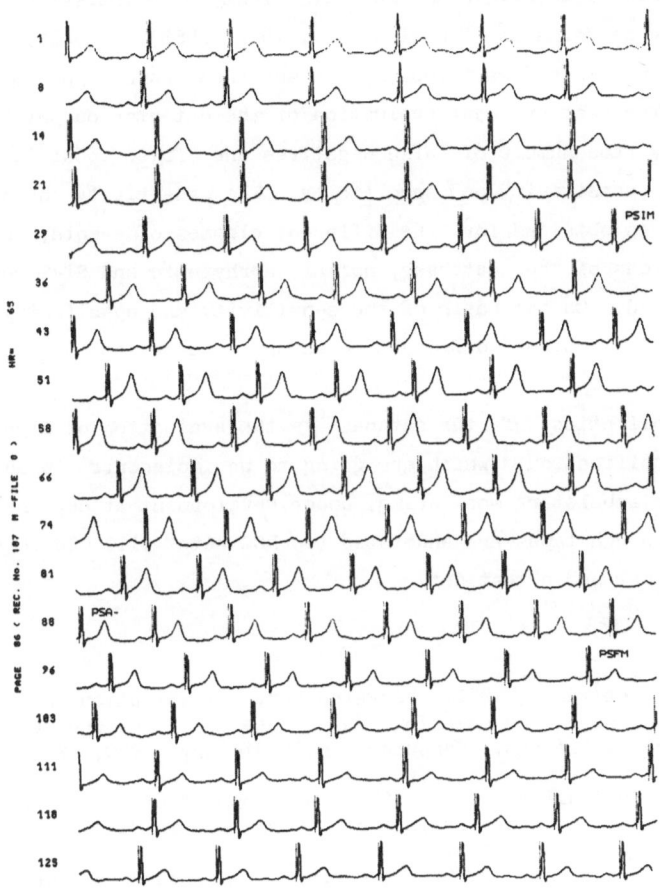

Fig.6   Episode of T wave amplitude variation.

APPLICATIONS

The ECG records, annotated and stored in the database, are available
for the beat by beat evaluation of the performance of the algorithms for
the analysis of arrhythmias and of the ST changes.   Moreover the ECG
database is useful in the clinical research for the determination of the
normal values of ECG parameters or for the standardization and improvement
of the classification criteria of the arrhythmias and of the ST-T changes.
Up to now 19 three hour cases have been selected and completely annotated:
a total of 240000 beats, 13000 arrhythmic and 17000 ST-T changes.   We

intend to extend the database to at least 50 cases.

The available data have been used at first in the evaluation of the QRS detector performance (Taddei et al., 1982; 1983). The QRS detector to be tested has been software implemented and has been applied to the ECG database. The beat by beat evaluation of the detector output has allowed to identify the number of false negatives and false positives and to derive the sensitivity and specificity. The sensitivity and specificity have been been obtained for the different classes of events, according to the annotations of the database; normal, arrhythmic and ST-T change beats are considered. On the basis of the sensitivity and specificity values it is possible to compare different detectors in order to individualize the best one.

The next application of the database is the evaluation of algorithms for the ECG classification, which are going to be implemented in an automatic analyzer for ambulatory monitoring, under development at our institute.

As soon as enough tapes are annotated two ECG sets will be defined: a development set and a test set.

REFERENCES

Hermes, R.E. et al. 1981. Development, distribution and use of the American Heart Association data base for ventricular arrhythmia detector evaluation. Computers in Cardiology 1980, 263-266. (IEEE Computer Society)

Ripley, K.L. and Oliver, G.C. 1977. Development of an ECG data base for arrhythmia detector evaluation. Computers in Cardiology, 203-209. (IEEE Computer Society).

Schluter, P. et al. 1981. Performance measures for arrhythmia detectors. Computers in Cardiology 1980, 267-270. (IEEE Computer Society).

Taddei, A. et al. 1982. Evaluation of QRS detectors based on sensitivity- specificity analysis. Proc. World congress on medical physics and biomedical engineering 1982, 18.22. (MPBE 1982 e.V., Hamburg).

Taddei, A. et al. 1983. Performance comparison of fast QRS detection algorithms. Proc. First Workshop on Ambulatory Monitoring (this volume). Pisa, April 11-12, 1983.

DISCUSSION

Chairman: B. McA Sayers

3.6 — Evaluation of ambulatory monitoring systems: experiences and perspectives.

BJERREGAARD: Could you tell me, Dr. Pahlm how long it takes to perform the analysis? You said a mean of 9 minutes I'm a little reluctant to accept such a small figure. We know for istance, that if you have a "difficult" tape it does require a large analysis.

PAHLM: I also showed there was a very wide distribution up to 25 minutes for 12 hour recordings. I suppose that the time could go up to 40 minutes for 24 hour recordings. We haven't evaluated that. So it's a very skewed distribution, with a very well defined maximum around a rather low figure, and a very long tail. With the computer processing and transfer time it takes about one hour and a half to perform all the procedure. We do a lot of the work at night, when the computer is idle. We have felt that the computer time is not the real critical thing, the critical thing is the human time, and that's where shortage is, at least for us.

ZYWIETZ: Particulalry for the morphology classification you, Dr. Marchesi, indicated, I feel that probably the computer should be used for analysis. It's very difficult, even if you have so many complexes as context, to see what the real differences are. So I propose, for a while to have a reproducibility study, and then you will see that, if you take a learning population of beats, and you calculate, something like the euclidian distances among the various feature you arc interested in it's much easier to detect in advance those deviating beats by the computer, and then to decide manually, because this is a very cumbersome work.

MARCHESI: In view of your experience, you have pointed out one of the major problems we have found out and one of the major causes of disagreement between doctors. We have actually considered of doing on automatic pre-classification. But we had decided to proceed manually in order to avoid possible bias.

If you leave free the doctor he can use his own attitude of recognizing only significant differences. When you use a numerical classification you can bias the doctor, convincing him that he has to account also for minor variations. We prefer to approach it in a practical way, leaving free the observer.

CHAPTER 4

FURTHER APPLICATIONS OF AMBULATORY MONITORING
AND TECHNOLOGICAL PERSPECTIVES

TOPIC: 4.1

Monitoring of non cardiovascular signals

AMBULATORY MONITORING OF NEUROPHYSIOLOGICAL SIGNALS, ART OR ARTEFACT.

Annalise Rosenfalck
Institute of Electronic Systems
Aalborg University Centre
Strandvejen 19
DK 9000 Aalborg, Denmark

INTRODUCTION

Long term monitoring of signals from muscle and brain play an increasing role in the prevention of occupational stress, for training of muscle control, in the prevention of sleep disorders and for the diagnosis and management of patients with seizures.

Recording of electromyogram (EMG) during static and dynamic activity is used for the analysis of work postures and movements that may be overstressing for the musculoskeletal system. Office and industry working processes require fast repeated movements which apparently stress the muscular system. The initial complaints of the workers are pain and muscle fatique, but these complaints often precede occupational musculotendon disorders.

Ambulatory monitoring of the electroencephalogram (EEG) is an important tool in the diagnosis of sleep disorders, in the evaluation of drugs in insomnia and for the diagnosis of patients with seizures.

The aim of this paper is to give inspiration for future collaboration. I have therefore only submitted a summary and a selective bibliography.

PROBLEMS

There are a number of problems which are common in long term recordings from muscle and brain.

1. Electrode problems

Ambulatory monitoring requires that the signals are recorded by surface electrodes. In long duration recordings over 6-10 hours the stability of condition and the placement of electrodes, changes in electrode impedance and lead displacement due to movement cause trouble when recording from muscles during work or from the scalp of a patient during seizures. There is an increasing need for small size preamplifiers with a single gain switch or active electrodes, in order to reduce artefacts.

2. Artefacts from neighbour tissue and environment

When recording with surface electrodes the distance between the electrodes and the generators (muscle or brain tissue) is large. The action potentials from the generators are volume conducted through the body which consists of tissue and solutes with highly different condution properties. The surface electrodes pick up the summated activity from all active generators within the body. Thus, even though the intention is to record from a single muscle the neighbouring muscles also contribute to the signal. Similarly when recording from the scalp the signal is often contaminated with signals from the heart, from muscles and from eye movements.

Signals from other body generators can in this connection be considered as artefacts.

Ambulatory monitoring is prefereably performed in the office, in industrial environment or in the patients home. Under these unrestrained conditions artefacts from ac-supply, sparks from high energy machines or pick-up from computers and from many other noise sources may cause severe artefacts in the recordings.

3. The need for quantitative methods and data reduction
EMG

In long term recordings of muscle activity there is a need for a quantitative analysis of the number of active motor units and their firing frequency. Neither of the following methods are really satisfactory although they are widely used and have been proven to be helpful. i) The calculation of the mean voltage is a relatively easy tool for the study of motor coordination in groups of muscle during voluntary movement. It allows the determination of the level of activity as a percentage of maximal activity, and to study work-rest cycles which are essential for the prevention of local fatigue and pain. ii) The center frequency of the spectrum of EMG has been shown to decrease with the development of muscle fatigue. However in occupational situations the force of contraction usually fluctuates over a wide range of contraction levels and findings are controversial. Recently the center frequency of the EMG has been found to depend also on the level of contraction; the temperature of the muscle and on the proportion of fast and slow muscle fibres in the individual muscles. iii) The Willison method (1964) which quantifies the pattern by counting the number of turns in 5 secs and by the mean voltage has proven to be an excellent method for the diagnosis of neuromuscolar disorders.

EEG

EEG is often monitored over 6-10 hours. The hard copy used for manual scoring is then 500-1000 m long. The manual scoring is thus time consuming but still more reliable than the scoring by automatic systems.

4. Cost of equipment

As mentioned previously artefacts from electrodes, leads, other organs and muscles and from the environment may contaminate the signals. Storing of the original signals on FM-tape-recorders and writing out as a hard copy with many channels is still necessary for control and verification of data analysis and data reduction. The cost of such equipment is high and new ideas are needed.

Signal analysis and data reduction can now be achieved by hardware devices combined with specially designed on-line computer systems. The power of microcomputer systems are just about sufficient for multichannel analysis. The development of hardware and software is often kept within research laboratories. There is a need for early exchange of ideas so that methods can be agreed and that programmes designed to be flexible so that they can be exchanged and used by several laboratories.

BIBLIOGRAPHY

The bibliography is selective but recent papers will through their own bibliographies lead the reader back to earlier work. The book: Recent advances in EEG and EMG data processing, 1981, Elsevier/North Holland Biomedical Press; the book: Motor unit types, recruitment and plasticity in health and disease, ed. J. E. Desmedt, 1981, Karger; Symposium 4 on muscle fatigue at Sixth International Congress of Electromyography, 1979, ed. A. Person; and the review: Kimmich, H. P. Modern patient care using biotelemetry. Its potential and technical relization at present and in the future. 1982. in Medical Progress through Technology 9, 85-93. contains much useful information not referred to below.

Andreassen, S. and Rosenfalck, A., 1981, Relationship of intracellular and extracellular action potentials of skeletal muscle fibers. CRC Critial Reviews in Bioengineering, 267-306.

Barlow, J.S. 1979. Computerized clinical electroencephalography in perspective. IEEE Trans. biomed. Engng. BME-26, 377-391.

Barlow, J.S. 1980. EEG transient detection by matched inverse digital filtering. Electroencephal. clin. neurophysiol. 48, 246-248.

Barlow, J.S., Creutzfeldt, O.D., Michael, D., Hauchin, J. and Epelbaum. 1981. Automatic adaptive segmentation of clinical EEG's. Electroench. clin. neurophysiol. 51, 512-525.

Bjelle, A., Hagberg, M. & Michaelsen, G. 1981. Occupational and individual factors in acute shoulder-neck disorders among industrial workers. Br. J. Indus. Med. 38, 356-363.

Björksten, M. & Jonsson, B. 1977. Endurance limit of force in longterm intermittent static contractions. Scand. J. Work Environ. & Health 3, 23-27.

Bourne, J.R., Jagannathan, V., Giese, B. and J.W. Ward. 1980. A software system for syntatic analysis of the EEG Computer Programs in Biomedicine. 11, 190-200.

Fuglsang-Frederiksen, A. 1981. Electrical activity and force during voluntary contraction of normal and diseased muscle. Acta neurol. scand. suppl. 83. 63, 60 p.

Gath, I. and Bar-On, E. 1980. Computerized method for scoring of polygraphic sleep recordings. Computer Programs in Biomedicine, 11, 217-223.

Gotman, J. 1982. Automatic recognition of epileptic seizures in the EEG. Electroenchephal. clin. neurophisiol. 54, 530-540.

Hagberg, M. 1981. Electromyographic signs of shoulder muscular fatigue in two elevated arm position. Am. J. Phys. Med. vol. 60, 3. 111-121.

380

Hagberg, M. & Jonsson, B. 1975. The amplitude distribution of
the myoelectric signal in an ergonomic study of the del-
toid muscle. Ergonomics vol. 18, 3. 311-319.
Hagberg, M. & Ericson, B-E. 1982. Myoelectric power spectrum
dependence on muscular contraction level of elbow flexors.
Eur. J. Appl. Physiol. 48, 147-156.
Herberts, P., Kadefors, R. & Broman, H. 1980. Arm positioning
in manual task. An electromyographic study of localized
muscle fatigue. Ergonomics vol. 23, 7. 655-665.
Isaksson, A., Wennberg, A. and Zetterberg, L.H. 1981. Compu-
ter analysis of EEG signals with parametric models. Proc.
IEEE. 69. 451-461.
Jonsson, B. 1978. Quantitative electromyographic evaluation
of muscular load during work. Scand. J. Rehab. Med.
Suppl. 6. 69-74.
Kadefors, R. 1978. Application of EMG in ergonomics. New
Vistas. Scand. J. Rehab. Med. 10. 127-133.
Komi, P.V. & Tesch, P. 1979. EMG frequency spectrum, muscle
structure and fatigue during dynamic contractions in man.
Eur. J. Appl. Physiol. 42. 41-50.
Lindström, L. Magnusson, R. & Petersén, I. 1970. Muscular
fatigue and action potential conduction velocity changes
studied with frequency analysis of EMG-signals. Electro-
myographics vol. 10, 4. 341-353.
Lindström, L., Magnusson, R. & Petersén, I. 1974. Muscle load
influence on myoelectric signal characteristics. Scand.
J. Rehab. Med. suppl. 3. 127-148.
Luopajärva, T., Kuorinka, I., Virolainen, M. & Holmberg, M.
1979. Prevalence of tenosynovitis and other injuries of
the upper extremities in repetitive work. Scand. J. Work
Environ. & Health suppl. 5, 3. 48-55.
Møller, E. 1981. The myogenic factor in headache and facial
pain. In Oral-facial and motor functions. (eds.) Kamura,
Y. and Dubner, R. Quintessence Publishing Co., 225-239.
Petrofsky, J.S. 1979. Frequency and amplitude analysis of the
EMG during exercise on the bicycle ergometer. Eur. J.
Appl. Physiol. 41, 1-15.
Petrofsky, J.S. & Lind, A.R. 1980. Frequency analysis of the
surface electromyogram during sustained isometric con-
tractions. Eur. J. Appl. Physiol. 43. 173-182.
Petrofsky, J.S. & Lind, A.R. 1980. The influence of tempera-
ture on the amplitude and frequency components of the
EMG during brief and sustained isometric contractions.
Eur. J. Appl. Physiol. 44. 189-200.
Principe, J.C. and Smith, J.R. 1982. Microcomputer based system for the detection and quantification of petit mal
epilepsy. Comp. Biol. Med. 12, 87-95.
Rosenfalck, P. 1968. Intra and extracellular potential fields
of active nerve and muscle fibres. Acta Physiol Scand.
(suppl. 321) 168 p.
Sterman, M.B. and Kovalensky, R.A. 1983. Baseline studies and
anticonvulsant drug effects on the sleep EEG power spectral response. Electroench. clin. neurophysiol. 55,
212-222.

Stulen, F.B. and De Luca, C.J. 1982. Muscle fatigue monitor:
A noninvasive device for observing localized muscle
fatigue. IEEE transactions of Biomed. Engen. BME-29,
No 12, 760-768.

Wickström, G. Hänninen, K. Lehtinen, M. & Riihimäki, H. 1978.
Previous back syndromes and present back symptomes in
concrete reinforcement workers. Scand. J. Work. Environ.
& Health. Suppl. 1, 4. 20-28.

Willison, R.G. 1964. Analysis of electrical activity in healthy and distrophic muscles in man. Journal of Neurology,
Neurosurgery and Psychiatry, 27, 386-394.

Whisler, J.W., ReMine, W.J., Leppik, I.E., McLain, L.W. Jr.
and R.J. Gumnit, 1982. Machine detection of spike-wave
activity in the EEG and its accuracy compared with visual
interpretation. Electroencephal. clin. neurophysiol. 54,
541-551.

Que, D., Fitch, D. and R.G. Willison. 1980. High speed automated analysis of EEG-spike and wave activity using an analogue detection and microcomputer plotting systems. Electroencephal. clin. neurophysiol. 49, 187-189.

Örtengren, R., Andersson, G., Bromann, H., Magnusson, R. and
Petersén, I. 1975. Vocational electromyography: Studies
of localized muscle fatigue at the assembly line. Ergonomics vol. 18, 2, 157-174.

LONG TERM RESPIRATION MONITORING AND
ITS RELEVANCE TO CARDIOVASCULAR MONITORING

F.D. Stott
Watford Road, Harrow, Middlesex, UK.

ABSTRACT

The principles, advantages, and other problems of the most frequently used systems of long-term non invasive respiratory monitoring are described and discussed, together with a summary of the method of calibrating such systems. The main relevance to study of a cardiovascular system is seen as the possible use of respiratory monitoring as a measure of physical work during a subject's normal daily activities, with application in the study of blood pressure variability and Ischaemic Heart Disease.

Long term non-invasive monitoring of respiration (i.e. without direct connection to the airway) has been possible by several different methods for many years now, but has found relatively little application because the volumetric accuracy has been poor, so that little more than respiratory rate has been obtainable from the recordings. One method that has been extensively used in electrical impedance pneumography, which depends on measuring the change in trans-thoracic impedance with inflation and deflation of lungs. Changes in tidal volume are reproduced with fair accuracy, but the calibration factor tends to be unstable, changing with posture, and even in constant posture changing with time, so that frequent recalibration is necessary.

All other methods attempt to determine the change in trunk volume with respiration, by measuring some geometrical factor which changes with trunk volume in a more or less predictable manner. Strain gauges, usually of the mercury-in-rubber type, have been used widely; these measure the circumference of the trunk at two (or occasionally more) sections. More recently, a magneto-metric method has been introduced; in this system, magnets are attached to the subject's back, and flux sensors to the front of the chest and abdomen. The parameter measured in this case is the A-P axis length.

The most recent technique introduced is the inductance plethysmograph which uses as transducers two elasticised bands which incorporate a strand of flexible wire. Each band thus forms a single-turn coil, which forms the inductance in the resonant circuit of an oscillator. Change of inductance is directly proportional to the area enclosed by the coil, so that the change of iscillator frequency directly reflects the change of cross-sectional area of the trunk. This parameter is more directly related to volume change than is circumference or A-P axis length.

These last three systems, unlike the impedance pneumograph, record abdominal and thoracic components separately, and are therefore able to distinguish between central and obstructive apnoea; in central apnoea signals from both thoracic and abdominal transducers are zero, while in obstructive apnoea, signals are still present on both channels, but in antiphase, so that they give a zero sum.

This is in some cases a great advantage but carries with it a compensatory disadvantage; volumetric calibration of these systems with two degrees of freedom is a more complex procedure than the calibration of systems with a single degree of freedom only. Two calibration factors have to be determined one for each transducer.

If the trunk is seen in terms of a model consisting of two cylinders, the thoracic cylinder of length L_T and the abdominal cylinder of length L_A, then $\delta V = L_T \, \delta A_T + L_A \, \delta A_A$ ....(1) where δA_T, δA_A are the changes of area of X-section with respiration of the thoracic and abdominal cylinders respectively.

The inductance plethysmograph measures δA_T and δA_A directly, so for this system we can rewrite (1) in the form

$$V = K_T \, U_T + K_a \, U_a \quad ....(2)$$

where V is the respired volume, U_T and U_a are the output voltage signals from the transducers, and K_T, K_a are constants having the dimensions of litres/volt. Practical methods of determining these constants are fully described by Watson (1981): he concludes that the inductance plethysmograph is nearly always within $\pm10\%$ of spirometry, even when the subjects posture changes.

The immediate relevance of this type of respiratory monitoring to circulatory studies lies in its use as a measure of physical work load.

It has been shown (Ford & Hellerstein 1959) that minute volume is a good measure of physical work, especially if the correct calibration factor for each individual case be determined by standard exercise tests. Direct measurement of O_2 uptake or CO_2 output would be a better measure than minute volume, but it is not at present possible by any method that is acceptable for long-term use on ambulatory subjects.

Fig. 1 shows simultaneous records by spirometry and inductance plethysmography on a subject exercising on a treadmill or three different work levels, and demonstrates that the Inductance plethysmograph can be used under such conditions with an acceptable level of movement artifact, as is demonstrated by the breath-hold periods, during which the subject continued walking or running while holding his breath.

384

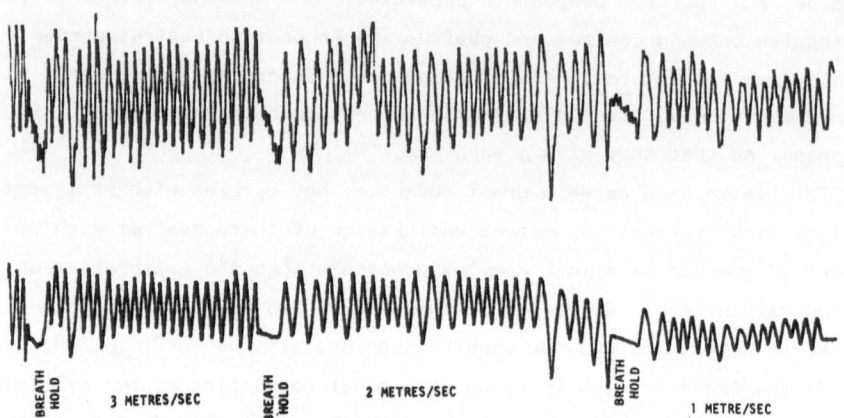

Fig 1   Simultaneous Spirometer (lower trace) and inductance
plethysmograph (upper trace) recordings during treadmill exercise.

If we can quantify physical work during a subjects normal activities,
this will remove one of the factors which affect blood pressure and heart
rate from the statistical analysis of blood pressure variability, and enable us instead to quantify the relationship and compare the results with
tests in the exercise laboratory.

This applies not only to studies of blood pressure variability but
also to studies of ischaemic heart disease. The work load required to
induce anginal pain and ST segment changes can be quantified directly in
the exercise laboratory, but the conditions are artificial, and not necessarily typical of the subjects normal activities. It would add valuable
extra information for the diagnosis and control of therapy of I.H.D. if we
were able to have available quantitative information on the physical effort
involved in the normal daily activities, at the same time as recording the
EKG for analysis of ST segment changes.

Another application of respiratory monitoring in cardiovascular research is to be found in the study of nocturnal fluctuations of heart rate
and blood pressure which are related to abnormalities of respiratory patterns during sleep. Fig. 2 shows a good example of this type of interaction
between the cardiovascular and respiratory system; the changes in blood
pressure and heart rate during episodes of periodic respiration are large;
much larger than the interaction between the two systems normally found
during the daytime recordings.

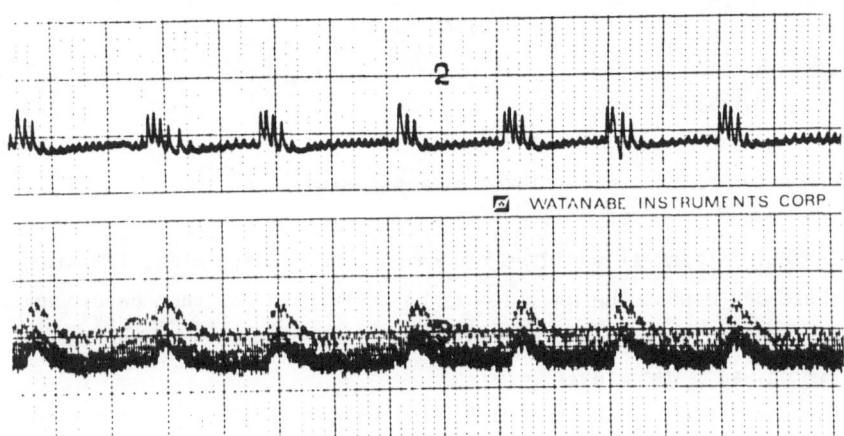

Fig. 2   Blood Pressure variation (lower trace) related to
nocturnal periodic respiration (upper trace)

Long-term ambulatory recording of respiration has been used very
little to date, in part because the systems available to do it have been
inadequate, both in respect of the transducers and the recording system.

The inductance plethysmograph is a great improvement on previously
available systems, especially in respect of calibration stability. The
carrier-type recording methods available on the ambulatory tape data recorders have not, to date, been fully adequate for respiratory recording,
which demands an exceptionally large dynamic range without loss of
linearity.

A digital recording system compatible with the inductance plethysmograph and the Oxford Medical Systems Mediolog 4-24 is now available which
overcomes this last problem, so that the way is now open for us to carry
out combined cardiovascular and respiratory studies on ambulatory subjects.

REFERENCES

Ford, A.B. and Hellerstein, H.K. 1959. J. Appl. Physiol., 14, 891
Watson, H. et al. 1981. ISAM - GENT - 1981. Proceedings of 4th
    International Symposium on Ambulatory Monitoring. Academic Press
    (London) Ltd. pp. 269-284.

DISCUSSION

Chairman: H.Wolff

4.1 - Monitoring of non cardiovascular signals.

VAN BEMMEL: I think it would be too narrow, Dr. Rosenfalck, if this group on ambulatory monitoring should only be restricted to the cardiovascular system. We could learn quite a lot of the experiences in other areas of monitoring, as I was myself.

For instance when I look at those pictures on the influence of the control mechanism on heart rate variability. I'm thinking at the same time of monitoring an infant during birth, pre-natal monitoring, and seeing exactly the same phenomena. When I'm looking at monitoring of patients carryng a tape-recorder, for instance, to be later on evaluated by a computer, I compare that with monitoring a patient during cardiac surgery, with Electroencephalogram, as Dr. Rosenfalck told us. And I think that from all these areas we can learn a lot. The experience is here, all in Europe, let's be happy. So I'd like to stimulate that all the experiences that are present in the institutes like the one in Copenhagen and others, is brought forward into this concerted action, or at least in this discussion. I have a short question for Dr. Rosenfalck: I know how many efforts she has put, herself, in to the analysis of EMG and EEG in the past twenty years or so: don't you feel a little bit sorry when you look at those "chewing" signals, as I call them, and you just look at the envelope of those signals, instead of looking to the frequency contents. Don't you lose too much of the information content in those signals?

ROSENFALCK: No. I don't think so, because most of the work on the frequency analysis is quite controversial right now. I've been through most of the literature recently, and it shows there is another method of analysing muscle signals during fatique, because frequency analysis depends on the level of muscle contraction. It has been shown you can not use that method below 20% of muscle contraction and what I really think is important is the pattern at rest and at various work conditions. The other thing on which the frequency-analysis depends heavily is on the temperature of the muscle. After these findings I would be afraid to put too much emphasis on the analysis of the frequency.

SAYERS: I too would like to support what Van Bemmel has just been saying.

I think there are important applications for monitoring other than cardiovascular variables, but not necessarily in isolation. There is some suggestions, for example the problem that I, not you, suffer from, as I get older and I can't hear so well, is in some sense linked to something cardiovascular. It's something we know nothing about. The second is that I'm quite sure that part of the quality of life is linked to one's capability of bringing sufficient neurological reaction, neurological tone to the normal every-day existence, that you can cope effectively as a human, and not just as a responding machine. This study could be done by evaluating the general effect of the environment on the individual and his quality of life. The only way you can do that is by monitoring accurately an adequate number of people under an adequate range of circumstances. This is not a trivial operation, it's not the sort of thing that you finish in a 3 year study, but really is something that should be put in hand for the next generation and, for the period after the year 2000, which as has hopefully been said is the year after which health for all is to be obtained. It isn't of course, and I think that will be the starting point of a more serious operation. May I make one other point: I understand, that 30% of the rural population suffer from balance disorders, vestibular disorders. If this is true, then we need to know something about the way it develops. I was refering to rural populations in England and Wales, where the studies have been done. If that is a true figure, then it is something serious that everyone has to be concerned with, in one way or another. We must find out some more about the way that sort of disability develops.

SANDOE: We would all be very glad if we could really monitor those triggering factors and the response and my question now is: can we monitor all those signals. Now we are working out of the free environment, but can we, in the free environment within 10 years, expect that we can monitor muscle potentials, EEG, and so on? You're touched upon the problem about the new work in the microvolt area, and we are now in the millivolt area. How is the future in that?

ROSENFALCK: I think the future is not too bad, because actually what we need is some kind of active electrodes for getting the signals up to the level where you are and where we can really get them away from the body without electrode movements, without electrodes artifacts. Most of those who make transducers do not consider electrodes as transducers. And I think it's very important that someone starts to say that the most important transducers actually are the electrodes, because they actually monitor something which is far away from the generator. If you think about the distance between a muscle fibre and a surface electrode, you are in a circumstance like you want to monitor the electrical activity here, with an electrode standing on the ninth floor. And with all the noise in between.

WOLFF: Doctors are only interested in symptoms and not in causes, and the fact that they want to measure only signals on the body, which are, is a sense, all symptoms, means that they lose one half of the equation, and this is the half of the equation I was trying to get them to take notice of. If you want to find out what makes people have this disease or be unstable on their legs, you have to look at what is their input, and not at what is their output, and people don't seem to think in those terms.

WALSH: I'd just like to point out to Dr. Rosenfalck that the problem of the active electrode at the site of measurement has been already thought of by others and in some ways tackled succesfully. There's one firm at least I know of in Cleveland, that makes a very successful EEG electrode, active at the skin, and there is also a body surface potential mapping group in Cleveland, another at Duke and one here in Italy which have all used active electrodes at the site of measurement. So this is not an unexplored area.

BALASUBRAMANIAN: I find it very fascinating that this method can be used to find the difference in response between the ST segment and the heart rate in the laboratory, which is controlled, to the peripherial environment. This leads us to the question Mr. Wolff put in: Under the monitoring environment how are you going to find out what are the differences between the ambulatory response outside the laboratory and within the laboratory.

STOTT: I think this is very relevant to what I was just saying just now, and I think it may seem to some of the pure scientists among us, that it's really unecessary that if you calibrate it in the laboratory, his responce to exercise test running for a bus should be exactly the same as his response to exercise tests running on a treadmill. But everybody in real life knows it doesn't work that way. Life isn't that simple.

BALASUBRAMANIAN: It doesn't work that way at all. Really, what we have found is that the heart-rate response in the environment outside, for the same amount of ST depression, is much less than in the laboratory. Something else which is acting outside the laboratory we are unable to quantitate. We don't know, whether it is food intake or peripheral temperature or whichever is happening. We need to monitor the environment outside.

STOTT: I think if at least we can get the respiration so we know how much he is doing in his every day activities, it would be a tremendous help. It would, at least, be a first stage on the journey. I'm quite sure it isn't the last stage. There are many other things we can monitor. The methods at our disposal are increasing all the time, but certainly I think now that respiratory monitoring has progressed from being more of a laboratory curiosity into being something that we can do on an ambulatory basis as a regular routine.

TOPIC: 4.2

Emerging technologies

THE POTENTIAL OF VLSI IN
AMBULATORY MONITORING

W. Sansen

Katholieke Universiteit Leuven, Elektrotechniek
94 K. Mercierlaan, B-3030 Leuven-Heverlee, Belgium

ABSTRACT

Several examples are given of integrated circuits which have been tailored to specific medical applications. They are a bone stimulator-telemetry system, a pressure telemetry system and a glucose monitoring telemetry chip . They all lack standardization whence they are not suited for mass production with (V) LSI techniques. The concept of the Internal Human Conditioning System is put forward as a possible solution to this problem. The IHCS can take up most existing medico-electronic functions. Still as standard chip it has to be tailored to each application by programming techniques. Some difficulties to realize the IHCS-chip are discussed.

INTRODUCTION

The advent of Very-Large-Scale-Integration (VLSI) will allow to integrate even more electronic functions on one chip than present day microprocessors. Such chips contain gate numbers in exces of 50.000 and require long development times. In order to be cheap they have to be mass-produced and find large markets.

In medicine however not many large markets can be found. Most medical devices are tailored either towards the patient or towards the medical doctor. Priority is given to the quality of the treatment above the potential reduction in cost due to the standardization of the device used. As a result it is not clear how VLSI, which essentially counts on massive use, could affect the discipline of custom medication.

In this text three examples are given, where integration of electronic functions has lead to custom made devices for medical diagnosis and therapy. These examples all carry out functions of ambulatory monitoring. They fully exploit the capability of integration to miniaturize the device such that it is easily implantable. However they are tailored (customized) to specific applications. As a result they provide only costly solutions to the problem. Also any change in specification would necessitate the development of another chip which even enhances the cost.

An alternative solution would consist of the development of one single chip which can be programmed to the needs of the doctor and of the patient as well. It would be the same chip for most applications and could be mass produced at a low cost. It would be programmed to fulfill the ever changing needs of users keeping touch of evolution in medical treatment.

Obviously such a standardized medical chip would have to be able to carry all basic function in medical treatment : ie measurement and stimulation.

In this text a general purpose medical chip is conceived which is called the Internal Human Conditioning System [1]. It is shown that most medical functions of measurement and stimulation can be carried with this chip. Also it is shown how programming the chip after fabrication allows to tailor its use to each kind of application as e.g. to ambulatory monitoring.

The IHCS chip has a complex structure and therefore necessitates VLSI techniques. Some of the difficulties will be described which have to be solved before this VLSI chip can be realized. Partial integration however is already been demonstrated. Full integration may lead to a revolution in medical practice.

Before the IHCS system is described, three LSI chips for ambulatory monitoring application are quoted. They are the bone stimulator telemetry system, the bladder pressure telemetry system and the glucose telemetry system .

BONE STIMULATOR TELEMETRY

For enhanced bone healing, small currents can be applied of 20...50 μA to the fracture site [2]. The healing proces can be shortened to three to five weeks. The healing proces however is largely unknown. Therefore a monitoring system has been added to the current stimulator and integrated on one chip for miniaturization.

The block diagram of the system is shown in figure 1 and the chip realization in figure 2. The stimulation current can be set by external resistances. The biopotentials are measured around the fracture site, multiplexed and transmitted to an external receiver where they are stored for subsequent analysis by computer.

PRESSURE TELEMETRY SYSTEM

For patients with incontinence a pressure pill has been developed to monitor pressure in the bladder. Its block diagram is shown in figure 3 [3]. The pressure is measured with a commercial pressure bridge. Its

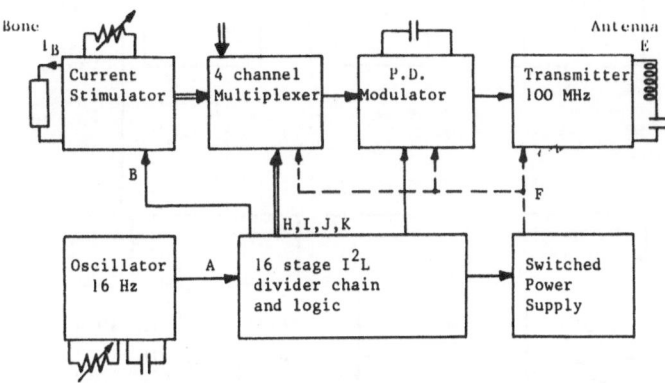

Fig.1 : Block diagram of Bone stimulator-telemetry system.

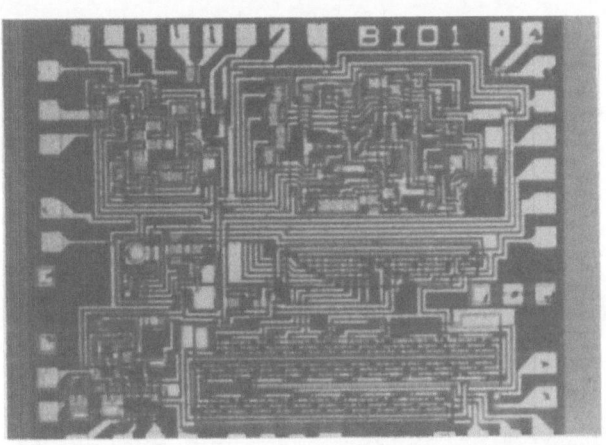

Fig.2 : Microphotograph of Bone stimulator chip

output signal is amplified and modulated on a carrier for wireless transmission to an external receiver-recorder. The chip which contains most
functions is shown in figure 4. The total size of the pill is about 24 x
3.5 mm. Again a custom chip had to be developed for this application.

394

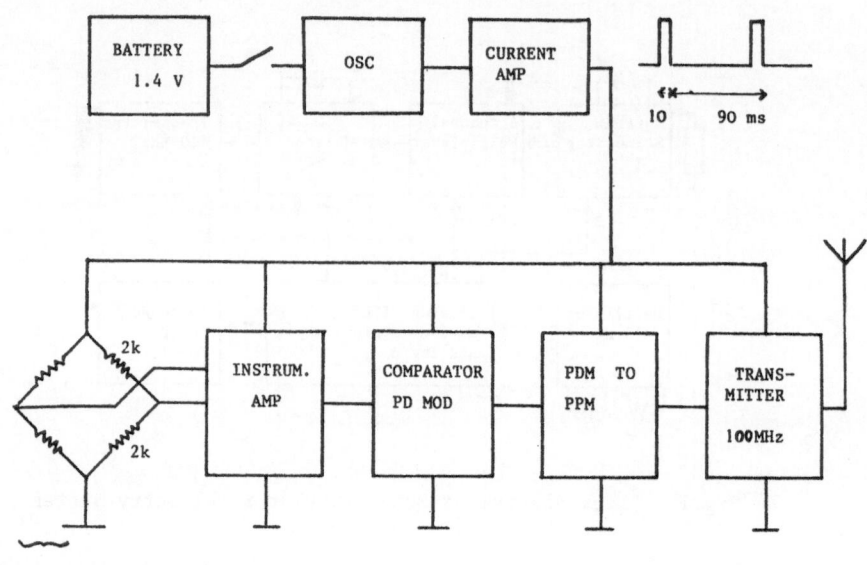

P Transducer

Fig.3 : Block diagram of pressure telemetry system.

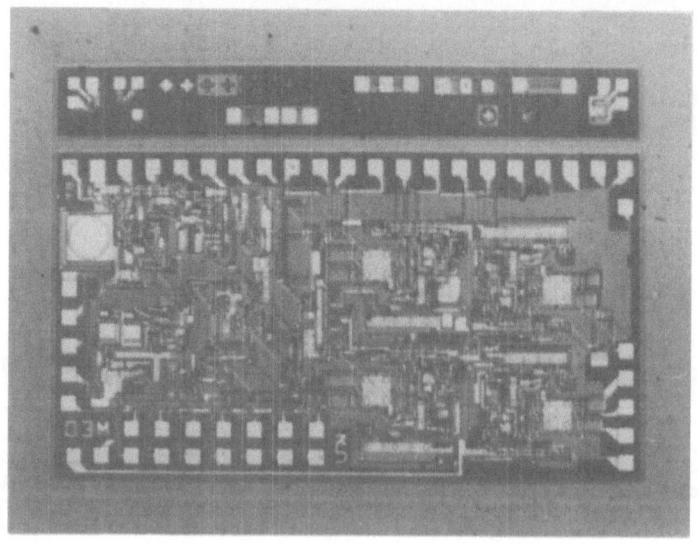

Fig.4 : Microphotograph of pressure measurement chip.

GLUCOSE TELEMETRY SYSTEM

For diabetics a glucose monitoring system has been developed in order to continuously monitor glucose concentration during several weeks [4]. It consists of a glucose sensor in addition to a telemetry system to carry out the measurement and to record the data. The block diagram is shown in figure 6. Both energy and drive voltage are radiated through the skin. The measured sensor current is sent back through the same channel. The chip which carries out all functions in the implant, is shown in figure 6. It is actually a bidirectional single-channel sensor monitoring chip which can be applied as well to other sensor applications.

The monitoring of more sensors however necessitates more complex acquisition circuitry. This is possible with the IHCS system depicted in figure 7 [1].

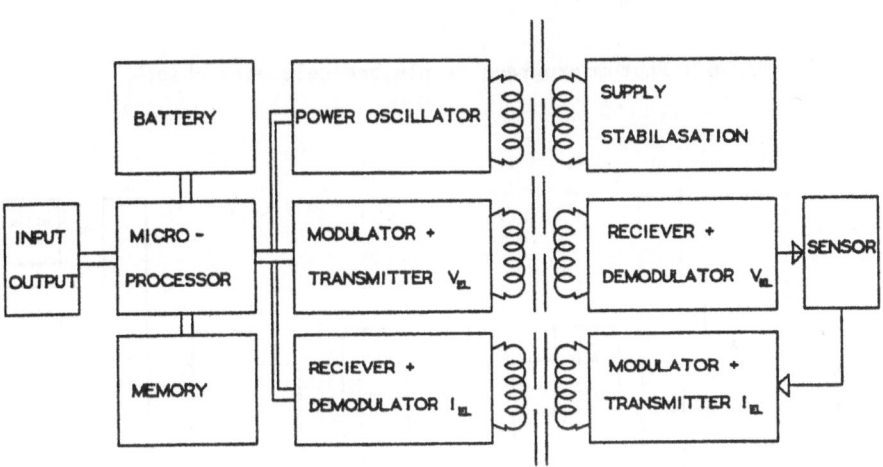

Fig.5 : Block diagram of glucose telemetry system.

IHCS SYSTEM

The IHCS system is a complete system (see fig.7) in the sense that it is able to carry out all necessary measurements and stimulations within the human body. It consists of a data acquisition part, a central processor and a general purpose stimulator. Also a telemetry telecommunication link is included.

In the data acquisition part, the signals from a number of sensors are amplified, filtered and multiplexed before A/D conversion. The sti-

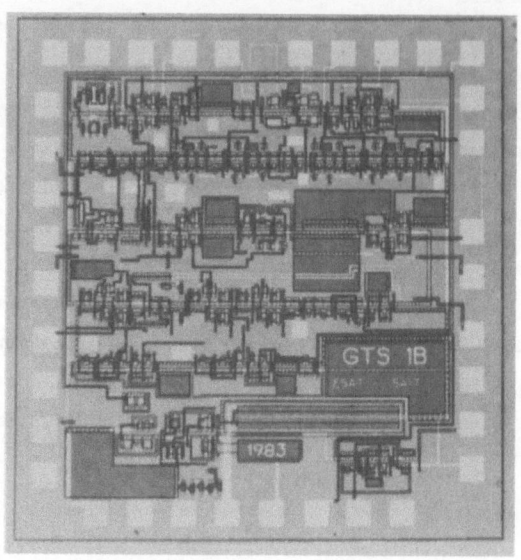

Fig.6 : Photomicrograph of glucose telemetry chip.

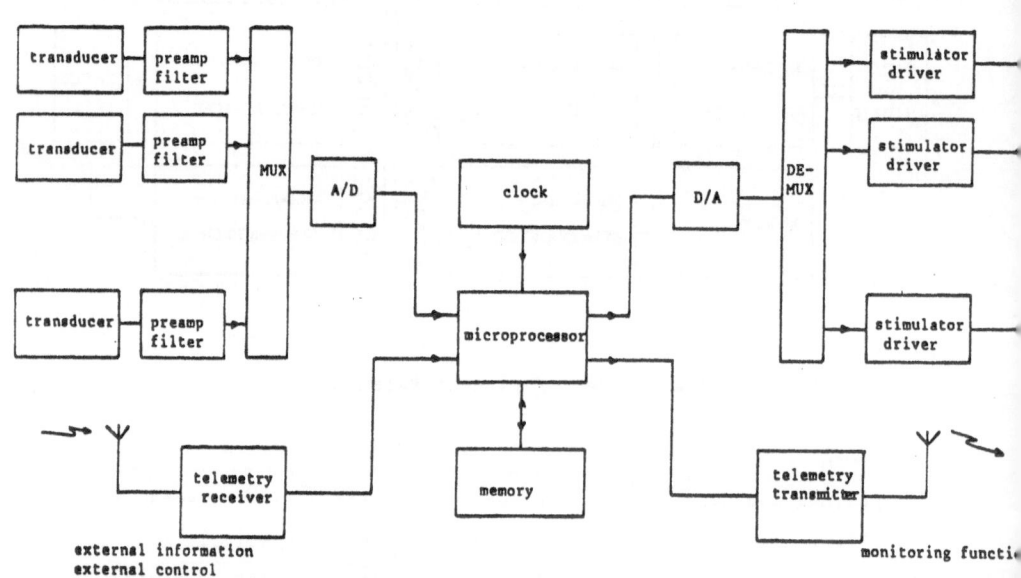

Fig.7 : The IHCS schematic.

mulator is programmable such that any stimulation waveform can be generated by the central processor and delivered by the stimulation drivers.

The central processor is the brain of the system. It analyses the incoming sensor signal and decides which stimulations have to be driven. It also applies more complicated signal analysis procedures including signal reduction and storage.

Most existing implantable devices are subsystem of an IHCS system. As an example consider a cardiac pacemaker (Figure 8). Simple pacemakers used to merely consist of a clock and one driver. Present day pacemakers however contain a microprocessor to synchronize the stimulation pattern to the biopotentials in the heart chambers. The stimulation pattern can be modified after implantation by means of a telemetry receiver. Continuous (ambulatory) monitoring is possible as well by means of a telemetry transmitter. The memory is used for two purposes. It stores the received information which determines the stimulation spike but it can also store ECG waveforms as in Holter monitoring.

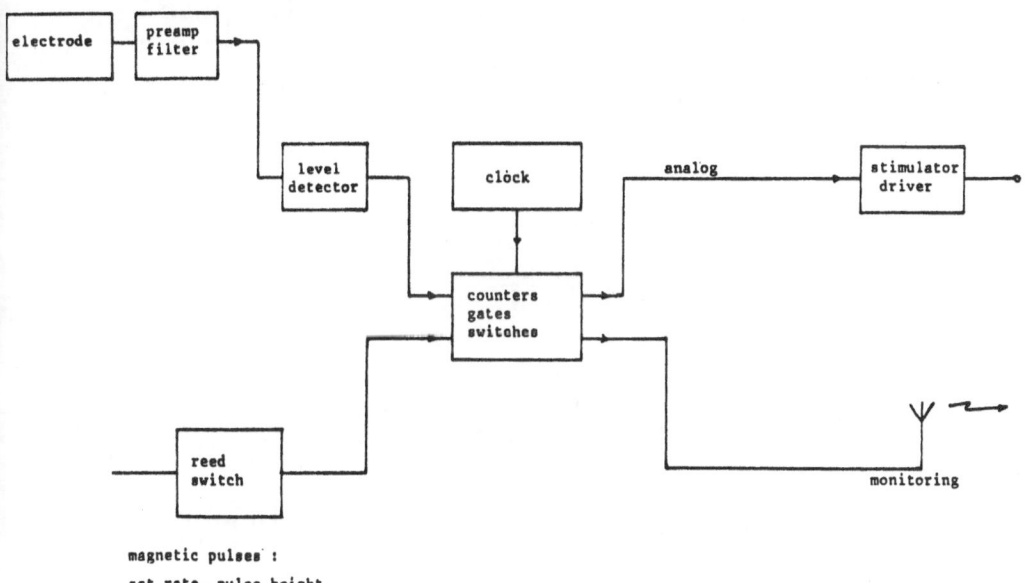

Fig.8 : Schematic of intelligent pacemakers.

398

In a Holter monitoring system, the IHCS system is simplified to a
limited number of transducers such as ECG, heart pressure and EMG in the
future (Fig.9). These signals are transmitted to a portable box containing
a reciever with a cassette recorder or solid-state memory. The task of
the microprocessor then mainly consists of the data compression to limit
the data to be stored. Ambulatory monitoring in this sense is of growing
importance for chronic health care, where patients take the monitoring
function home rather than to spend long periods in the hospital for observation.

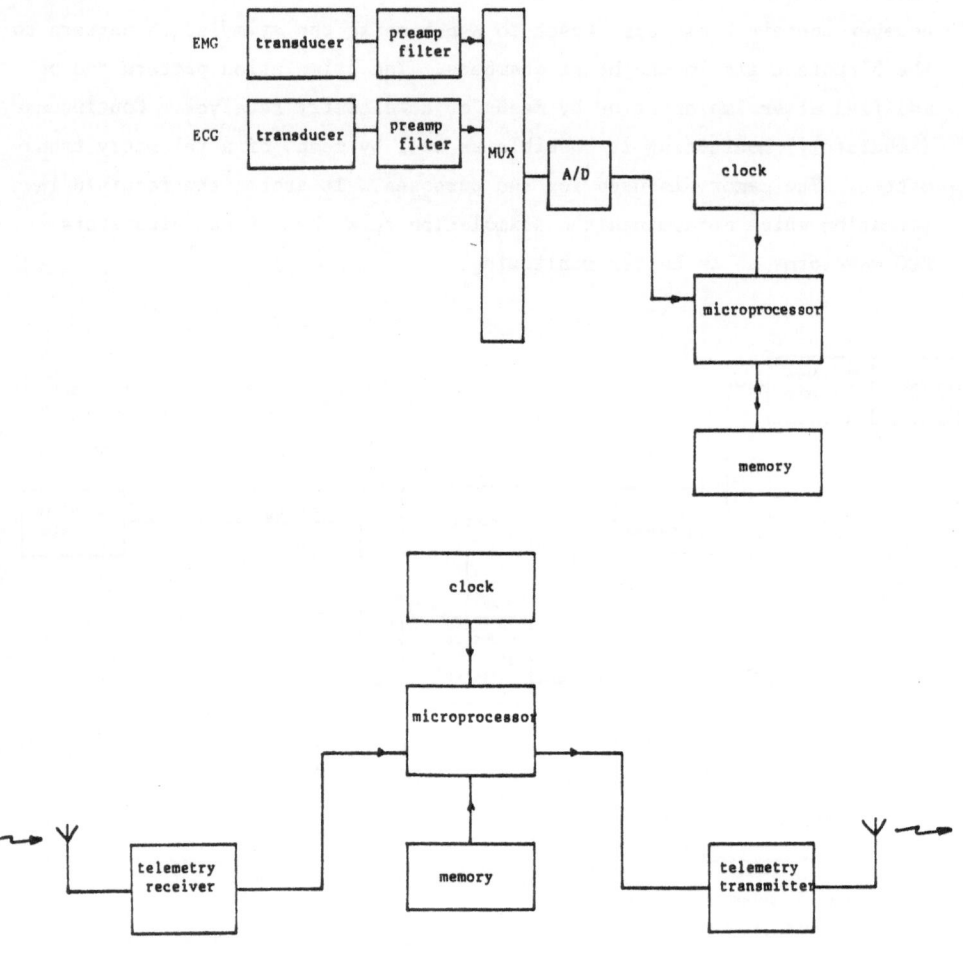

Fig.9 : Holter monitoring system.

Other examples of IHCS subsystems are general purpose telemetry and stimulation systems. In biotelemetry (fig.10) pressure, temperature, pH, biopotentials etc. are measured and multiplexed on one signal line before
being transmitted [5]. A microprocessor is included only if signal analysis is required.

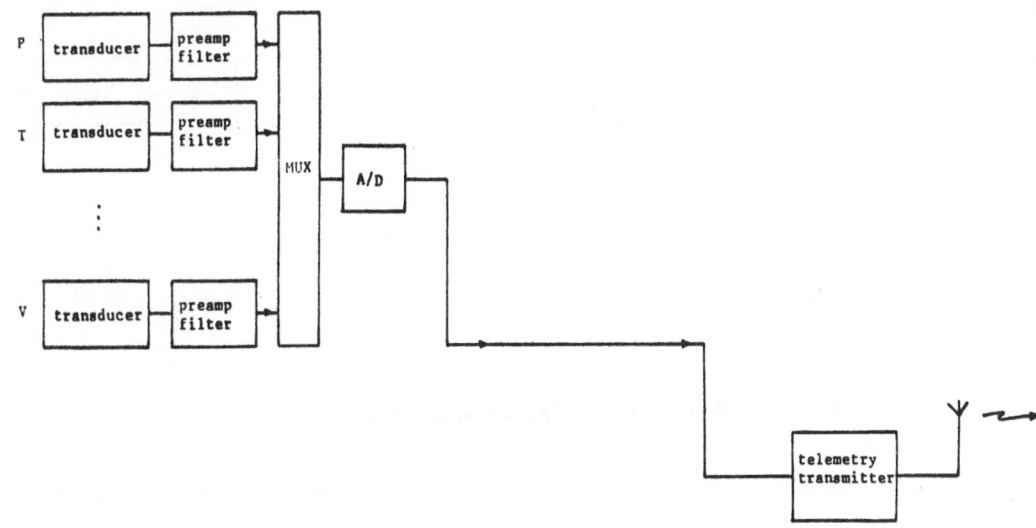

Fig.10 : Schematic of biotelemetry system.

In an ear stimulator for deaf (fig.11) up to eight bipolar electrodes
have to be driven [6]. The microprocessor is required to convert speech
information from a telemetry receiver to the eight channels positioned at
different frequencies in the cockled.

In this way several more examples of subsections of a universal IHCS
can be quoted. Not a single IHCS has been realized hitherto because of
lack of integration power. VLSI is expected to change this. Some of the
difficulties to realize a monochip IHCS chip are explained next.

THE VLSI-IHCS CHIP

A full IHCS system includes all blocks of figure 1 from sensors to
stimulation drivers. The difficulties to integrate these blocks are
shortly discussed in order to   examine the feasability of the IHCS chip.

Transducers have traditionally not been realized in silicon material

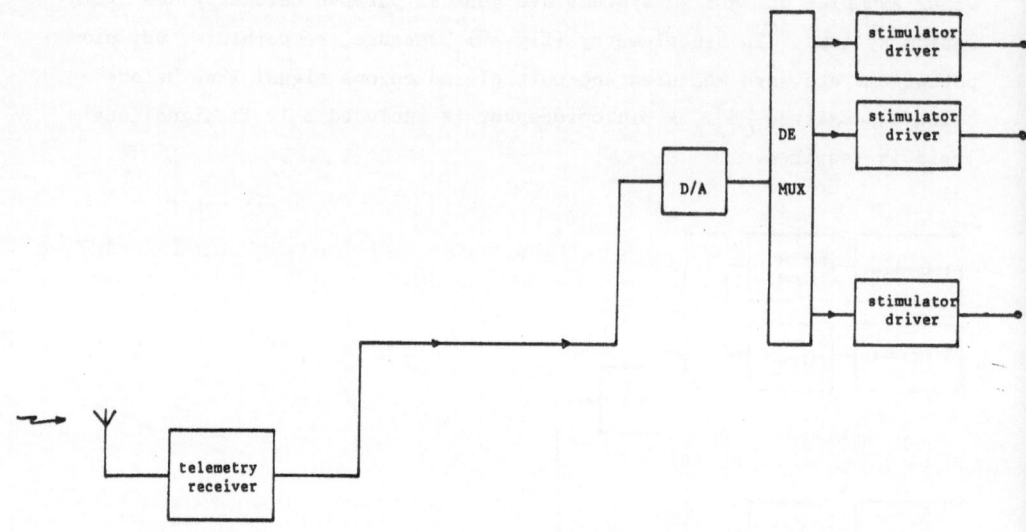

Fig.11 : Schematic of implantable stimulator.

and are therefore not compatible with VLSI processing. Exceptions however are pressure sensors and some chemical sensors [7]. IHCS integration thus leads to problems of compatibility of materials. Preamplifiers and filters have to handle signals of widely varying amplitude and bandwidth (see fig. 12). As a result both will have to be made programmable in order to provide best performance for the power required. This complicates the electronics and leads to more chip area.

Nature signal	Amplitude range μV	Bandwidth Hz
EEG	10-200	0.5-100
ECG	100-10.000	0.5-200
EMG	10-2000	2-1000
respiration vol.	-0.36.m³/min.	0.1-2
pressure blood	-300.mm Hg	(DC) 0.1-20

Fig.12 : List of some physiological signals.

On chip filters with programmable filter frequencies can only be realized with switched capacitor techniques [8]. Multiplexers with programmable sampling rates have already been demonstrated [9].

The main problem besides programmability however, is power dissipation. For implantable devices low power drain is directly translated in long lifetime. The main sources of power are batteries and RF couplers. Batteries are heavy and have limited lifetime. RF couplers and therefore preferred for long life implants. Conventional ways to save power in the implant is the use of low clock frequencies, low duty cycles for both measurement and stimulation, and all other techniques which are common to VLSI design such as low supply voltage and the use of CMOS technology [1].

CONCLUSION

It has been shown that the IHCS chip is the only viable VLSI chip for implantable applications. Difficulties in material compatibility, in complexity and power dissipation have to be solved before VLSI will allow the realization of the IHCS chip.

REFERENCES

1   Sansen, W. June 1982. On the integration of an internal human conditioning system, IEEE Journal Solid-State Circuits, SC-17, N°3, p. 513-521.
2   Sansen, W., De Dijcker, F. 1980, Implantable stimulator and biotelemetry system for enhanced bone healing, Biotelemetry V, p. 43-46.
3   Puers, R., Sansen, W. A low voltage micropower monolithic signal conditioning and central chip for pressure telemetry, IEEE Journal Solid-State Circuits, to be published.
4   Sansen, W., Celen, J., Colin, F., Garcia, O. Sept. 1983, Implantable glucose measurement system, 5th Ann. conf. IEEE Eng. Med. Biol. Soc., Columbus, Ohio.
5   1979, Implanted telemetry systems based on integrated circuits, Biotelemetry and Patient Monitoring, Vol.6, N°3.
6   Sansen, W., Peeters, S., Van Paemel, M. 1981, Programmable auditory prosthesis for sensorial deaf, Proc. 5th Nordic Meeting on Med. Biol. Eng. Linköping, Sweden, p. 450-452.
7   June 1983, Solid-State Transducers Conference, Delft.
8   Hosticka, B., Broderson, R., Gray, P. December 1977, MOS sampled data recursive filters using switched capacitor integrators, IEEE Journal Solid-State Circuits, SC-12, p. 600-608.
9   Sansen, W., Wouters, J., Busshaert, H., Slabbaert, J. 1983. Monochip eight-channel sensor interface with A/D conversion, Solid-State Transducers, Delft, Abstracts p. 90-91.

DISCUSSION

Chairman: H.Wolff

4.2 - Emerging technologies

RIPLEY: I'd like to add an additional comment to what Dr. Sansen has told you. I don't think that the technology for VLSI is completely away from the individual research developer. In the United States, there already is what you might call a concerted action in VLSI development through the research community and by this I mean the government has set up facilities where individual chips can be manufactured for the individual research. As Dr. Sansen has told you the way you design these chips is with a computer so anybody basically can have design tools in their shop, can sit down at the terminal and design a chip, and send the specifications to a fabrication facility and get a chip back. Now, I know in fact that one centre in the United States is looking into the design of an arrhythmias processing algorithm using only single VLSI chip. So I think we can see that happening in the very near future, maybe in the next two years.

SANSEN: I don't agree with that because I think it's misleading to say that VLSI is within the grasp of everybody. I think VLSI is whithin the grasp of many people but there is quite a difference between conceiving a chip, even with computer design tools and having it working in the medical field. That means that when you've made your 1st design, you'll spend or lose much more time afterwards. As in the U.S. and as in many countries of Europe, they go to the first stage, they make something on paper, and there you are with your 1st chip, but of course your problems still have to start, and this is especially time if you talk about ULSR. But of course as a sub part of the USLR circuit, I agree.

VAN BEMMEL: I should like to take part in the discussion. I find it very interesting. What Doctor Ripley mentioned of course is not the designing of a VLSI chip from the very beginning. It's like what we do now with our software, and with our computers. The modules are there. They have been standardized and what the user does is to construct a VLSI from those modules the way he likes it. In fact you have shown it yourself, in your very general set-up. The user could select himself, even taking into account the saving of power, could select those sub-functions he likes. And I think it is coming, maybe not in two years.

SANSEN: Oh yes, if this is what you meant, yes, but I think we understimate the difficulty to make a full VLSI circuit working. Which is not going to be work for a University laboratory of any kind, and that's why I dind't agree with the fact that every student can make a chip and make it work on a VLSI chip.

ROSENFALCK: I'm somewhat in doubt as to whether it's wise to solve all problems in one chip, as you suggest. Whether you should really be able to reach the wide frequency range and the wide range of amplification. Is that really the right way to do it? Dont't you think it's better to have less complicated and one goal directed circuits?

SANSEN: You say that's complicated but I think the complication is not in the electronics but in interfacing with the tissue, which is therefore the same for one electrode as it'is for ten electrodes, so now if you put in there a very simple chip or a complicated chip, that's the same problem.

ROSENFALCK: It is a question of cost, because it would be cheaper to make a simple chip which could solve our interface problems, and then have that on. I mean, they don't take up so much room, so if for each different interface problem you could make a simple chip, wouldn't that be a better way to go?

SANSEN: Don't forget that manufactures have to mantain each chip for each customer, so you have to repeat the work all the time with each different chip. I think it's a waste of effort. I think it is not possible to make one chip for everybody. That's my point. It is possible to make one complicated chip for everybody, and then there is at least a chance that a company may make it for you. Let's assume that each particular chip has been made in samples of one hundred. What's the cost of that? It's 20000 dollars, divided by 100, without development. But people are not willing to pay; that you oan pay that once, only at the beginning of each project, then after three years they stop the project the chips are dead, you throw them away and that's it. I don't think there is a solution is making a separate chip for each application, because you have to montain so many different chips, and you have development and this is an enormous cost. I think we have to make a chip that can be programmed or changed afterwards.

DAMGAARD ANDERSEN: What do you think about the future of very high speed integrated circuit in medicine? You know, those are emerging, they can process signals at a very high speed and can be programmed from the exterior.

SANSEN: As long as you stay on the curve of the constant power delay is no problem, but if you deviate from that so you use more power than you need for that speed, then you are in problems because you need more power than necessary. So I think there are applications for circuits of any speed, very slow and very fast ones, if the energy per function per unit time is the same.

APPENDIX

**PRESENTATION AND DISCUSSION OF A PROPOSAL FOR A
CONCERTED ACTION ON AMBULATORY MONITORING**

The following draft text, prepared by C. Marchesi, was been distributed to all the participants the day before the discussion:

"The use of ambulant recording of physiological variables for diagnosis and monitoring is expanding so rapidly that its cost to the community has attained important figures. On the other hand, several aspects concerning its effective role and criteria for application are still controversial. Some of these controversial items will be solved only through further progress in research and knowledge. Some others might be substantially clarified by a joint effort performed by several institutions: these latter include the definition of a standard of quality for the instrumentation performances, the definition of criteria for application, and the identification of limiting factors of the technique. These issues might thus constitute an appropriate set of questions to be tackled by a concerted action approach.

1. PROBLEMS IN AMBULATORY MONITORING.

The critical problems in ambulatory monitoring can be grouped around 4 topics, (observability, accuracy, precision, and optimization) which represent the various aspects of uncertainty of the procedure.

1.1 OBSERVABILITY OF THE CARDIOVASCULAR SYSTEM.
The problem of observability concerns the definition of the minimal set of variables that should be simultaneously monitored to assess the cardiovascular system performances in various conditions.
It is an open research topic and it doesn't seem to fit to the concerted action requirements.

1.2 ACCURACY OF THE AVAILABLE SIGNALS IN THE ASSESSMENT OF THE PERFORMANCE OF THE CARDIOVASCULAR SYSTEM.
The available signals are 1 + 3 ECG leads, invasive peripheral pressures, non invasive indicators of pump function.
The question of accuracy concerns the sensitivity/specificity of the information derived from these signals (rhythm abnormalities, ST-T changes, peripheral pressure parameters, systolic time intervals, etc.) in discriminating between different abnormalities of the cardiovascular system.

The experience in this field seems to be sufficiently advanced to make possible and profitable a joint research effort, that could probably solve most of the current uncertainty. Such an effort should be concentrated on the adoption of a standard protocol by cooperating groups to evaluate the degree of correspondance between abnormal signs and pathological status by an appropriate follow up study. It should be noted that the outcome of this action could also lead to better insight into some of the observability problems, such as the optimal number of ECG leads, the mechanical signals to be monitored, and the duration of the continuous observation.

1.3. PRECISION OF THE ALGORITHMS AND OF THE PROCEDURES FOR ANALYSIS. This topic refers to the problem of the sensitivity/specificity of the methods of analysis in detecting, measuring, classifying relevant events, independently from their pathophysiological meaning.

The approach to this evaluation is represented by the annotated data base to be adopted and proposed as the gold standard by the cooperating groups. The American Heart Association and the Massachusetts Institute of Technology together with other institutions have developed annotated data bases for the evaluation of arrhythmia detectors: they cover an important aspect of the global problem, but additional ones should be considered.

An important outcome of this study could be a recommendation to manufacturers to recognize the produced data base as a quality standard for the single algorithms or also for the whole system. To this end manufacturers participation to the concerted action, or other forms of interaction with them in the course of the action, should be considered.

1.4 OPTIMIZATION OF THE CLINICAL APPLICATIONS OF AMBULATORY MONITORING.

A large series of problems, so far approached in a purely empirical manner, belongs to the level of optimization. They include:

. indication for ambulatory monitoring, in relation to the three phases of patient conditions: at risk, suspected disease, post-acute;

. graduation of indication with reference to the different disease status;

. indication to the use of different signals and number of leads;

. geographical distribution of specialized centers;

. graduation of instrumentation complexity levels in relation to aim and cost;

. effectiveness in reducing the need for hospital admissions or shortening its duration.

These problems could be approached by a preliminary systematic enquiry in order to outline the present experiences of the participating groups and the results of the enquiry should constitute a reference for the identification of the limiting factors of the presently available instrumentation and procedures, and planning the study.

2. ORGANIZATION.

A working group of the experts should be constituted for each of the three topics of accuracy, precision and optimization in ambulatory monitoring. A steering committee with medical, engineering, and statistical expertise should coordinate their action. The activity of the working groups should proceed according to predetermined time limits associated with scheduled "success criteria".

3. SCHEDULE AND FUNDS.

To be effective the action should have a duration as short as possible. A three years duration seems to be adequate to the scope.

The first, as preparatory year, should be devoted to the planning and attainment of practical working agreements between the cooperating centers; the second year should represent the actual starting year for the execution of the planned procedures at highest priority;

the third year should be devoted to the analysis, distribution and discussion of the preliminary results and to the starting of other subjects presently at lower level of priority.

After the third year the concerted action should be reconsidered: in case of success it could be useful to maintain only the activity of the steering commitee for the coordination of the work in progress and the distribution of results.

The budget for the action should cover the expenses for travel and meeting of both steering committee and working groups, and those for central management of the action".

DISCUSSION

Chairman: C. Marchesi

MARCHESI: I'd like to add only a few words, and leave to you the opportunity of expressing fully your ideas, to point out what is, in my opinion, a major problem. I served for several years in the group at the EEC, called Monitoring the Seriously Ill with a number of you, and the result of this experience is that it is very difficult to produce common results, for the simple and obvious reason that we must add new work to our usual work. Thus, we have to consider quite honestly this practical problem and decide which are the lines where we are ready to serve toward a common effort. I think that ambulatory monitoring of the cardiovascular system is in such a position. We have in fact many open questions which can be solved only by joint effort and many people with enough enthusiasm to afford them. I propose, if you like, that each of you answer to the question whether the draft document is a suitable frame work to deal with. In the positive case, let me know your particular positions about or against the various points described in my proposal. In this way my work of summarizing your views will be quite easy.

DEGANI: I'm not directly involved in ambulatory monitoring. I'm mainly involved in EKG analysis. I have some experience of concerted action because I have been working for several years in the Common Standard for quantitative Electrocardiography (CSE) concerted action. There are four words which are the key words in the document produced by Carlo Marchesi I would change the order in which you have written your words in the document, because I have tried to see an order of complexity of the different programmes. So, in my opinion, the lowest complexity is given by the programme you call "precision". By precision you mean, the accuracy that existing algorithms perform when working on a number of signals which are presently analyzed, let's say EKG, pressures and a few others. This means that you have to use an annotated data-base where you have events annotated. The clinical significance of these events is not well known. There is something which is different from the context, which must be detected by the computer system. So this is the precision of the systems, and it is at the lowest grade of complexty. Then there's "accuracy", and here we move to the clinical part. The accuracy is a sort of estimate of the capability in detecting what really is physiologically or clinically significant. For example whether the EKG only, or the EKG plus the pressure or the EKG plus pressure plus respiration and whatever also, is able in fact to monitor the condition of the patient. Then the problem of "observability", and this is a very difficult problem. This is because, I think observability means in fact whether all the signals which are present to be analysized, are enough to monitor in a proper way the patient. And finally, "optimization" which is closely related to the observability and also refers to various problems such as appropriate diffusion of this technology, economic impact, etc. I should say that almost everybody has spoken about "precision" in these two days. What is my feeling is that this subject is very well at hand for a concerted action. This is the first thing that the concerted action should investigate. Precision of existing systems independently of any clinical evidence. Obviously the concerted action should include technical people as well as physicians, because it needs an annotated database. Moreover we heard a lot of people talking about "accuracy" and we have heard problems, and possible solutions, but mainly problems. This is a more complicated problem than the first one, but still I think it can be in the reach of concerted action. As regards the third and fourth point, we have heard different positions about observability from Wolff, Rosenfalck, Sansen and Sayers. Somebody was saying we need to monitor more, and some saying we can monitor less, so this is really a big problem and I wonder from my experience, whether this is the aim of a concerted action, if only some critical points can be brought up. I think that this should be the aim of an Indirect Research, if I remember correctly what Professor Donato said in the opening address. And finally, about optimization, I haven't heard a lot. I mean, it's quite difficult to understand what optimization can be, but probably for example, the use of real time processor can, in some sense, be interpreted as "optimization". My overall feeling is that the document prepared by Carlo Marchesi is just an outline. It should consider also practical problems, it's a sort of philosophical document. It does not seem to me to be ready to be presented to the CEE for a decision.

MARCHESI: I have to clarify some possible misunderstandings. When I say that I have prepared a draft document, I mean this document is not ready for a decision to the Community, and exactly I take your point: it is a general introduction. But I think there is some more than a philosophy, because I have precisely indicated some practical lines that are useful for a concerted action. They certainly have to be further discussed; it is not up to me to make anything concrete before this discussion.

SANSEN: May I ask Dr. Degani one question?: there are four topics mentioned in this document, and they seem part of the existing concerted action on the ECG. Can I ask her the following question: which one of those topics is closest to the content of the existing concerted action? And which one is most remote from it.

DEGANI: " Precision" is very common. We, in fact, are evaluating already existing EKG processing systems. And we have already an annotated data base of events which in our case are waveforms which are marked without any consideration of clinical significance of the signal. And then we have just started wondering what we can do, in the few years we have to work with, in the field of, "accuracy". So we need now to set up an annotated data base, but from the point of view of clinical significance. This means having signals annotated on indipendent EKG data. We will end up our action with suggestions and standards, we hope standards, as regards "precision", and we hope with suggestions as regards "accuracy" .

TALMON: I can add a little more about the CSE project. When Jos Willems was comparing performance of different EKG analysis programmes, on the same digital data, he came out that considerable differences were found in measurements that are considered to be clnically relevant, like QRS durations, and there seemed to be some confusion in the developers of these systems on what you really should measure. Well, this was, I think, a very good starting point for looking to precision. When you're talking about accuracy of diagnostic procedures, that's one step further. Then it becomes more difficult to define a common aim for the study. As soon as it's really very practical and you can decide an existing problem, from a technical point of view, most programme developers can be involved is this kind of studies. As soon as it becomes broader, and more uncertainty is involved in the goal of your study, then it can get little more difficulty. It's also important that when you really want to start a project on ambulatory monitoring, you define in a very practical way, the common problems. And only later to extend the project in a further phase.

ZYWIETZ: I think Dr. Donato has explained already at the beginning of this conference what a concerted action should be. If we look at this conference and if we look at the future, we have first to ask which of the problems we have discussed may be of common interest and can be solved better commonly than separately. So what I foresee is that during the next years we'll get more equipment, even intelligent records, available on the market, and to have a centre where we analyse the performance of those systems. There are already methods described how to do that. For example the MIT data-base, the AHA data-base, and I wonder whether it was worthwhile to start this job at zero-level again. So my proposal is to take or to use these data-base and maybe to add something, what seems to be more relevant to Europe or to our problems. So this would be the system evaluation in terms of assessment of the precision of the systems. It could be a major task for this concerted action. Another point that it is not quite clear, was brought up yesterday in the discussion by Dr. Rosenfalck and Van Bemmel. Heinz Wolff has pointed out that we have taken snap-shots for many years, and we still do that in clinical examinations. Now we are going on to continuously measure many parameters, that means we follow more the dynamic behaviour. I wonder whether there are, besides the blood-pressure measurement, besides the EKG, other signals like the EEG and others, worthwhile to be monitored, and whether it is possible to find, a common set of problems inherent in all these methods, to be tackled in a concerted action. We should just stay on ambulatory monitoring of cardiovascular parameters, or we should think for a while to general principles to be applied in other continuous measurements.

ROSENFALCK: As far as I understand, we have no choice because there's no doubt that ambulatory monitoring of the cardiovascular signals is the most important item to be considered. On the contrary it's written in an official document of the CEE that the goal of the work which we're going to do here, is the development of devices and procedures for ambulatory monitoring of physical variables of diagnostic importance to rehabilitation, therapeutical needs, drug use and occupational health. And since it's written there, we are asked to widen the subject and this is probably why Dr. Wolff and I are here. That it's not sufficient to keep ourselves to the cardiovascular system, we're not ever going to have approved the action about ambulatory monitoring, unless we widen the scope to other variables. We have to write a proposal which includes more variables, more physiological variables, than EKG and pressure. So I don't think i's so bad, to try to look at different problems. I mean, for istance, seizures or attacks of dizziness, or something that might widen the scope of your measurements on the cardiovascular system.

EEG plus the EMG, plus the EOG is certainly emough to classify the sleep stages, but probably it would be of equal importance to evaluate the EKG parameters at the same time here. I know for example that a Finnish group is working in restricting parameters to only being movement parameters, and once they have stated how they relate to the EEG, they might be concerned in knowing something about movement and temperature, for instance during sleep. If we look at drug use, then EKG and EEG are important parameters. So I think we are simply forced to allow that Dr. Marchesi will have to try to make more broad proposals, which do include more parameters. And I think that it's not so bad, because what all of us could be interested in what we have said previously, the sensors we are all interested in quantification and in data reduction, and I am not in doubt that all of us who work is EMG and EEG can gain, for instance, from looking at the reduction system by Dr. Pahlm, and from other people who have shown us excellent data reduction systems here. And then again we have common problems with telemetry and with storing the signals.

MARCHESI: I'd like to spend just one word about this, because I'm really sorry that with Dr. Rosenfalck it's really difficult to establish a sort of agreement. We spent a lot of discussion with you and Dr. Wolff and Dr. Sansen in Brussels, and I thought, we agreed that one thing is to assess priority, and a different thing is to speak in terms of scientific or social interest. What is convenient to do is not the same thing as what is convenient to do immediately, and our effort should be oriented to, something we can afford together immediately. Perhaps you remember that I am now working on EEG analysis in relation with EKG and hemodynamic variables. For that reason I can say honestly that it is a research topic at the moment, and you can prove that if you consider that very few papers are published on these matters. That's what I'd like to clarify. It is of course open to discussion, but it is my view and. I thought we were in agreement about that point when we discussed this subject in Brussels.

ROSENFALCK: We were in agreement that it was the only possible thing, because you have sent such an excellent proposal for this topic, and that since it did cover a part of the goal of ambulatory monitoring and then, this workshop should take place. At the same time an effort should be made to broaden the subject to take into account what was written in the official document, and there was a kind of problem in getting your proposal through the CRM because it was too narrow a subject, and it was not the goal of the EEC to have an exclusive club.

MARCHESI: But do you think we have to start with so broad a proposal, covering eveything? That's the point. What's important? What do we have to start with immediately?

GHIONE: I would make a comment on blood-pressure measurements because I think it's not completely correct to put on the same level EKG and blood-pressure measurement. EKG is quite developed and we've seen a lot of very nice devices to monitor and to extract information. As regards blood-pressure measurements, thing are much worse, they are not so advanced. But the speakers about this topic brought up some very interesting information. For instance, the fact that measuring blood pressure for 3 hours at rest gives us us quite a good idea of the blood-pressures in general. This is very provoking information. And I think that an important issue should be tackled, such as the problem of the reference method. The method by clinical characterization can be performed on limited amounts of subjects, so I think that a single institute would not be able to validate this kind of information by itself. And maybe this kind of information could be better collected if people performing invasive blood-pressure monitoring would come together to compare different ways of measuring invasively and not invasively by putting information of more centres together. It should be possible to have enough data, maybe, to obtain some real good information. Blood pressure and EKG are, two very different things, and for blood pressure, we need to start very basically.

SANSEN: I in principle agree with what Dr. Rosenfalck has said. But of course there are some problems with that, because if we have to monitor ECG and EMG and everything, then it's going to be a problem to find equipment, because nobody makes equipment to be used so that people can record and compare data. That's one problem. Another problem is that indeed I remenber that there was a discussion on how to start a concerted action and I do remember the fact that the priority would go to the ECG monitoring. So the compromise that we will have to discuss is, I think, how to start the concerted action on ECG, and add something on all the parameters, and it's something that will have to be discussed. There was some suggestion by Dr. Zywietz, there may be other suggestions. Certainly I don't know of any equipment which is able to provide data on EEG and ECG and EMG, and for sure this is one problem we have to face if we want to expand.

ZYWIETZ: I would like to make myself clear. It was yesterday mentioned that we should gather all the experience from other monitoring systems, but we should also be aware that there is a very large difference, a very different level of state of technology between ECG monitoring and EEG or EMG monitoring. So if we want to achieve any practical results in a small interval of time, we have to restrict ourselves to practical things such as standardisation, user protection, and those things which we can achieve now with ECG monitorig systems. I have not clear to what extent we can stimulate research in the monitoring of signals. One major aspect of the Rome Treaty was that we should have in Europe standardization, common standards for many things, and I think this was the reason to create concerted action, while research on a more basic level is still to be done at single country level. We may have to find some common interests with groups which monitor other signals. But to reach practical results, we have to limit ourselves.

SANDOE: It has been stated here several times that ECG monitoring is a sort of high level technique we debate it daily, we are not so convinced about that. We had some very impressive data from U.S. during this meeting. How much they used their laboratories, how much money is involved in them? When I had to write my paper for this workshop, I was sitting down and thinking about what I was using for, this ambulatory monitoring technique in my daily work. I think that we have to propose a concerted action able to consider deeply the clinical aspects. In other words we should promote the study of the "accuracy" of the ECG monitoring, its capability as diagnostic tool. For instance it should be very interesting to make a point effort to study cronocardiology, to collect a library of tapes about cardiocronogy and not limit ourselves to only the study of etpotic beats, which are not so important.

WALSH: As was pointed out by many of the speakers, I think the problem of EKG versus blood-pressure monitoring is totally different. EKG is an enormous effort involving many centres around the world and it's highly evolved, so that this is perhaps the major thrust of this conference. Where my experience is more concerned in, is the area of blood pressure. I think a very practical topic to which this kind of commission can be addressed, as was pointed out by Dr. Cashman, is that standards could be written by which people could report the performances of invasive blood-pressure systems. It might not seem to be so important because the actual scope of invasive monitoring in the world is small. However, as the market begins to get flooded, and to some extent is already flooded, with non invasive blood-pressure recorders, the invasive recorders are going to be the only standard by which the non invasive records can be evaluated. So I think a first priority would be to write a set of standards by which the performance of the Oxford and other invasive recorders that might be developed, and associated computing systems, can be evaluated. And then,

in conjunction with that, writing protocols for the way in which non
invasive systems could be compared to the more reliable invasive data, to
make some sensible clinical impact ultimately. This is quite a reasonable
function for an international symposium such as this.

SAYERS: Can I remark that there are, generally speaking, two sort of things
the European Community does well. First of all, it can agree things. It
doesn't happen very often, admittedly, but when it does it is rather
spectacular. The sort of thing I have in mind is agreeing standards of
signal quality, and I support what'has been said, just recently. And
secondly, agreeing the basis on which you can pool data, that is, from
different populations, and different environemeants. I must confess to
being rather bored with the ECG. There's been so much effort poured in on
it, that I'm rather dubious if we're going to get a vast amount out of
looking at that. When it comes to blood-pressure, however, I think the
situation has been correctly stated. There's a lot we don't know, we do
not know a great deal about the pathological features we don't know very
much about what typically happens in normal individuals. And for example,
how many episodes of low blood-pressure that accur during the day in normal
individuals can be ultimately related, as I was muttering yesterday, to the
general deterioration of hearing capability, in the population as it ages?
And is this related to noise environement? And what about activity levels?
They might be postural movement levels, the general neurological tone, how
rapidly are the eyes buzzing oround, taking note of what's happening in the
outside world, and so on. All these sort of things are appropriate, but
they do require common standards to be agreed, as a basis on which analysis
can be brought forward. So I think establishing bases that are commonly
agreed as acceptable, for recognizing that you're dealing with similar
populations, gives you the opportunity to pool populations. After all,
when you think about what the EEG has got to offer, it's just a lot of
people, and a large number of centres with a lot of experience. So you can
pool experience or add numbers, and these are the two things that I think
one should pay most attention to. I'm suggesting we don't deal any more
with the expanding activity on a multi centre basis on ECG, but we might
look again at blood-pressure. We don't have emough information about what
the common standards are, to know, first of all, the quality of the signal
you're getting, the quality that I'm getting, and somebody else, in order
to make valid comparisons. So I would suggest that we bend our minds a
little bit, to what we can agree in general, and how agreement can be

brought forward. I would also suggest that we try and encourage different centres to be exploring different sort of variables. It may be that the EMG is a good one to work with, I rather shirk from trying it my self, I must admit, but the EOG is perhaps one stage less complex, maybe. I can imagine there would be some sense for somebody to set up a trial in which you have a large number of people walking around not with things attached to them, but acting as portable collectors of ambient noise. We don't know anything about that either. And if you want to expand the range of monitoring and I think you should at least consider this, then I think that's one thing you might do, and if at same time you looked at it in the light of blood-pressure, that would be useful. We could get a number of people, and take a snap-shot across the cross section of the population, of different age groups, and get some sort of picture about what sort of things they typically exhibit, what sort of environement they typically experience, then you're got the very first stages of deciding whether there's any sense in exploring whether the noise environement is linked to any of these physiologycal deteriorations.

MARCHESI: May I ask you a question: I certainly have considered the problem of broadening our interests, of course, but I'd like to know whether a concerted action is the possible environment to host this sort of not well defined problems. In other words, in case a concerted action can afford the pooling of these sort of experiencs, I would agree with you and Prof. Rosenfalck. But under this point of view, do you think that it is really possible to afford at the same level of priority all these enormous problems you were suggesting?

SAYERS: No, I wouldn't have said they could all be held on the same level of priority. But I do think that it is perfectly proper to think about common objectives to gain experience with a number of these variables. And it would be perfectly reasonable for us to agree that in a number of centres there will be different variables measured. Standards have to be agreed, then we would be pooling experience which admittedly I suppose could be done in any one centre, if there were emough centres in any one country to make it possible. If there aren't, you must get experience multinationally. I would certainly have thought that you could make a case for trying to agree common standards, exchanging experience of a quantitative kind on blood pressure, and secondly trying at the same time to encourage a development of experience with different sort of variables for the reasons I've just been saying.

MARK: I'm not aware that we (in U.S.A.) have anything that could be called concerted action, unless you would call conferences held by NIH and other groups from time to time to living together working groups to share ideas and publish memoranda. Another form which exists is the Cardiology bodies of the manufactures of medical instruments, the ME group which worries about trying to establish standards in instrumentation. And I'm not sure that this is the same group that would do that, but someone somewhere has got to establish a language by which people communicate how things work. And how that information should be expressed. I'm not familiar enough with what a concerted action is, to know whether that's the appropriate body, to involve manufacturers. If it's a subject that has to do with, for example, how a device should work, what the standards should be, or how a system should be evaluated and how the results should be published, yes, (we do involve the manufacturer in this kind of common effort) I think you really need to have the manufactures involved in that.

MARCHESI: Not very many manufacturers were using the standards you are proposing, is that true?

MARK: No, they do use it, but they haven't talked about it yet. And one of the reasons is because, as I mentioned, the appropriate format for expressing results isn't generally accepted, so they tend to be protective of their secrecy. The users, which is what I think this group would represent, could conceivally do it yourself, or could drive in terms of demanding that kind of information, I should think very powerfully.

RIPLEY: I offer this as a bit of informations which I think is relevant to what you're approaching to do here. A number of years ago the American Heart Association got together and wrote a paper which put together a set of recommendations on reporting diagnostic electrocardiography performance. I think mostly everyone here has seen that paper, and knows what is involved with that. I know that the American Heart Association is at this point initiating another effort to write recommendations for ambulatory monitoring, and I think that what you're trying to do here is something similar to that. And it might be important if we could coordinate, if the Europeans procede.

DEGANI: In our concerted action we have some consultants who are from the States. I think that the main participants are European centres and we have, for example, also some connection with manufacturers, with IBM with Hewlett-Packard, etc. Obviously all those firms are interested in standardization and I think that the broader the audence the best that can be the results. In any case, I don't know exactly if there can be some accepted official connection between Europe and United States. I have some doubt about that.

ZYWIETZ: As far as industry is concerned, in this CSE concerted action, the manufacturers or the developers of ECG programmes are interested in having their programmes tested by standards or by the data base we have collected within the CSE project. There's like we try to remain independent from industry, however, we analyse the product itself. United States have, the FTA and NIH and they have very strong recommendations particularly FDA. We do not have any comparable institutions in Europe. It may be helpful to create in a number of concerted action in Europe, such type of quality control institutions.

TALMON: With respect to the CSE project, there are at this moment no formal relations with American Heart Association and World Health Organization. We have some personal contacts with the people over there, and what we want to do is, in the second half of this year to get into discussion with those people, trying to get the effort we have made accepted by those people, so that there can be some integration between what has been done in the past by the American Heart Association and the work we are doing which is more directly related to the processing of the data.

CERUTTI: I have only two short comments. The first one is that I am not very happy about your key words, in your draft, and especially "observability" and "optimization". I realize that in the field of the science of control and in the field of signal processing they have a precise meaning and they may be misleading in a general assumption, like the one you mentioned. The second comment is that I'm concerned with signal processing, with biomedical signal processing, so I think a particular topic for the concerted action would be the evaluation of algorithms for biomedical signal processing for ECG, EEG, evoked potential. We have a common background for approaching this problem, and I think, due to your review and the review from Professor Marck and Ripely, the equipments have not too many algorithms of p-wave recognition, for example, or t-wave recognition. I think my proposal is that we have to make a standardization of these algorithms, find out all the possible and well functioning algorithms presently available and the ones that seem promising in pattern recognition, in parameter extraction. They should be evaluated on a larger basis not in one site, but in many sites in Europe.

DAMGAARD ANDERSEN: I would suggest the following: why don't we send a paper, which should be delivered within two weeks, containing our suggestions to Dr. Marchesi? He gets proposals or contributions from interested persons, and then he tries to work it together and make a real proposal which may be commented by the interested people.

MARCHESI: It's exactly the sort of thing I have in mind. To make my work less hard, try to follow the scheme I have proposed. You can go against every word, but in that order. If there are no further comments, I would ask Dr. Rosenfalck to close the session with her recommendations.

ROSENFALCK: I think it's a very good idea that all of you who really are interested in continuing this work, really write to Dr. Marchesi and have the chance to reach the goal of the proposal. But I think one thing that's rather important is that many of you that are here today belong to another concerted action and you have to be sure that there's no overlap, between these two groups. Because CRM is not going to make two concerted actions with the same people. So you have to schedule exactly what is the goal of this group different from the goal of the CSE concerted action. Since you have asked me to close the session, and we are not going on, then I'll use the opportunity to thank you, Dr. Marchesi for extremely nice time here in Pisa. When I came to Milan I went out, and found Galvani Road, and turned around a road, and this was Via Volta, and then I thought this should be the right start of coming to Italy. And certainly it has been a nice time here, Italy is so different from the Nordic Countries. It's nice, it's warm, it's old: time is different you don't care so much about time as we do in Demnark, where we always are in a hurry you have plenty of time which made us feel more relaxed and life more enjoyable I think we all want to thank you for having received us so heartly, and for having given us so excellent opportunity for discussing the subject we were so interested in. Thank you very much.

MARCHESI: I am really very glad to have all of you here. Our workshop would not have been so successful without your contribution, so deep and so important. Thank you very much, and let's hope it is the first start—point of something to build up together.